# Augmentative and Alternative Communication: European Perspectives

# Augmentative and Alternative Communication: European Perspectives

### Edited by

## Stephen von Tetzchner and Mogens Hygum Jensen

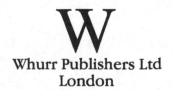

**Whurr Publishers Ltd**
London

© 1996 Whurr Publishers Ltd
First published 1996
Whurr Publishers Ltd
19B Compton Terrace, London N1 2UN, England

Reprinted 1997

**British Library Cataloguing-in-Publication Data**
A catalogue record for this book is available from the
British Library.

ISBN 1-897635-591

# Contents

# Contributors

**Rosa Afonso**
Centre for Habilitation of Cerebral
Palsy
Tr. Maceda, 160
P-4300 Porto
Portugal

**Norman Alm**
Microcomputer Centre
Department of Mathematics and
Computer Science
The University
Dundee DD1 4HN
United Kingdom

**Anne E. Baker-Mills**
Institute for General Linguistics
University of Amsterdam
Spuistraat 210
NL-1012 VT Amsterdam
Nederland

**Sarah Barnett**
Academic Department of Child
Health
Chelsea and Westminster Hospital
369 Fulham Road
London SW10 9NH
United Kingdom

**Carmen Basil**
Department of Developmental
and Educational Psychology
University of Barcelona
Campus Vall d'Hebron
Passeig Vall d'Hebron 171
E-08035 Barcelona
Spain

**Serenella Besio**
Institute for Educational
Technology
National Research Council
Via De Marini 6
Torre de Francia
I-16149 Genova
Italy

**Eva Björck-Åkesson**
Forskningsinstitutionen
Jönköping University
Postbox 1026
S-551 11 Jönköping
Sweden

**Jane Brodin**
Stockholm Insitute of Education
Department of Special Education
Post box 47308
S-100 74 Stockholm
Sweden

**Maria Grazia Chinato**
Cooperativa L'Albero
Via Camozzoni 1
Verona
Italy

**John Clibbens**
Department of Psychology
Plymouth University
Drakes Circus
Plymouth
Devon PL4 8AA
United Kingdom

**Sarah Collins**
Department of Psychology
University of Stirling
Stirling FK9 4LA
United Kingdom

**Julie Dockrell**
Department of Child Develop-
ment and Primary Education
Institute of Education
London University
20 Bedford Way
London WC1
United Kingdom

**Joaquim Faias**
Centre for Habilitation of Cerebral
Palsy
Tr. Maceda, 160
P-4300 Porto
Portugal

**José M. Ferreira**
Centre for Habilitation of Cerebral
Palsy
Tr. Maceda, 160
P-4300 Porto
Portugal

**Manfred Gangkofer**
Steinfeldstrasse 6

D-27299 Langwedel
Germany

**Juan Carlos Gómez**
School of Psychology
University of St. Andrews
St. Andrews
Fife KY16 9JU
United Kingdom

**Mats Granlund**
ALA Research Foundation
Sibyllegatan 7 1 tr.
S-114 51 Stockholm
Sweden

**Nicola Grove**
Department of Educational
Psychology and Special Education
Needs
Institute of Education
London University
20 Bedford Way
London WC1
United Kingdom

**Margriet Heim**
Institute for General Linguistics
University of Amsterdam
Spuistraat 210
NL-1012 VT Amsterdam
Nederland

**Erland Hjelmquist**
Department of Psychology
University of Gothenburg
Postbox 14158
S-400 20 Gothenburg
Sweden

**Mogens Hygum Jensen**
The Royal Danish School of
Education Studies
Skolebakken 171
DK-6705-Esbjerg Ø
Denmark

**Sophia L. Kalman**
Helping Communication Method-
ological Centre
Damjanch u 28/b
H-1071 Budapest VII
Hungary

**Kaisa Launonen**
Social Services Department of the
City of Helsinki
Vammaisneuvola
Sofianlehdonkatu 8
SF-00610 Helsinki
Finland

**Filip Loncke**
Orthopedagogishe Centrum
Sint-Gregorius Institute
Jules Destreelaan 67
B-9050 Gent-Gentbrügge
Belgium

**Lourdes Lourenço**
Centre for Habilitation of Cerebral
Palsy
Tr. Maceda, 160
P-4300 Porto
Portugal

**Harald Martinsen**
Department of Psychology
University of Oslo
Postbox 1094 Blindern
N-0317 Oslo
Norway

**Elisabete Mendes**
National Federation of Institutes
for Education and Rehabilitation
of Disabled Children
Rua Padre Américo 7c
P-1600 Lisboa
Portugal

**Susanne Møller**
Egedammen Adult Education
Centre
Skovledet 14
DK-3400 Hillerød
Denmark

**Ana Moreira**
Centre for Habilitation of Cerebral
Palsy
Tr. Maceda, 160
P-4300 Porto
Portugal

**Alan F. Newell**
Microcomputer Centre
Department of Mathematics and
Computer Science
The University
Dundee DD1 4HN
United Kingdom

**Cecilia Olsson**
ALA Research Foundation
Sibyllegatan 7 1 tr.
S-114 51 Stockholm
Sweden

**Andras Pajor**
Helping Communication
Methodological Centre
Damjanch u 28/b
H-1071 Budapest VII
Hungary

**Jorge Rato**
National Federation of Institutes
for Education and Rehabilitation
of Disabled Children
Rua Padre Américo 7c
P-1600 Lisboa
Portugal

**Annika Dahlgren Sandberg**
Department of Psychology
University of Gothenburg
Postbox 14158
S-400 20 Gothenburg
Sweden

**Encarnación Sarriá**
Faculty of Psychology
National University of Distance
Education,
Ciudad Universitaria, s/n
E-28040 Madrid
Spain

**Martine M. Smith**
School of Clinical Speech and
Language Studies
Trinity College
Dublin 2
Ireland

**Emili Soro-Camats**
Department of Developmental
and Educational Psychology
University of Barcelona
Campus Vall d'Hebron
Passeig Vall d'Hebron 171
E-08035 Barcelona
Spain

**Javier Tamarit**
CEPRI
Avda. de la Victoria, 63

El Plantio
E-28023 Madrid
Spain

**Hans van Balkom**
Institute for Rehabilitational
Research
Zandbergsweg 111
NL-6432 CC Hoensbroek
The Netherlands

**Stephen von Tetzchner**
Department of Psychology
University of Oslo
Postbox 1094 Blindern
N-0317 Oslo
Norway

**Marguerite Welle Donker-Gimbrère**
Institute for Rehabilitational
Research
Zandbergsweg 111
NL-6432 CC Hoensbroek
The Netherlands

**Bencie Woll**
Centre of Clinical Communication
Studies
City University
Northampton Square
London EC10 0HB
United Kingdom

# Introduction

## STEPHEN VON TETZCHNER AND MOGENS HYGUM JENSEN

Augmentative and alternative communication involves the use of non-speech modes as a supplement to, or a substitute for, spoken language. The main focus here is the usage of manual and graphic communication systems in interventions for populations with developmental disorders of speech and language, including children, adolescents and adults with autism, dysphasia, intellectual impairment and motor impairment. The models of language and communication applied by interventionists are the basis for their understanding of acquisition and use of normal and atypical language and communication forms. In designing interventions, this understanding is essential for defining goals and selecting strategies to be applied.

This volume is a first attempt to establish a distinctive alternative to complement the predominantly behavioural orientation within the field of augmentative and alternative communication. The perspectives presented here build on, or are influenced by, transactional models of development (Sameroff and Chandler, 1975; Sameroff and Fiese, 1990); the psycholinguistic tradition of studying the mental processes underlying the normal and atypical acquisition and use of language (e.g. Bates, Bretherton and Snyder, 1988; Brown, 1970; Crystal, 1987; Slobin, 1979; Tager-Flusberg, 1994; Yamada, 1990); and social-constructivist models of language and communication, which claim that 'an individual's abilities do not arise from the exercise of individually possessed "cognitive processes", but are constructed out of the social interactions an individual is immersed in' (Service, Lock and Chandler, 1989, p. 23; Bruner, 1983; Lock, 1980; Marková, Graumann and Foppa, 1995; Vygotsky, 1962).

The present chapters reflect the professional discourse within this field in Europe. They include theoretical descriptions and discussions, and experimental and clinical empirical studies. Clinical studies include case studies and group studies, as well as broader depictions of clinical practices within individual countries. The authors present different perspectives and insights, apparent in how theories of language and communication are integrated with models of habilitation, clinical

1

knowledge of non-speech communication and intervention, and understanding of the human and cultural situation of users of augmentative and alternative communication. In addition to clinical issues, the contribution of research on atypical language development and use to the understanding of language and communication in general is addressed.

Due to the existence of different languages and political and cultural traditions, Europe is far from being a unified continent. These differences underlie the relatively large variability in the development and implementation of services concerned with augmentative and alternative communication. Some countries have a longer tradition in this area than others, and the approaches applied differ. The political conditions may have played a significant role (cf. Kalman and Pajor, this volume; Mendes and Rato, this volume; Zangari, Lloyd and Vicker, 1994), but it is notable that many of the same major problems and barriers arise across countries and systems, but at different points in time. Thus, although theories and intervention approaches vary, the main issues addressed in this volume appear to be the same.

Terminology, notation and alternative communication systems referred to in this volume are presented at the end of this chapter.

## Augmentative and alternative communication in Europe

There have always been people with limited or no functional speech, but the written history of augmentative and alternative communication is both short and limited in scope. The Irish author Jonathan Swift may have been the first to describe an 'aided language system'. His fable of nearly 300 years ago seems to parallel present-day descriptions of the inconvenience of having to depend on a communication aid and the need for assistance in using this communication form:

> '... since Words are only Names for THINGS, it would be more convenient for all men to carry about with them, such THINGS as were necessary to express the particular Business they are to discourse on ... which hath only this Inconvenience attending it; that if a man's Business be very great, and of various Kinds, he must carry a greater Bundle of THINGS upon his Back, unless he can afford one or two strong Servants to attend him. I have often beheld two of those Sages almost sinking under the Weights of their Packs, like pedlars among us; who when they met in the Streets would lay down their loads, open their Sacks, and hold Conversation for an hour together; then put up their Implements, help each other to resume their Burthens and take their leave.' (Swift, 1726/1970, p. 158).

Lines may be drawn from present-day practices of augmentative and alternative communication intervention to the work of de L'Epée and Itard 200 years ago in France (cf. Lane, 1977), and to the various attempts through history to alleviate the grave communication problems and break the isolation of people with dual sensory impairment. The first may have been Diderot's *Letters on the blind, for use by those who can see* in 1749, followed by professionals for example in Belgium, England, Germany, Sweden and Switzerland in the nineteenth century (Meshcheryakov, 1979; van Dijk, 1966). Still, except for the use of manual signing in the education of deaf and deaf-blind children, the singular role of speech in language intervention remained unchallenged until the middle of this century (cf. O'Neill, 1980; Rockey, 1980; Weiner, 1986). Early use of pictures and traditional orthography have been documented in the autobiographies of people with motor impairments (cf. Brown, 1954; Steenbuch, 1957), but systematic use of non-speech communication for hearing populations did not really take hold until the end of the sixties (Bonvillian and Nelson, 1982; Kiernan, Reid and Jones, 1982; LaCour, Freund and Nielsen, 1979; McNaughton, 1990; von Tetzchner, 1990; Zangari et al., 1994).

European and North American traditions differ in several ways. North American researchers and practitioners tend to publish more than their European colleagues. For example, 70–75 per cent of all scientific publications within developmental psychology stems from North American researchers (Weinert, 1990). North American research also appears to receive considerably more attention than research conducted in other parts of the world. The fact that the English language is read by a large part of the professional society may partly explain this, but Weingart (1989) found that American journals were cited much more frequently than European journals published in English, which again were cited more often than scientific journals published in German.

The North American influence is also strong in the field of augmentative and alternative communication. The major scientific journal in this field is *Augmentative and Alternative Communication*, published by the International Society for Augmentative and Alternative Communication. In the eight issues of 1993 and 1994, 52 articles (including letters to the editor) by 97 different authors (some authors appeared in more than one article) were published in this journal. Of these, 41 articles were written by authors with a North American affiliation (some authors were not originally from North America, but attended a university there), seven articles were by European authors, and one article was by Japanese authors. Three articles were co-authored by researchers from North America and a non-American country. Eighty-two authors had a North American affiliation, ten gave a European address, and five came from Japan and Australia. Of the two thousand references listed in these articles, only eight titles referred to publications in a language other than English.

The empirical knowledge gathered by North American researchers has been invaluable for European researchers and practitioners, as indicated by the large number of references to North American literature in the European literature, including the present volume. However, scientific evolution depends on diversity and selectivity (Plotkin, 1994), and the result of the North American dominance has been less diversity in theoretical bases and intervention approaches than would be optimal for the development of the field. Moreover, for most European countries, the national language is not English. In addition to text books for parents and professionals, research reports published in the country's national language are important for building up competence and disseminating information nationally (cf. Mendes and Rato, this volume). However, such reports, which might have been a supplement to the North American studies, are often only known locally.

In addition, cross-cultural studies may be an important source of information about the consequences of different organisational structures and use of intervention strategies. This kind of knowledge is important both for understanding the development of individuals who use augmentative and alternative communication in various settings, and for planning and organising habilitation services.

Different European countries have not given the same degree of attention to all groups who might need augmentative and alternative communication. Some potential users have normal language comprehension and need mainly an expressive means (cf. Martinsen and von Tetzchner, this volume). This group is typically associated with communication aids and graphic representations. The situation prior to the present-day approaches is not well documented, but communication boards were produced by F. Hall Roe in the USA at the beginning of this century (Goldberg and Fenton, 1960). Similar devices based on written language were probably in use in other countries as well. However, for children and others belonging to this group who were unable to read, descriptions given by pioneers in Europe and North America are very similar, indicating a lack of systematic material for making expressive language available through graphic means. Picture boards were used, but not in a systematic manner, typically produced with material from magazines and the like (McNaughton, 1990; von Tetzchner, 1990). The introduction of Blissymbols was a true revolution, not only because it made expressive language available to motor-impaired and non-reading individuals with good comprehension of spoken language, but also because it opened up the systematic use of graphic sign systems in general. The significance of this influence can hardly be overestimated. It is relevant for the history of alternative communication systems that Lenneberg in 1962 published a study that demonstrated comprehension of spoken language by a person unable to speak. The results are not surprising, but the fact that this study was published in a scientific journal mirrors the beliefs usually held at the time about the potential competence of non-speaking people.

The other important innovation was the application of alternative communication systems also for hearing individuals with severe or profound linguistic and intellectual impairment. The first published studies were to a large extent motivated by the discussion of the biological bases of language and the question whether language is specific to the human species (cf. Chomsky, 1959, 1968; Lenneberg, 1967; Skinner, 1957). Strategies which had been used for teaching manual and graphic signs to primates in order to demonstrate language in these species were extended to humans with limited cognitive function (e.g. Deich and Hodges, 1977; Fulwiler and Fouts, 1976; Premack, 1974).

Augmentative and alternative communication intervention for both groups expanded fast in some European countries, like the Scandinavian countries and the United Kingdom (cf. Bjerregaard and Nygaard, 1975; Kiernan et al., 1982; von Tetzchner, 1990). A survey in 1978 indicated that 53 per cent of the special schools for intellectually impaired, autistic, and language impaired children in the United Kingdom used manual and/or graphic signs (Kiernan et al., 1982). Blissymbols were used in The Netherlands first in 1973 (Koerselman, 1994), shortly after these were first introduced to non-speaking individuals in Canada (McNaughton and Kates, 1974). In Norway and Sweden, Blissymbols came into use around 1976. A Swedish device based on Blissymbols and synthetic speech was ready in 1981, and in 1983 the number of Blissymbols users in Sweden was estimated at 1000 persons. A Nordic Blissymbolics Committee, comprising Denmark, Finland, Iceland, Norway and Sweden, was formed in 1978 (Holgersen, 1996, December 1995; Björck-Åkesson, 1983; Jaroma, 1992). Other European countries did not get started until the eighties, but are catching up (cf. Braun, 1994; Kalman and Pajor, this volume; Mendes and Rato, this volume). In some countries, like Greece, France and Austria, augmentative and alternative communication seems to have had little influence on research and intervention practices.

The introduction of manual signs for hearing individuals was mainly directed at people with intellectual impairments, and this took place simultaneously with the general sign language revolution in the seventies (Berg and Sørhuglen, 1980; Bjerregaard and Nygaard, 1975; Grove and Walker, 1990; Kiernan et al., 1982). A number of books on the sign languages of deaf people appeared between 1975 and 1985 (e.g. Engberg-Pedersen, Hansen and Sørensen, 1981; Friedman, 1977; Klima and Bellugi, 1979; Martinsen, Nordeng and von Tetzchner, 1985; Schlesinger and Namir, 1978; Woll, Kyle and Deuchar, 1981). However, European countries differ significantly with regard to how much they use manual signing. A positive attitude toward manual signing for deaf people was probably an important factor for beginning to teach manual signs to hearing, intellectually impaired people. Such attitudes were found in North America, Scandinavia and the United Kingdom, and in these countries, manual signs have been more commonly used than graphic systems (Bonvillian and Nelson, 1982; Grove and Walker, 1990; Kiernan et al., 1982; von Tetzchner, 1993a; Zangari et al., 1994).

In countries with a primarily oral approach to the education of deaf children, for example, Germany, Hungary and Portugal, systematic alternative language intervention seems to have started with Blissymbols in the early eighties (Ursula Braun, personal communication, October 1995; Kalman and Pajor, this volume; Mendes and Rato, this volume). As a form of written language parallel to Chinese, the Blissymbolics system may have been more acceptable than pictures and manual signs, while at the same time in fact preparing the ground for the development and wider use of pictographic systems, because it contributed to making the possibilities of graphic systems clear, as well as the shortcomings of a too advanced system (cf. Kalman and Pajor, this volume). It may be noted, however, that the countries who took up manual signing early also tended to adopt the use of graphic signs quickly.

The first electronic communication aid was made by the British company Possum (Copeland, 1974), but more recently much of the North American technology has been adopted in Europe. However, systems like Minspeak (Baker, 1986) have not been readily available outside English-speaking countries, due to lack of synthetic speech technology or because an incompatible technology was used. Because there is no competition in developing speech technology for languages used by a comparatively small number of people, these technologies have tended to be developed late, and, like synthesised Norwegian, to have poor quality. There is, for example, still no speech synthesiser available for Irish (Martine Smith, personal communication, August 1995; see also Kallen and Smith, 1992). Being language independent, devices with digitised speech became popular in several European countries.

In many countries, the new technologies created optimism, and there is little doubt that the technology used in modern communication aids has been a decisive factor in creating the interest in aided communication of the last ten years. However, it also led to an emphasis on technology rather than intervention and communication. This was unfortunate, because expectations were not fulfilled and economy instead of function became the main focus, in particular in countries where communication aids are not provided free by the state. In some instances, the technological focus became a barrier to other intervention strategies. The attraction of technology and the fact that communication aid users include individuals with good comprehension of spoken language, compared to manual signing which usually is directed at people with cognitive impairments, may have contributed to the relatively greater interest in aided rather than in non-aided forms of alternative communication.

# Main themes

Two main themes pervade this volume. Both are related to a need felt by professionals for intervention based on a more thorough understanding of non-speech communication, as well as of the processes involved in habilitative work. One theme thus relates to communicative interaction with non-speech communicative means, with an emphasis on linguistic complexity and interaction. The understanding of these issues may be enhanced by investigating the details of dialogues, and many of the authors present excerpts of real communicative exchanges. To our knowledge, there are more such excerpts in this volume than in all published books on augmentative and alternative communication combined.

Most of the earlier studies focused on the acquisition of individual manual and graphic signs, and to a lesser degree on multi-sign utterances. Discussions of communicative exchanges were almost non-existent. This was true for both manual and graphic signs. After 1985, communicative processes of aided language use have received some attention (cf. Alm, Arnott and Newell, 1989; Blau, 1986; Kraat, 1985; Light, 1985, 1988), but analyses of dialogues and conversational interactions have remained rare. Such analyses are even less frequent in studies of manual signing, probably related to the fact that many aided language users have primarily motor impairments and normal intellectual skills, while nearly all hearing people who depend on manual signing are severely or profoundly intellectually impaired with extremely limited language and communication skills.

A number of the chapters in the present volume are concerned with multi-sign utterances and dialogues. For example, Grove, Dockrell and Woll investigate multi-sign utterances and productive grammar among intellectually impaired children. Sarriá, Gómez and Tamarit discuss how autistic children may be helped in overcoming their special problems in establishing and maintaining social interaction. The collaborative nature of interactions involving the use of communication aids is demonstrated by several authors (Collins; van Balkom and Welle Donker-Gimbrère; von Tetzchner and Martinsen). Similar collaborations may be apparent in interactions involving manual signing as well (Møller and von Tetzchner). The communication form may in itself play a crucial role (cf. Alm and Newell; Heim and Baker-Mills; Smith), and several authors address the particular multimodal situation of people who understand spoken language, but express themselves by alternative non-speech means (Gangkofer and von Tetzchner; Grove et al.; Martinsen and von Tetzchner; Møller and von Tetzchner; von Tetzchner et al.). However, in addition to reflecting the children's impairments and the functional characteristics of communication aids, the unique dialogue contributions of young aided language users may also, through transactional processes, influence the conversations and their parents' interactional styles (von Tetzchner and Martinsen).

Heim and Baker-Mills suggest that intervention for children may be indirect only, based on models present in the environment and feedback on own production, similar to children who develop speech normally. Hjelmquist and Sandberg, on the other hand, maintain that adolescents who use Blissymbols may fail to utilise the metalinguistic competence they actually have. One may speculate whether this may be a result of insufficient explicit teaching, and that young aided speakers will benefit from a mixture of implicit and explicit teaching (cf. Martinsen and von Tetzchner).

The other main theme approached is the question of how to involve parents and professionals in the creation of a language-supportive environment. This theme is related to the previous one through a common focus on the interactional context, which is central for understanding the changes taking place in intervention practices. These changes are necessary in order to address the diverse contexts of the total environment and the life quality of the communication impaired person. The historical processes constitute a clear undercurrent in many chapters, reflecting the cultural diversity of present-day practices and the professional situation in various countries (Basil and Soro-Camats; Björck-Åkesson, Granlund and Olsson; Gangkofer and von Tetzchner; Kalman and Pajor; Launonen; Lourenço et al.; Mendes and Rato; Møller and von Tetzchner). In spite of the cultural differences and the more extensive theoretical framework for example presented by Björck-Åkesson and her associates compared with the clinical observations presented by Kalman and Pajor, Mendes and Rato, and Lourenço and her associates, similar processes are apparent in Sweden, Portugal and Hungary.

Alternative communication systems are still to a large extent regarded as educational tools rather than as everyday means of communication (Gangkofer and von Tetzchner, this volume; Lourenço et al., this volume; Smith 1991; von Tetzchner, in press). There is a gradual change of focus, from the educational setting alone to a more comprehensive view of the total life situation of the individual in question. There also seems to be a change toward an earlier onset of alternative language intervention, and from augmentative and alternative communication intervention being a strategy for an exclusive group to a general prophylactic strategy for individuals at risk for severe language impairment. Crucial issues within the second theme are the training of professionals, parents and other significant people, and the creation of a fully language-supportive environment. Due to the fact that augmentative and alternative communication represents a new approach for many professionals, training and supervision of those who are responsible is imperative in order to implement appropriate intervention strategies. There is increased attention to the home situation and other non-educational settings, but in some countries, influencing the awareness of professionals has been the primary goal, with inclusion of parents still lagging behind (cf. Basil and Soro-Camats; Björck-Åkesson et al.; Heim and Baker-Mills; Kalman and Pajor; Launonen; Lourenço et al.; Mendes and Rato).

In spite of the fact that the growth of the field of augmentative and alternative communication has been closely related to the general development of information technology, there are few technically oriented chapters. This may mirror the fact that the technology probably is more advanced than is necessary for the applications of the technology. The two chapters with a main focus on technological development (Alm and Newell; Brodin and von Tetzchner) are more concerned with interaction and dialogues than with the technology itself, and thus reflect the fact that the main barrier to the development of more functional communication aids is not the state of available technology, but rather insufficient understanding of communicative and linguistic processes. The same view is apparent in the discussion of models (von Tetzchner et al.).

Many of the chapters present a case study or use one or several individual cases to illustrate theoretical or practical points. A number of case studies exist in the professional literature and some authors believe these have outplayed their role (e.g. Iacono, 1994). However, the case studies presented here clearly demonstrate a need for the reflection and awareness that can only grow from a basis of detailed descriptions. Case studies are a method of record keeping to document diagnostic and interventional practices (Yin, 1989) and '... do seem to have a pivotal role to play in the early years of a behavioural science' (Crystal, 1986, p. 143).

The main function of early case studies was to demonstrate that augmentative and alternative communication intervention may be useful for people with various impairments. This is no longer important, and present-day case studies have a different function, namely to focus on processes of communication and intervention that may not easily be explored by quantitative studies with a single individual or a group of subjects. The strength of the experimental approach is that the contribution of particular factors can be isolated by controlling for other factors that may influence the course of intervention. The strength of case studies lies in their 'degree of freedom' and the inclusion of rich contextual information typical of real intervention situations (cf. Campbell, 1975). There is actually a dearth of such descriptions within a communication framework. Most studies describe intervention in rather loose terms without including the interactions that result from the same interventions.

Moreover, without detailed descriptions of everyday practice and the resulting communication skills, the implications of theory and empirical studies for practice may sometimes be difficult to interpret, and consequently hard for professionals to relate the knowledge these studies provide to their own practice. 'In high utilization environments research producers and users belong to overlapping professional networks with ongoing communication ... the objective (of which) is to assure that researchers and users are exposed to each other's worlds and ideas – producing a rich marketplace of ideas' (Yin, 1993, pp. 19-20). Case studies may thus fulfil the function of facilitating the transfer of knowledge from theoretical reflections and experimental studies to everyday practice, thus contributing to a foundation for expert and non-expert professional discourse (cf. Habermas, 1984, 1987).

The cases presented in this volume are exemplary, not because they demonstrate the best possible practice, but because it is possible to learn from them. Some of them demonstrate the difficulties encountered when attempting to transform theoretical notions and empirical research into the practical everyday life, or when intervention strategies are developed without sufficient understanding of the possibilities and limitations of alternative communication systems and the various impairments people who are using them may have (cf., Soro-Camats, Basil,Gangkofer and von Tetzchner; Kalman and Pajor; Møller and von Tetzchner)

## Terminology

We have attempted to employ terminology used in the modern professional literature, though allowing for a certain variety. However, at one point the terminology of the present volume differs from most of the literature within the field. The term 'sign' is used as a generic term for linguistic forms that are not speech and includes all kinds of manual and graphic forms. The reason for this is that although in the literature on augmentative and alternative communication graphic signs have often been described as 'symbols', in the field of linguistics, both vocal (speech), manual and graphic signs are referred to as language symbols (Lyons, 1977). From a semiological perspective, Peirce (1931-1958), among others, distinguishes between 'symbolic' and 'iconic' signs. According to Peirce, a symbol is an arbitrary sign while non-arbitrary signs are 'icons'. The majority of the graphic signs of the 'symbol' systems (PCS, PIC, etc.) would not have been regarded as symbols by Peirce. Using the term 'symbol' to describe only one type of communication system seems imprudent. Because it refers to the actual form of the expression, 'sign' appears to be a more neutral concept.

Distinctions are made between *manual* and *graphic* systems (see below), as well as between *aided* and *non-aided* communication forms (cf. Lloyd and Fuller, 1986). The term *non-speaking* is used to indicate that an alternative language form is used, while use of the term *nonverbal* will indicate that the person in question lacks any kind of language; spoken, manual or graphic.

A distinction is made between habilitation and rehabilitation (von Tetzchner, 1992, p. 13):

*Habilitation* means to build up and support functions, interaction and life quality for people with congenital or early acquired impairments.

*Rehabilitation* means to rebuild previously mastered but lost functions, and recreate possibilities for interaction and life quality for people with acquired impairments.

An important reason for making this distinction is that there may be large differences between the consequences of congenital and early acquired impairments on the one hand, and impairments acquired at a later age on the other. A congenital or early acquired impairment may make it difficult to develop skills which are only indirectly related to the impairment. For example, people who lose sight and hearing at an adult age can usually still speak and write, while people born deaf and blind rarely learn these skills. Many children with motor and speech impairments develop reading and writing difficulties, while adults who get comparable motor and speech impairments rarely acquire such difficulties. These differences have important implications for intervention goals and strategies. Moreover, due to the diverse developmental experiences of the two groups, their cultures and life forms will also differ. The present volume is mainly concerned with habilitation.

The term *significant people* is used to refer to family, friends, daily carers in sheltered housing, and others who are close to the person or responsible for his or her interests. It does not usually comprise teachers and other educators. Age is indicated with years;months. If Tom is five years and three months old, this may be expressed as 'Tom is 5;3' or 'Tom is aged 5;3'.

# Notation

A throng of notational systems has been used by various authors. It is now a generally accepted convention to use capital letters for manual signs (SIGNS), but there is no generally accepted notational system comprising all or most forms of non-speech language expressions. The conventions used here are based on the professional literature and suggestions made by authors of the present volume (Table 0.1). There may be room for improvement, but we urge other authors to adopt these or suggest improvements referring to the notations used here. We also want to emphasise that personal preferences should not play a major role when adopting one or another notational system. One convention is as good as another, as long as most authors adhere to it, and it will probably take quite a long time for any notation to become truly conventional.

Table 0.1: Notations

*Naturally spoken utterances* are italicised.

'*Words and sentences produced with digitised or synthesised speech*' are italicised and in quotation marks.

MANUAL SIGNS are in capital letters.

*GRAPHIC SIGNS* and *PICTURES* are in capital letters and italicised.

Some manual or graphic signs need more than one word in translation. When the gloss of a single sign contains two or more words, these will be hyphenated, for example YOU-AND-ME.

<u>Indications of whole words and written ready-made sentences</u> are underlined.

<u>S-p-e-l-l-i-n-g</u> is underlined and has hyphens between letters.

'Interpretations or translations of meaning' is used for interpretations of manual or graphic sign utterances. It is also used when giving the meaning of facial expressions, gestures, pointing,etc., for example, 'yes' (nodding) and 'no' (shaking the head).

{ ... } indicates simultaneous expressive forms, for example speech and manual signs, or manual and graphic signs. {GLAD *I am glad*} means that the manual sign GLAD is produced simultaneously with the naturally spoken sentence *I am glad*.

## Communication systems

### Manual signs

There are two types of manual signs. The national sign languages have developed through use by the deaf population, for example British, Catalan, Danish, French and Norwegian Sign Language. They have grammars that are different from the national spoken languages. These also differ from each other and there may be dialectal variation within the national language (Engberg-Pedersen, Hansen and Sørensen, 1981; Martinsen et al., 1985; Woll, Kyle and Deuchar, 1981). The other type consists of manual sign systems, that is, systems of manual signs which are designed to reflect the spoken languages. They may to a lesser or greater degree be based on the vocabulary of the national sign language, but the syntax and eventual inflections are derived from the spoken language. Also these systems differ from one country to the other, and include for example *Signed Norwegian* (Norsk tegnordbok, 1986), and *The Paget Gorman Sign System* (Paget, 1936; Paget, Gorman and Paget, 1976), as well as the *Methodological Signs* introduced by de L'Epée (1776). For hearing, language-impaired populations, manual sign systems rather than sign languages are applied.

## Graphic signs

Graphic sign systems are often linked to the use of communication aids, ranging from simple pointing boards to devices based on advanced computer technology. Blissymbols (Bliss, 1965) and Premack's plastic shapes (Premack and Premack, 1972) were two of the first systems to be used, but quite a number of systems have come into existence in the course of time. Only the systems represented in the current volume will be illustrated here (for overviews, see Vanderheiden and Lloyd, 1986; von Tetzchner and Martinsen, 1992; Welle Donker-Gimbrère and van Balkom, 1995). Examples are shown in Figure 0.1.

### *Blissymbols*

Blissymbols are a form of logographic writing, that is, written signs that are not based on the alphabetic principle. This means that the word, not the letter, becomes the smallest unit in the written language (Downing, 1973). It was first used in Toronto as a system of writing for physically disabled children unable to speak and with additional difficulties in learning to read and write (McNaughton and Kates, 1974).

The Blissymbolics system consists of 100 basic signs that can be combined to form words for which there are no basic signs. A number of these sign combinations are conventional, but a specific Blissymbol or a given combination may be used slightly dissimilarly in different countries, in the same way as a word in the spoken language when translated is not exactly the same in another language. Where a conventional combination has not been decided upon, there may be several ways of expressing the same word in Blissymbols.

Communication boards with Blissymbols usually consist of both basic signs and combinations that the user often needs. For the majority of words in the spoken languages, however, there are no established conventions, and in many cases, users of Blissymbols may either not know the accepted form or lack the necessary basic signs. Thus, it will be up to the user to find a suitable sign combination to express what he or she wishes to say.

The Blissymbols that form a combination may be regarded as semantic elements. The single signs are combined and given meaning through analogy. For example, *ELEPHANT* usually consists of *ANIMAL+LONG+NOSE*. *HOME* is *HOUSE+FEELINGS*. *TOILET* is *CHAIR+WATER*. *HAPPY* is *FEELING+UP*. In addition to the graphic signs that correspond to whole words, there are also a number of Blissymbols that constitute grammatical inflections and denote parts of speech, such as *PAST, PLURAL, ACTION, OPPOSITE-MEANING*, etc. Thus the Blissymbolics system has a fairly complex construction, based on combinations of signs, including grammatical elements.

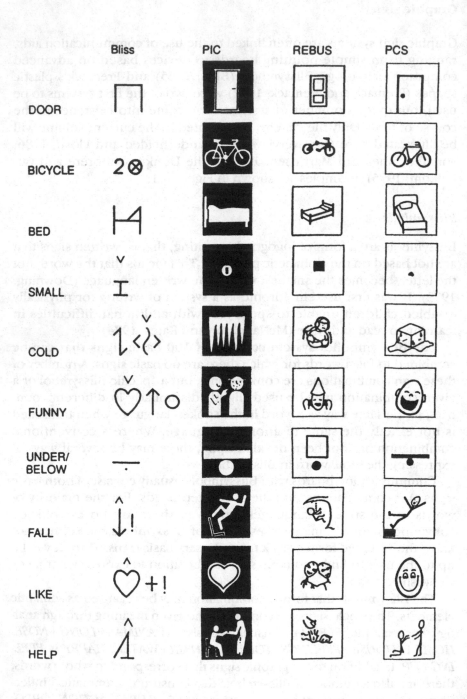

**Figure 0.1:** Systems referred to in this volume: Blissymbols, PIC, Rebus and PCS.

The basic signs and sign combinations may also be joined together to form sentences. Bliss (1965) gives information about syntax but in principle any word order may be used. In most countries, the word order taught will resemble that of the spoken language.

## PIC

The Picture Ideogram Communication System (PIC) originated from Canada (Maharaj, 1980). This system has become very popular in the Nordic countries and Portugal, and has to a great extent replaced the use of Blissymbols for people with intellectual impairment or extensive language difficulties. PIC consists of stylised drawings which form white silhouettes on a black background. The gloss is always written in white lettering above the drawing. The number of PIC signs vary between countries. There are 563 Norwegian (1989), 705 Danish (1995), and 400 Portuguese PIC signs (1989). The Dutch system *Vijfhoek Pictogrammen Systeem* is based on PIC (Welle Donker-Gimbrère and van Balkom, 1995). Also PIC signs may be used to form sentences, as well as new words, but this is not a usual practice (von Tetzchner and Martinsen, this volume).

## PCS

Picture Communication Symbols (PCS, Johnson, 1981, 1985) consists of approximately 1800 signs. These are simple black and white line-drawings with the gloss written above. Some function words, such as articles and prepositions, for example *OF, FOR* and *WITH* are represented in traditional orthography without any line-drawing. The signs are easy to draw, and PCS can therefore be easily copied by hand. PCS is common in the United Kingdom, Ireland and Spain, and is growing in popularity in Denmark.

## Rebus

As with Blissymbols, the Peabody Rebus Reading Program (Woodcock, Clark and Davies, 1969) was devised as a system of logographic writing (Clark, 1984). A British version, closely linked with the Makaton project, has been developed (van Oosterom and Devereux, 1985; Walker et al., 1985).

The Rebus system to a certain extent represents a different approach to that of Blissymbols, PIC and PCS. The system consists of 950 graphic signs, the majority of which are iconic. It is possible to combine these in the usual way; *STREET+LIGHT* becomes *STREETLIGHT*. In addition to the usual combinations of words, the pronunciation of the sign's gloss may also be used. For example, *LIGHT* can mean both 'bright' and 'not

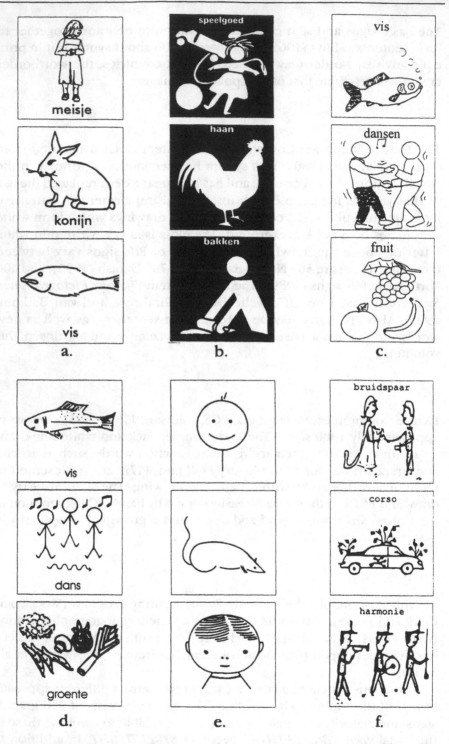

**Figure 0.2:** Six Dutch graphic sign systems: a) Taalzakboek, b) Vijfhoek Pictogrammen systeem, C) Beta Beeldtaal, d)Maria Roepaan Beeldlezen, e) Picto and f)Van Geijtenbeek Beeldplaatjes.

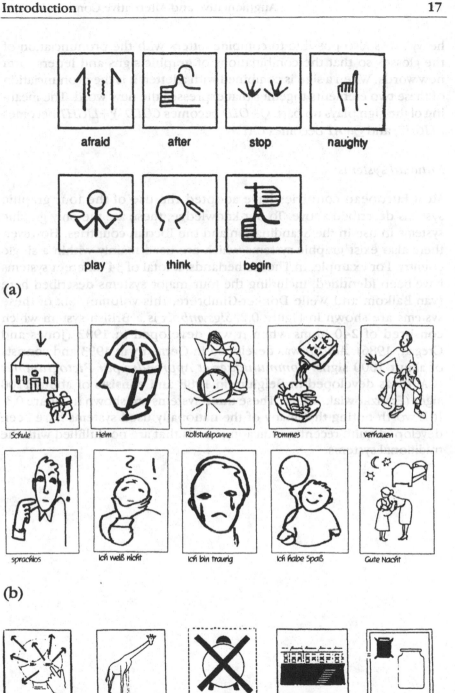

(a)

(b)

(c)

**Figure 0.3:** a) Sigsymbols from United Kingdom, b) Alladin from Germany, and c) Communiquer et Apprendre par Pictogrammes (CAP) from Belgium.

heavy'. It is also possible to combine letters with the pronunciation of the glosses so that the combinations of graphic signs and letters form new words. When a sign is combined with a letter, it is the pronunciation of these two elements together that expresses the new word. The meaning of the sign plays no part. C+*OLD* becomes *COLD*. P+*LIGHT* becomes *PLIGHT*, and C+*AT* becomes *CAT*.

## National systems

Most European countries have adopted the use of the four graphic systems described above. To our knowledge, these are the only graphic systems in use in the Scandinavian and the Iberian countries. However, there also exist graphic systems which are used mainly within a single country. For example, in The Netherlands, a total of 34 different systems have been identified, including the four major systems described here (van Balkom and Welle Donker-Gimbrère, this volume). Six of these systems are shown in Figure 0.2. *Sigsymbols* is a British system which consisted of 240 items when it was developed in 1982 (Jones and Cregan, 1986). *Aladin* was developed in Germany in 1993 and consists of about 1000 signs. *Communiquer et Apprendre par Pictogrammes* (CAP) was developed in Belgium in 1988 and consists of about 1200 signs (Franzkowiak, 1994). These three systems are shown in Figure 0.3. It is worth noting that many of the nationally used systems have been developed quite recently, indicating needs that are not fulfilled with the traditional systems.

# Chapter 1
# Preliminaries to a comprehensive model of augmentative and alternative communication

STEPHEN VON TETZCHNER, NICOLA GROVE, FILIP LONCKE,
SARAH BARNETT, BENCIE WOLL AND JOHN CLIBBENS

Researchers and practitioners alike depend on a theoretical framework
for their work, whether it is explicitly formulated or not. A model represents a formalisation of a perspective which might serve as a guide to
develop hypotheses and scientific inquiry, as well as the individual interventions of practitioners. It may help to make the implicit assumptions
of research and practice explicit, public and open to scrutiny and
change, and thereby aid in generating new knowledge and avoiding
unwarranted positions. However, explicit theoretical models are lacking
within the field of augmentative and alternative communication. One
consequence of this is a lack of theoretical coherence. This makes it difficult to explain the positive or negative results of interventions, or to
generate theoretically based predictions which might improve subsequent interventions. For practitioners a model may help in selecting
appropriate systems and modes for communication, and – equally
important – in seeing the complex interrelationships between an individual's skills and modes of communication and conversational
processes and standing in the community.

Although language can be used for other purposes than communication, such as the regulation of own behaviour described by Vygotsky and
Luria (Luria and Yudovich, 1959; Vygotsky, 1962), it is the processes
underlying conversational exchanges that are the main focus here. The
essence may be depicted as a conversation between two individuals
taking turns expressing and perceiving messages, thereby creating and
negotiating meaning in order to make themselves understood and to
understand the other.

A number of models have been designed to describe some or all
aspects of the production and reception of vocal language and the
communicative exchanges in various conversational settings (for
reviews, see Miller and Eimas, 1995). However, it is not clear whether

these models fully capture the special instances of multimodal and coproductive conversations involving augmentative and alternative language users.

For the purpose of this chapter, considerations are mainly directed at developmental disorders. To include aphasia as well as amyotrophic lateral sclerosis, Batten disease and other acquired or negatively progressing conditions, additional considerations would apply.

In this chapter, it is not our intention to advance one specific model but to focus on issues which must be attended to when using existing models or attempting to develop and apply new models for the processes underlying the acquisition, comprehension and use of alternative and augmentative communication. Three different perspectives will be discussed: from written language, bilingualism, and the theory of relevance.

## General and specific models

The first question is whether a special model of augmentative and alternative communication is needed or whether a more general model would suffice. One problem with a special model is that one may lose contact with mainstream developments in the study of language and communication. The literature in the field of augmentative and alternative communication already seems quite self-referential and narrow in focus, often citing minor authors within this field instead of authors who are central within the main literature. In addition, introducing augmentative and alternative communication into general models may actually broaden the scope of these models, in the same way as the definition presented by Hockett (1960), which specified that language should be 'vocal', had to be modified as a result of the sign language revolution in the seventies (Schlesinger, 1970).

On the other hand, distinctive characteristics of augmentative and alternative communication may make special treatment necessary, first and foremost the multimodal and coproductive situation discussed below. There also seems to be a fundamental difference between communication where the articulatory process is integrated with the form of the utterance (as in speech and manual signs), and communication where graphic or tactile signs are selected from a static display and the planned movements involved in articulating the message may consist of indicating with hand or eye, or activating a switch with the head. Languages which have evolved naturally, in face-to-face communication, are spoken or signed – although in theory, a graphic language could evolve in a similar way (Donaldson, 1993; Welle Donker-Grimbrère, 1994). The difference may only be one of automaticity – once the communicator has attained technical and procedural competence, language is processed in an ordinary manner. Alternatively, the language mode may have an impact on the way linguistic information is represented and processed. Further, in ordinary linguistic interactions, the same mode of communication is used by the individual for both producing and perceiving language. Thus, even if a general model is used, in order for it to account for the special characteristics of augmentative communication, it may be necessary to integrate special adaptations as suggested by Lloyd, Quist and Windsor (1990). In that case, the difference between a special model and an adapted general model is a practical rather than a theoretical issue and may depend on the extent of the modifications.

## Multimodal communication

An overriding issue is the relationship between non-speech forms and speech, and the asymmetrical relation between the language modes of the disabled communicator and the spoken language of the environment. People in the environment may adapt to the alternative communication user in three main ways (Martinsen and von Tetzchner, this volume).

Firstly, they may adopt the alternative mode and use this in all communications with the person, in this way creating an enclave of alternative communication use within an environment of natural speakers. Such enclaves may consist of the school, home, institution and similarly restricted environments. This would make communication symmetric and pose few problems for traditional communication models, making modifications necessary only to allow for new forms of signs (manual, graphic and tactile) and slower communication.

Secondly, people in the environment may speak normally when responding to the user of alternative or augmented modes. This would imply that both of the partners use different modes of communication for comprehension and production. Except for professional translators, it is unusual even for bilingual people to find themselves in situations where they have to simultaneously comprehend one system and produce another. This is, however, often the case for users of augmentative and alternative language, and a model would have to account for this multimodal situation.

Thirdly, people in the environment may speak normally, perceive the alternative form when used and translate what the disabled person has said into speech. Such translations may consist in reading traditional orthographic script or be quite similar to traditional translation between cultural languages such as Norwegian and English. The translation may not even be made for the non-vocal communicator but for the conversational partner's own benefit. Other translations may go beyond the ordinary processes of interpretation and formulation, involving, to use a statistical metaphor, a higher 'degree of freedom' in interpretation. The disabled communicator may be asked to acknowledge the translation and in some cases, the translation may involve a long negotiation process before the message is phrased or paraphrased (cf. Collins, this volume). The nature of these translations implies that the natural speaker will be responsible for speaking the messages of both parties and for providing back-channel conversational devices (Blau, 1986). These behaviours are typical of dialogues between aided language users and natural speakers, but are also apparent in other kinds of interaction where messages are perceived as incomplete or ambiguous, for example people with learning disabilities whose speech or manual signing is unintelligible.

People in the environment of a non-vocal communicator may not adhere to one of these main strategies but mix them. Significant people in an individual's environment may not use the same set of strategies, and the communication impaired individual may not have the same degree of competence in different modes or systems. For example, a person may be more competent in one mode or system for teasing, swearing and 'chatting-up', but have greater competence in another mode or system for discussing theoretical physics.

The code model proposed by Lloyd, Quist and Windsor (1990) offers one perspective on multimodal communication. The proposition is that the original message is formulated as a spoken representation by both partners, and subsequently coded into an alternative or augmentative modality as required for effective communication. This position is challenged by recent findings which suggest that although the code model may account for the behaviour of the natural speaker, the disabled communicator may realise meaning directly into an alternative modality (e.g. manual or graphic sign) rather than translating a spoken representation (Fuller and Wright, 1994; Grove, Dockrell and Woll, this volume; Smith, this volume). It may therefore be appropriate to consider other perspectives, on both the psychological and the sociological impact of multimodal communication. Two relevant approaches are suggested by the study of language acquisition and use in bilinguals, and by the study of the relationship between primary forms of language (spoken or signed) and their written derivatives (text). These approaches may be viewed as metaphors, or analogies, for looking at augmentative and alternative communication.

# Primary and derived languages

The analogy of written text rests on a distinction between primary and derived languages. Primary language systems have evolved, seemingly as a biological adaptation which is species-specific (Darwin, 1871; Lenneberg, 1967). The distinction between primary and derived modes is basically a distinction between what came first and what has been the result of a subsequent recoding. It implies that each manual, graphic and tactile sign corresponds to a spoken word - a gloss - and that putting together the glosses of the signs will produce a spoken message, as when reading aloud. The only problem in the 'reading' may be that some words are lacking due to a telegraphic style. This metaphor is probably implicit in the work of many practitioners.

Manually coded speech, finger spelling and Morse code are derived from the primary-form speech. By contrast, British Sign Language, Catalan Sign Language and other national sign languages are primary languages in their own right. Although essentially a form of script, claims have been made that Blissymbols may function independently from spoken languages (Besio and Chinato, this volume). However, the same may be said about signed variants of speech which in practice rarely follow the spoken form. Keyword signing and cued speech are not really derived forms but devices for augmenting the partner's comprehension of speech, and as an input to language production, the result may be a mapping that is different from the primary mode (cf. Grove et al., this volume). This may shed some doubt about the tendency to use terms 'augmentative' and 'alternative' as if they were equivalent: the consequences for language development may be very different if a modality augments a primary language, or serves as the primary language.

The basic distinction between what comes first and what follows from a recoding also often mirrors the sequence of acquisition. For example, most people acquire speech (the primary mode) prior to learning to read and write (the derived mode). For access to written language, people need more than just an environment that exposes them to print – they need to learn the rules which match phonological and orthographic codes. It is possible for high levels of fluency to develop so that eventually the process of expressing oneself in a derived language is automatic, but many people never obtain this level of literacy. Donaldson (1993) argues that learning to write could be as natural as learning to speak if script were used as the mother-tongue, that is, functioned as a primary language. Further, variation of the canonical acquisition order is possible. Individuals with motor impairments may learn graphic signs or traditional orthography before they learn to speak (Koerselman, 1994; vander Beken et al, 1994).

The perspective offered by the acquisition of literacy suggests that research and practice in augmentative and alternative communication should take account of the relationship between primary and derived forms of language and their interaction with the learning sequence for individuals. Attention needs to be paid to the way in which one language form maps onto another, and the potential effects on learning and use.

# Bilingualism and bilinguality

For the purpose of simplification, the term 'bilingual' is used in this context to refer to both bilingual and multilingual situations. The use of two or more forms of language may have consequences for processing skills of the individual as well as for social structures and community structures. The sociolinguistic literature has adopted a multidimensional approach, distinguishing bilinguality and bilingualism (Hamers and Blanc, 1989). *Bilinguality* is concerned with cognitive aspects of the competence of an individual, such as differences between receptive and productive skills, cognitive organisation and stage of learning. *Bilingualism* is concerned with socio-cultural aspects affecting the different language groups within a community, such as diglossia, differences related to language use and cultural identity. The issues related to bilinguality and bilingualism demonstrate the interaction of dimensions to be included in a comprehensive model.

Relative to bilinguality, an alternative language form may be the first or the second language learned, depending on the relationship between reception and production. If the relationship is asymmetric, as for children with a good comprehension of speech using aided communication who tend to get expressive means only after their comprehension is assessed (von Tetzchner, 1988), acquisition strategies may be similar to second language learning even if it is their first mode of expression. If the relationship is symmetric, with the child needing the augmentative language for both reception and production, strategies will be similar to first language acquisition (Martinsen and von Tetzchner, this volume).

Relative to bilingualism, the analogy rests on the similarity between a multilingual or bilingual situation and the asymmetrical relation between the language modes of some users of alternative language. A major difference, however, is that people belonging to a linguistic minority interact with other people using the same language, including communities of deaf people using sign languages (cf. Lane, 1984). Users of augmentative and alternative communication perform multilingually within a monolingual setting, with speech therapists or teachers attempting to introduce one or more, often lower status, 'linguae francae'. (Of course, a user of alternative communication may also live in a true bilingual situation, e.g. a member of an immigrant or refugee community).

The bilingual perspective suggests that attention should be directed to the way in which people process information in more than one mode, influences from one mode to another, and the effects of the attitudes towards alternative communication modes held by users and their partners. For example, hardly anything is known about communication aid users' ability to comprehend messages constructed by others with their own system.

Applying a bilingual perspective as an analogy for understanding the multimodal situation of many alternative language users raises the question of the linguistic status of alternative modes of communication. People who use different modes for reception and expression may not be considered truly bilingual. This issue seems to be important for both individual cognitive processing and the communication process itself.

## Linguistic status

Questions regarding the nature of language have traditionally been approached by listing the structural characteristics which are deemed to be universal to all natural languages, and evaluating prospective candidates to see if they meet these criteria. Three features are widely thought to be fundamental, though not sufficient: arbitrariness, productivity and duality of patterning (Crystal, 1991; Wasow, 1973).

*Arbitrariness*. Languages have a conventionalised relationship between form and meaning, that is, between the *signifier* and the *signified* (de Saussure, 1977). This raises the issue of iconicity in language. It used to be thought that manual signs, for example, were icons, and thus did not function in an abstract way (Myklebust, 1960). Bellugi and Fischer (1972) showed that although cues to the meaning can be discerned in the form of manual signs, they are processed as linguistic symbols. More recently, researchers have suggested that iconicity is pervasive in spoken language as well as sign language, although it takes a less obvious form (Hiraga, 1994). Arguably, it is not the presence of iconicity which disqualifies the linguistic status of a system, but the absence of arbitrariness.

*Productivity*. Languages must have a discrete set of rules that allow an infinite number of meanings to be generated from a finite set of units. The rules which govern combinations of units constitute the grammar of the language. However, the criterion of grammatical rules is more stringent. For example, it appears that it is possible to have a productive set of lexical concepts (which will allow novel combinations to be generated) without necessarily developing a grammar (cf. Grove et al., this volume). The early word combinations of young children seem to be pre-grammatical, and the division into form classes or semantic classes is not relevant until the child begins to set up conditions of reference (Bates, Shore, Brethertod and McNew, 1983; Radford, 1992).

*Duality of patterning*. Languages have two levels of structure, which operate independently of one another. At the higher level, combinations of meaningful units occur (words and morphemes). At the lower level, sequences consist of segments which are meaningless in themselves (phonemes, or *cheremes* for manual signs), but combine to form meaningful units. These segmental, hierarchical properties of language underlie the systems of rules for generating new combinations. Evidence that children are segmenting language into its component bits suggests that they are mastering an abstract system, rather than simply stringing together semantic concepts.

There is ample evidence that children who learn a primary language experiment with formal patterns, and manipulate linguistic segments from early in development (Leonard, Schwarz, Folger and Wolcox, 1978; Weir, 1962). Iconic gestalts, such as Rebus and PCS signs, can be recombined productively at the higher level of structure (meaningful elements) but do not have duality of patterning – there is no level of meaningless segments which can be analysed, broken up and reassembled (although combinations where letters are combined with the phonetic form of the graphic sign's gloss to create new word forms, unrelated in meaning to the sign, have this function). The result is less flexibility and variety of expression, but the consequences for cognitive and linguistic processing are not known.

It is possible to analyse the extent to which various alternative communication systems meet these three criteria (cf. Besio and Chinato, this volume). Not everything which looks like language is language. Symbols belonging to a linguistic system may not always be used in a linguistic way. For example, the few spoken words or manual signs of a language impaired individual may be processed as separate gestalts in the same way as some early words in development seem to be processed as separate gestalts by young children rather than as elements of a lexical network (Harris, 1992). On the other hand, in the same way as children's first words develop into a complex linguistic system, symbols that are part of a non-linguistic system may eventually be processed as linguistic symbols. The nature of this transition, however, has not received much attention and remains obscure.

In the current taxonomy of augmentative and alternative communication systems, distinctions are drawn between linguistic and non-linguistic systems on the basis of symbolic status, iconicity and productivity (Fuller, Lloyd and Schlosser, 1992). A productive line of research might involve exploring the extent to which these distinctions affect the child's ability to learn language (see Smith, this volume).

# Theory of relevance

The distinction between an act of language and an act of communication is exemplified in *relevance theory* (Sperber and Wilson, 1986). The term originated with the maxim 'Be relevant' suggested by Grice (1975). According to this theory, comprehending the meaning of an utterance cannot be derived by a process of linguistic decoding, since an utterance can have many distinct interpretations depending on such features of the communicative context as the identity of the speaker and the audience, their shared assumptions, the physical surroundings and the immediately preceding discourse. Relevance theory suggests that linguistic processing is enhanced by inferential processing. It is implicit that the communicator has to determine how to ensure that the message will be relevant to the receiver. Ensuring relevance involves a trade-off between the effort expended in interpreting the utterance, and the information gained. It may be noted that it has been suggested that this form of processing may be impaired in autistic people (Tager-Flusberg, 1993), resulting in misunderstanding and communication breakdowns. Since many autistic people use augmentative and alternative communication, a model should be able to incorporate this and similar processes. Relevance theory offers another perspective for exploring the interactional dynamics of augmentative and alternative communication (Happé, 1993).

## Aspects of a model

The content of a comprehensive model designed to include both traditional and augmentative communication may for practical purposes be divided into four dimensions of the communication process: physical, cognitive, interactional and socio-cultural aspects. They represent different viewpoints for describing communication processes but are not independent and it may sometimes be difficult to keep them separate. For example, transmission may be difficult to distinguish from cognitive processes of production and perception; physical aspects like production time may influence both the interactional aspects and the status in society; a multimodal situation may influence both interactional aspects and cognitive processing. Another example, the problem of non-use of systems can be usefully addressed from the perspective of cognitive processing, interactional processes, or bilinguality which explores the effect of socio-linguistic status on acquisition and use.

On the other hand, they may only be superficially described in one synergetic model (cf. Prutting and Elliott, 1979). A comprehensive model may in fact be an overview or a metamodel of different models. Metaphorically, these may be regarded as interactive models, levels or modules where new developments in one field can lead to modifications of that particular model as well as in the relationship between modules and thus the total structure of the model (these modules should not be confounded with modular theories of the mind, cf. Fodor, 1983).

A number of models for augmentative and alternative communication have been proposed, typically focusing on the transmission aspect. For example, Shane (1980) bases his model on characteristics of the signs (vocal, non-vocal and representational). Lloyd, Quist and Windsor (1990), building on Sanders (1976), emphasise the function of different sensory modalities and motor skills, and, superficially, neurological processing. Other aspects, including linguistic and cognitive processing, are not specified in any detail. Schiefelbusch and Hollis (1980), building on the theoretical framework of Osgood (1957), focus on the processing of different systems and modes of communication, and possible processing deficits.

In the sections which follow, these critical dimensions of communication will be discussed with reference to the application of perspectives from literacy, bilingualism and the theory of relevance.

## Physical aspects

The physical aspect encompasses the physical energies of making and transmitting signs from one person to another. These aspects may be the easiest to model. The signal-transmission model of Shannon and Weaver (1949) represents a model of physical aspects in its most basic form. When specified for normal speech and alternative forms of language alike, the most important issues concerning physical aspects are motor skills involved in articulation of vocal and manual signs, and indication of graphic signs, on the production side. Noise and light conditions in the environment are crucial for adequate transmission and reception of acoustic and visual modes of communication.

One significant modification introduced by Lloyd and his associates is a sub-model for aided communication where the production of graphic modes of communication is accounted for by distinguishing between the act of selecting and indicating signs (pointing, scanning, etc.) and their transmission (visual or synthetic vocal) which is perceived by the communication partner at the receiving end. This sub-model, however, includes only the aided communicator and thus fails to include those instances where the natural speaker translates and formulates the message of the aid user in spoken language and the processes of acknowledgement and negotiation discussed above.

Physical aspects of communication tend to be considered of less theoretical interest than cognitive, linguistic and interactional processes. However, a significant amount of research is concerned with this aspect, including, for example, visibility of cued speech (Kipila and Williams-Scott, 1988), perceptual cues used in recognition of manual and graphic signs (Poizner, 1983; Yovetich and Young, 1988), intelligibility of synthetic speech (Scherz and Beer, 1995; Venkatagiri, 1994), functionality of prediction devices (Alm and Newell, this volume; Newell et al., 1992) and motor requirements for manual signing (Dennis, Reichle, Williams and Vogelsberg, 1982; Grove, 1990; McEwen and Lloyd, 1990; McIntire, 1977). Adaptations of communication aids, teaching imitation and good articulation of manual signs, and techniques for eliciting vocalisations and speech sounds take a significant part of practitioners' attention, in fact, probably more than many language related tasks.

If it can be extended to production as well as interpretation, relevance theory appears to have a particular application to the study of physical aspects, since it makes predictions about the relationship between effort and effects within an act of communication.

## Cognitive aspects

The cognitive aspects include traditional psycholinguistic issues: the perception and comprehension of signs, representation, generation of ideas and production of messages (McNeill, 1987; Slobin, 1979). They also include the cognitive frames underlying the comprehension and production of messages (Goffman, 1974; Schank and Abelson, 1977). Linguistically, there seems to be evidence for distinguishing phonological, lexical and grammatical processing (e.g. Dockrell and McShane, 1993; Pinker, 1994; Smith and Tsimpli, 1995; Yamada, 1990;) but other categories have been suggested, for example to distinguish between phonological, syntactic, thematic and semantic representations (Frazier, 1995). In addition, as discussed above, processes in speech and non-speech modes may not be analogous, and processing may differ with regard to whether the use of manual, graphic or tactile signs is grounded in speech comprehension or not, and whether they have been acquired as a first or second language.

A number of cognitive models exist, describing the hypothetical processes of speech and manual signing (cf. Bellugi and Studdert-Kennedy, 1980; Miller and Eimas, 1995; Siple and Fischer, 1991). The role of production for perceptual categories of speech has been a central discussion (cf. Wathen-Dunn, 1967). There is also a large literature on the processing of pictures and words written with alphabetic and non-alphabetic script and tactile perception, mainly in normal but also in disabled populations (Kavanagh and Venezsky, 1980; Kikuchi, Yamashita, Sagawa and Wake, 1979; Paivio, 1986; Seidenberg, 1995). Less is known, however, of the processing of pictographic signs used for communicative purposes. A model should not be biased to any particular modality or mode of communication. It should separate receptive and expressive modes, be able to take into account the existence of processing differences due to impairments of the nervous system, and allow specification of the extent to which uptake and output by an individual will be affected by a particular combination of impairments (cf. Bishop and Mogford, 1993; Tager-Flusberg, 1994).

Pictorial graphic signs (e.g. PIC, PCS and Rebus) may be learned in a very different way from less pictographic ones such as Blissymbols. They seem to be difficult to assimilate into a linguistic system (Soto and Olmstead, 1993) and may be perceived and reacted to more as pictures than words by people in the environment (Basil, 1992; Smith, this volume; von Tetzchner and Martinsen, this volume). In a communication task involving printed words and PIC signs, Raanaas (1993) found that college students tended to interpret the PIC signs more as pictures than as word meanings corresponding to the written glosses. When the same printed words were used without the graphic sign, metaphorical interpretations were more frequent. This tendency to understand graphic communication in a more literal and underextended way than the glosses written on them is likely to influence communicative interactions and the acquisition process. This is also reflected in the design of pictographic systems. For example, pictorial similarity seems to have been negatively perceived as a potential source of interference in learning by the developers of PCS. In this system (as in others) the same word may have several pictorial representations, for instance *WORK* and *HELP*.

In a model, it may be necessary to distinguish input, that is, the production of the communication partner, from uptake – that part of the message which is selectively attended to and processed (cf. Harris, 1992). In the comprehension of a spoken message, speech sounds are perceived by the auditory receptors, decoded as words and sentences, and assigned meaning. In the production of a message, the speaker conceives of some communicative intention and prepares an utterance which will make this intention recognisable by the interlocutor. This implies the use of abstract lexical and grammatical representations and phonological forms, to which phonetic rules are applied. At the motor level, a neuromuscular programme specifies the articulatory configurations of the output. It is hypothesised that each component functions in a modular, automatic fashion – no conscious cognitive effort needs to be expended in the linguistic formulation of a spoken or signed message (Levelt, 1994). While there is usually enough flexibility in the interaction of inferential and linguistic processing to accommodate problems of use, for a user of augmentative and alternative communication, the balance may be different. Using a graphic system may on occasion require more effort than the communication warrants, and this may help to explain why graphic communication systems and communication aids are not always fully used. This explanation is consistent with the theory of relevance, and the same theory can be used to explain why linguistic messages tend to have telegraphic structure, suggesting that this is a pragmatic accommodation minimising cognitive effort, and maximising the cognitive effect (von Tetzchner, 1985). The problem may not be specific to aided communicators – motor impaired signers and people who stutter or have unintelligible speech may also find the cost high compared with the benefit.

Knowledge about cognitive and linguistic processing among bilingual people may be useful but is still not well understood (Vaid, 1986). The underlying mental representation for systems may vary in bilingual people along a continuum from compound to co-ordinate. In *compound* cognitive organisation, the individual constructs a single concept which is represented by tokens of both systems. For example, the manual sign HOUSE, the spoken word /haus/ and the written word house might form a single representation, accessed by any of the three. With co-ordinate organisation, the sign HOUSE would access a separate representation from the written word house. There might be a partial overlap, or the representations might be entirely different, depending on the learning process. A person may show more compound organisation for some concepts, and more co-ordinate for others (cf. Kirsner, 1986).

Relative to the relationship between primary and derived languages, understanding the cognitive organisation of different modes is particularly important for people where there is limited correspondence in the mapping of the language forms, unlike speech and orthographic script where one corresponds closely to the other. Intervention seems to a large degree to be based on a tacit assumption that the child understands what is said and learns signs with reference to the spoken word (Grove et al., this volume; von Tetzchner and Martinsen, this volume). Even if the assumption were correct, that the receptive language determines the fundamental organisation of the linguistic system, children would have to learn the correspondence between the two systems, and it is not known how a child develops a mapping system between a receptive system in one modality and a productive system in another modality, with different vocabularies. There may not in fact be a direct conceptual mapping between spoken and alternative language use. The intervention guiding the acquisition process of communication aid users does not usually seem to make explicit how the same meaning or idea may be expressed in different language forms (von Tetzchner, 1993b). The often-used strategy of keyword manual signing may provide limited information concerning the relationship between signs and the utterances spoken (cf. Grove et al., this volume). Thus, one may question the opportunities for children to learn manual or graphic signs if they don't understand speech (cf. Fuller and Wright, 1994).

Having to rely on insufficient input for production may not be an easy task. The language produced by alternative language users, whether in graphic or signed form, may bear more resemblance to a 'protolanguage' (Bickerton, 1990) or pidgin (Mills, 1994; von Tetzchner, 1985) than to the fluent models with which they are surrounded in everyday life: a limited, apparently truncated syntax whose meanings need to be amplified and negotiated by interlocutors. Deaf children faced with limited sign input based on spoken language seem to effectively 'creolise' the input, producing language that is more grammatical than the input (Singleton and Newport, 1993). There is not enough evidence about children's spontaneous use of aided communication to know whether this also happens with graphic systems. Von Tetzchner (1985) and Mills (1994) have suggested that many of the characteristics of expressive language produced by primary users of these systems may be like those of pidgin languages – though whether the similarities result accidentally, or from economy of effort, or due to other factors is at present unknown. In an experiment where PCS was used in a communication task, normally speaking children did not map the graphic sign utterances directly on spoken language even if they had all the necessary signs available (Smith, this volume). The productions of a child who communicated through drawings suggest consistent elaborations of meaning (Fuller and Wright, 1994).

Issues related to cognitive aspects play a significant role for both theory development and clinical practice. For example, it is not clear what to look for in the assessment of cognition, nor whether it is appropriate to use standardised measures in this context. Knowledge about the relationship between cognitive processing and alternative and augmentative language functions is limited and the construction of a comprehensive model may function to highlight this.

## Interactional aspects

The interactional aspects may be considered the basic level of the model. They include communication functions and the structure of conversational exchanges of communication involving users of augmentative and alternative communication. The environmental strategies outlined above will have interactional consequences but whatever strategies are applied in the environment, additional factors may influence the communication process. Many manual signs may not be understood due to poor articulation or lack of competence among people in the environment. Indications of graphic signs may only be approximate and difficult to interpret. Additionally, use of overextensions and unconventional analogies and metaphors due to limited vocabularies and divergent thinking may lead to difficulties in interpretation and translation (von Tetzchner and Martinsen, 1992).

Communication with an aid is usually slow, and puts a heavy demand on attention maintenance in both partners, and users often experience misunderstandings and conversational breakdowns. There is an asymmetry between the aided speaker and the naturally speaking communication partner, who often has to articulate the contributions from both (Collins, this volume; Kraat, 1985; Marková, 1995; von Tetzchner and Martinsen, this volume). Conversational analyses show the importance of distinguishing between coproductive turns and turns expressing the partner's own messages. Blau (1986) found back-channel communication played a primary role in dialogues between communication aid users and naturally speaking people. She describes five conversational back-channel devices typical of such dialogues: *restatement, expansion, query, correction* and *acknowledgement*. She also describes speaker feedback as a back-back-channel device. Similar conversational devices are also frequent in conversations between speaking people and manual signers they believe have good comprehension of spoken language. They may also be attempted by the speaking person even if the manual speaker gives little evidence of speech comprehension.

From a different perspective, von Tetzchner and Martinsen (this volume) suggest that the graphic signs in aided language conversations may function more as strategies for making the partner formulate a message than as linguistic signs that may be combined in multi-sign utterances, even if the aid user were in principle able to produce sentences.

Lastly, non-verbal devices such as pointing, gesturing and pantomime may play a wider and more significant role in everyday communication for individuals using augmentative communication than for normally speaking people. These devices may also have a different distribution; for example there may be a higher proportion of gestures that may substitute for words, such as emblems, language-like gestures and pantomime compared to illustrators, gestures used to emphasise or highlight particular parts of the flow of speech (Ekman, 1975; McNeill, 1992). Being able to depict and make these processes open for analysis is an important requirement for a comprehensive model of augmentative and alternative communication.

## Socio-cultural aspects

Socio-cultural aspects will include the relationship between the individual and society, for example how use of diverse communication modes may influence social standing and opportunities within the community at large. Models concerned with participation in various social and cultural settings (e.g. Beukelman and Mirenda, 1992) and concepts from bilingualism are particularly applicable in this context.

For people living in traditional bilingual situations, there may be a large group or only a few people using the minority language. A person using non-speech forms of communication may hardly ever see them used in the environment, and will thus be deprived of language models outside structured teaching. This is typical of the environments both of people using communication aids and of people who rely on manual signs, who are exposed to signing only in planned routines or a limited number of situations (Bryen and McGinley, 1991; Grove and McDougall, 1991; Kiernan, Reid and Jones, 1982). Frequently, one or more systems may not be used by anyone else in the environment – for example at home with the family, or in a school where many different systems are used. From a bilingual perspective, a speaker of a language who finds himself isolated as the only fluent speaker of that language in the community (e.g. through emigration) is unlikely to be able to sustain skills in that language. This can result in language loss, which in turn can leave the speaker with only limited fluency.

Alternatively, there may be several individuals using the same graphic system, e.g. PCS, PIC or Blissymbols, in a school or institution, communicating mainly with the natural speakers. However, even if they communicate with each other, they may be unable to do so directly and will depend on a speaking person translating and formulating their messages in speech.

The standing of the language form is important for both intervention and social functioning. Low status may lead to small expectations and satisfaction with limited linguistic achievement and little social participation. Being unable to speak is in itself a low-status attribute. Even so there is great variation in standing depending on the mode of language used. Graphic and tactile language forms have lower status than speech. Similar attitudes toward different writing systems as those expressed by Rousseau in 1791 are probably still present:

'The depicting of objects is appropriate to a savage people; signs of words and of propositions to a barbaric people, and the alphabet to civilized people' (cited in Olson, 1993, p. 1).

Many parents and professionals do not seem to regard non-speaking children as having a language before they have learned traditional orthography. Manual signing also has lower status than speech in spite of the heightened standing resulting from the sign language revolution in some countries.

Acknowledgement of the minor language form may lead to an increased standing of the individual in the community. The standing of both deaf people and sign language for hearing language impaired people increased significantly in Norway after a 16-week sign course in prime time on the national television at a time when most of the population could receive only this station. On a smaller scale, when a staff member was assigned the role of interpreter for an intellectually impaired woman who was the only one dependent on signing in the sheltered housing, her status increased among the other inhabitants (von Tetzchner and Martinsen, 1992).

There are also significant differences in status among communication aids: high-technology systems may be perceived as higher in status than low-technology systems, even when used in a context where this is a less efficient form of communication. There are strong parallels here with bilingualism. A native speaker of French or Welsh in England is usually regarded as advantaged, whilst a native speaker of British Sign Language or Turkish may be seen as disadvantaged.

The term *diglossia* which relates to status differences between variations of the same language (Ferguson, 1959) may be used to describe the differences between various manual and graphic systems and communication aids. In a horizontal relationship, the languages are perceived as separate systems with equal status (e.g. English, Dutch and German). Where languages are varieties within the same system, but with one higher in status than the other, they are described as vertically related (e.g. High-German and Swiss-German, or British Sign Language and Signed English). A diagonal relationship occurs between languages that are not only from different communication systems, but are accorded different status across these systems, such as Blissymbols and PCS.

While it is relatively straightforward to see how members of a community may have multicultural identities related to language use, as well as being disabled (Abberley, 1987; Oliver, 1986), this notion appears somewhat novel in relation to the use of augmentative and alternative communication. So far, there has not been any movement of signing culture among intellectually and linguistically impaired people using sign language, in the same way as in the deaf communities, probably reflecting the fundamental differences between these two populations of manual signers.

Similarly, users of graphic systems do not tend to form language communities and the fact that direct communication between graphic language users is not usually promoted makes this unlikely to happen. They may still have preferences with regard to mode of communication, and identify themselves with one form rather than another (Blau, 1986, p.1):

(1)    A communication aid user (C) is talking to a natural speaker (N)
       C:    'Myself, I prefer a communication board as to a machine'.
       N:    *Uh huh. Why?*
       C:    'I feel it takes away my personality, if you know what I mean'.
       N:    'Yes' (Nods head).

It may be noted that (1) represents a short version of the actual conversation. In reality, the natural speaker had to formulate the messages of both communication partners, and it took 50 individual acts to complete the five message units. In another case known to us, a girl with cerebral palsy, although perfectly able to communicate in spoken English, requested that she too be given a communication aid, to be more like her peers in a specialist centre where this was the norm.

In order for researchers and practitioners to see the interrelationships between socio-cultural aspects, and developmental and interactional aspects, and to include them in their understanding of the social situation of users of augmentative and alternative language, a comprehensive model must incorporate this kind of process.

# Conclusions

The construction of a comprehensive model of augmentative and alternative communication raises a number of questions, and the nature of the model applied has implications for theoretical and practical issues discussed. It is important to be open to current theoretical perspectives rather than to attempt to produce a model of limited scope. Using and understanding an alternative communication system is not only a matter of learning a set of word forms different from the sound images of speech and then matching the forms. As pointed out by de Saussure in the beginning of this century, signs get their meaning through opposition to other signs in the language, and the two parts of signs, the *signifier* and the *signified*, are inseparable (de Saussure, 1977).

It should also be noted that the perspectives outlined here have not fully incorporated those dynamic features which would be necessary to account for developmental processes. Consideration of these issues lies beyond the scope of this chapter, but it is recognised that communication, by its very nature, is dynamic and changeable, rather than static and fixed. These qualities need to be reflected in any model which is proposed.

The four different aspects suggested in the present chapter are intertwined in complex manners. It may be a Sisyphean task to attempt to make one model that includes all relevant aspects, and if anyone managed to do it, others would probably not be able to decipher it. This is one reason for not attempting even a sketch of one here. The viable solution will probably be to make sub-models, depicting an aspect or part of an aspect. The main recommendation resulting from these preliminaries is that model builders should try to take the whole into account even when constructing only a smaller part of it, and that clinicians should have the totality in mind when they plan intervention for an individual.

### Acknowledgement

This chapter is based on several informal workshops held in Belgium and the UK. The authors want to thank Helen Cockerill, Janet Larcher, Gilliam Nelms, Keith Park, Alice Thacker, Koen vander Beken and Mark Williams for their contributions to the discussions.

# Chapter 2
# Situating augmentative and alternative language intervention

HARALD MARTINSEN AND STEPHEN VON TETZCHNER

Strategies used by professionals for assessing children with language and communication impairment, and for creating conditions for language learning, are usually based on diagnostic categories and assumptions about how particular child characteristics influence development. In the present chapter it is suggested that in order to make intervention optimal, professionals should focus not only on the characteristics of the child, but also on practical considerations, such as the feasibility of the teaching involved and the potential for creating adequate conditions for learning. It is further suggested that the process of intervention planning may be facilitated by distinguishing between three main functional groups in need of augmentative and alternative communication; the *expressive, supportive* and *alternative* language groups. The purpose of distinguishing between these three groups is to highlight the fact that the objectives of augmentative and alternative communication intervention vary. Focusing on the conditions needed for learning in the three groups may be helpful both in identifying the individuals in question, and for motivating the use of an alternative form of communication.

## Background

When children fail to speak at the normal age, professionals will have to choose between intervention based on speech or on an alternative form of communication. In most countries, however, there is still considerable resistance against non-vocal communication forms. The choice of communication intervention is often made on an ideological basis rather than according to a set of rational criteria (cf. Gangkofer and von Tetzchner, this volume; Kalman and Pajor, this volume). The number of professionals who regard non-speech forms of communication as an option is rather limited. There is a long tradition linking language intervention to speech training (cf. O'Neill, 1980; Weiner, 1986), and for example in

Britain, treatment for stuttering was the basis for development of speech therapy (Rockey, 1980). There also seems to be an ideological linkage between speech training and behaviour analysis, although there is no theoretical reason formulated within the behaviourist tradition which should cause such a bias.

Another characteristic of the language intervention strategies and methods applied is that they are often based on a Piagetian understanding of linguistic and cognitive development. The central notion is that the child's interactions with the physical world form the basis of intellectual development which in turn determines language development (Piaget, 1952). Hence, recommendations for introducing non-speech communication systems are usually based solely on characteristics of the individual (e.g. Lombardino and Langley, 1989; Shane and Bashir, 1980). Although there is considerable disagreement with regard to which cognitive, motivational and social skills are required for various forms of intervention (Kahn, 1975; Lloyd and Karlan, 1984; Reichle and Karlan, 1985), decision criteria within this field have been more concerned with specifying what the child can do than with what it may be able to learn under various conditions of intervention (cf. also Hamers, Sijtsma and Ruijssenaars, 1993).

Individual characteristics will always be an important basis of intervention decisions, since the child must have unintelligible or extremely limited spoken language skills for alternative language intervention to be considered. However, within a social constructivist perspective of language acquisition, it is the child's interactions with both the physical and the social world that determine the course of its intellectual development and language acquisition (Lock, 1980; Service, Lock and Chandler, 1989). The role of adults – for some children, interventionists (teachers, speech therapists, psychologists, etc.) – in the acquisition process itself is one of the main differences between what may be termed cognitive and social constructivist traditions:

> 'Studying child thought apart from the influence of instruction, as Piaget did, excludes a very important source of change and bars the researcher from posing the question of interaction of development and instruction peculiar to each age level. Our own approach focuses on this interaction' (Vygotsky, 1962, p. 117).

The focus of intervention within a social constructivist and transactional perspective is the context of teaching. It is not the presence or lack of particular skills in itself that is decisive, but how this may affect the ability of the interventionist to create a situation with suitable conditions for learning.

Assessments used in individual-oriented intervention (cognitive skills, attention, language comprehension, preferences, attributions of pre-communicative intentions, etc.) are useful. However, instead of asking which characteristics a child must have in order for a particular programme to be introduced, one might ask how situations can be constructed in such a way that the child can learn to use some kind of language form in a communicative manner. By letting the interactive context determine the communication modes one may reduce the bias towards selection of only one system (cf. Lombardino and Langley, 1989). Speech should be chosen whenever it can be shown to be functional. Non-vocal communication forms should be chosen when they seem to create better conditions for intervention.

## Deciding on a language form

In order to provide optimal intervention and give children the best opportunities for developing language and communication, it is critical to identify the individuals for whom speech-based intervention alone may be attempted and those who may benefit more from augmentative and alternative language intervention. The main language forms – speech, manual signs and graphic signs – can be distinguished from each other by the way they are taught. The intervention programme for each child can be assessed in relation to the difficulties involved in its arrangement and implementation. Since there is no set of proven and knowledge-based criteria for the choice of communication form, pragmatic guidelines should be searched for. It is our suggestion that such guidelines may be found not solely in the child's characteristics, but by considering the contextual prerequisites for teaching the expressive use of the communication form. When teaching comprehension, it is necessary to ensure that the input appears under conditions that make it salient and meaningful, and to assess whether the child is able to take in, react to, and learn from the input given.

### Speech

There is one critical prerequisite that all kinds of speech training depend on and try to manipulate: that the language impaired child can be influenced to produce vocal sounds. Without a means for eliciting vocalisations, speech training cannot be carried out. If the child habitually vocalises – say, babbles or displays delayed echolalia – one basic prerequisite for speech training is present. The productions can in principle be reinforced, shaped, put under control of situational conditions, or given meaning by other people's reactions and environmental manipulations; that is, through designing social contexts in which the child's utterances are meaningful.

If the child does not vocalise, speech training will depend on the teacher's ability to make it do so. In traditional forms of speech training, vocalising was often facilitated by first encouraging the child to breathe voluntarily through the mouth – for instance, by making the flame of a candle flutter – and thereafter to voice the breath to make a sound (Luchsinger and Arnold, 1965). Such methods are still in use, but most forms of speech training depend on the teacher being able to make the child imitate sounds (cf. Reichle, Piché-Cragoe, Sigafoss and Doss, 1988; Yoder and Warren, 1993).

For children who do not easily imitate sounds, the usual way of starting speech therapy is first to teach them how to imitate motor acts; that is, to follow the general instruction 'Do as I do' when some motor act is performed (e.g. the teacher lifting her right arm), or a specific instruction such as 'Point at your nose', while the teacher is performing this act. In these instances, the effectiveness of the intervention depends on how long the imitation pretraining period lasts before learning is achieved, and whether imitation is achieved at all.

If a motor act is not imitated, the teacher usually guides the child's hands through the appropriate movements. Since young children initially seem able only to imitate acts which they are already able to perform (Guillaume, 1971), this procedure may increase the number of acts the child masters and thus can imitate, but may not lead to the acquisition of imitation as a metaskill applicable to all forms of motor actions. Many people with communication and language problems have particular problems in learning to imitate. There are examples of children and adults who have been trained in imitation for years in preparation for subsequent speech training. In one Norwegian case, imitation was used for 17 years without any success.

In conclusion, speech training should be initiated only when the child vocalises or is easily taught to imitate vocal sounds. However, a child's ability to imitate vocal sounds should be regarded as a necessary but not sufficient condition for language intervention based on speech training. Lately, doubts have been raised with regard to whether vocal imitation will increase the intelligibility and functionality of speech (Gibbon and Grunwell, 1990). The production of speech is regarded less as a matter of being able to physically produce a word form than of being able to activate a word that is appropriate in the context. Word-finding problems are considered a major element of language disorders, indicating the need for an approach based on conceptual networks, situated learning and contextual cues. The fact that a child imitates speech sounds should be included in the design of the intervention programme. However, whether imitation should be used as a training strategy will depend on the teacher's ability to elicit such behaviour in a context where the child's imitations become meaningful from a communication perspective and lead to spontaneous language use.

## Manual signing

Prerequisites for teaching manual signs should also be addressed with regard to the feasibility of creating practical intervention situations. Manual signs are usually taught in one of two ways. Firstly, the teacher may hold the hands of the child, mould the appropriate hand shape, and guide the hands through the articulation of the sign (e.g. Schaeffer, Musil and Kollinzas, 1980). Secondly, the teacher may demonstrate the articulation of the sign and encourage the disabled child to imitate it (e.g. Reichle, 1991). In both strategies, the meaning of the manual sign is taught through the teacher's and other people's reactions and by designing social situations for intervention where the manual signs function meaningfully.

The ability to use the hands is a necessary but not sufficient indication for choosing manual sign intervention. With hand-guidance, the practical arrangement of the intervention situations depends on the child not reacting too negatively to having the hands guided. However, many children and adults with pervasive communication and language problems have good hand motor skills but dislike being touched, especially if their hands are restrained. They may react to this by struggling against the teacher, even fighting with her, or by freezing or slipping down to the floor as a kind of non-violent protest. Even if the teacher is able to force the child's hands through the movements, these kinds of reactions to the hands being held may make it impossible to create a situation where manual signs are actually used to fulfil communicative functions. The teacher might try for some time in case the child habituates to the situation and the problem diminishes. However, if the negative reactions persist, successful teaching of manual signs by this method is not likely to be achieved.

The second strategy depends on the teacher's ability to make the child imitate hand movements. As discussed above, although it has proven successful in some cases, in many cases imitation may not be feasible. However, most people do learn to imitate at least simple motor acts, and the main issue is whether a learning situation based on imitation will facilitate functional use of manual signing. In a simple choice-making task, Iacono and Parsons (1986) found hand-guidance to be more efficient in manual sign instruction than imitation even for a subject who had some imitation skills. One reason may be that the common focus in imitation-based intervention is the teacher's movements rather than the choices and other forms of communicative acts that the learner is supposed to perform. This focus on form instead of function may make it an interactive motor-learning condition rather than a condition for learning functional language. In order for the situation to be successful for teaching language and communication, the teacher must be able to make the child attend simultaneously to the particular object, person or event chosen, and the movements of the teacher. Moreover, when using imitation, the teacher may lose the possibility of synchronising the production of the manual sign with those moments when the child is attentive to the referent of the sign. The possibility to do this is otherwise one of the advantages of teaching manual signs compared to other communication forms.

### Graphic signs

Intervention situations with graphic communication systems have two main components: to pay attention to and indicate a graphic sign; and the communicative consequence related to these acts. Arranging and carrying through an intervention programme depends on the teacher being able to control the child's direction of attention. In order for the child to be able to understand the relation between the graphic signs and their references, it must look at and attend to the graphic signs within the communicative framework established by the teacher. If the intervention is comprehension-oriented, this means that the teacher has to control the child's direction of attention either through physical intervention, for example, by turning its head in the direction of the graphic sign or highlighting the graphic sign in the child's visual field. Graphic signs may also be placed in locations where the child naturally looks. If the teacher cannot control and direct the attention of the child towards graphic signs in the course of communicative interactions, this form of intervention is not likely to be successful.

If the focus of the intervention is production, the teacher has to react to the child's gaze, or assist the child in pointing, or in another way physically indicating the graphic sign within a communicative context. Many children and adults in need of communication and language intervention display unusual attentional styles and oppose being directed. For people with autism, lack of attention to other people and difficulties connected with direction of attention are prominent features of the syndrome (cf. Sarriá, Gómez and Tamarit, this volume). Similar problems are found in various other clinical groups. For these children, meeting the requirements for effective expressive teaching of graphic signs may be difficult to achieve. Thus, when planning intervention with graphic signs, the possibility of controlling the child's direction of attention and of teaching it to use an appropriate way of indicating should be assessed.

## Three functional groups

Children who need an alternative form of communication may be divided into three main groups, *the expressive, supportive* and *alternative* language groups, according to the functions that the augmentative and alternative communication is assumed to fill. The motivation for this division is to bring out the fact that the objectives of implementing alternative communication intervention vary. The three groups differ with regard to the size of the gap between expressive speech and spoken language comprehension, the role spoken language plays in intervention, how long the child is expected to depend on the alternative communication system, the range of situations in which the alternative system is needed, and various other dimensions relevant for intervention (cf. von Tetzchner et al., this volume; von Tetzchner and Martinsen, 1992).

## Expressive language group

Children and adults who belong to the expressive language group have a large gap between their understanding of other people's speech and their ability to express themselves through spoken language. Typical members of this group are children with cerebral palsy who do not have sufficient control of the speech organs to be able to articulate speech sounds intelligibly (anarthria). Their language comprehension may, however, be good. In addition, they often have motor impairments that affect all or most of their movements, making graphic sign systems the obvious choice.

For the expressive language group, the purpose of the alternative communication intervention is to provide them with a communication form which will become their permanent means of expression, that is, to be used in all kinds of situations and for the rest of their lives. Comprehension is not usually a significant goal of the intervention. The main focus is the relationship between the spoken language used in the environment and the alternative language form used by the child to express itself. However, intervention may include teaching comprehension of complex graphic signs (e.g. Blissymbols) and traditional orthographic reading. If manual signing is used, unless the child is living in a signing environment (e.g. with deaf parents), sign comprehension is usually included in the teaching.

## The supportive language group

The supportive language group consists of children who are taught an alternative language form as a temporary intervention measure, and children who have learned to speak but who have difficulty in making themselves understood with the help of speech. The first subgroup comprises children who are expected to begin to speak but whose language development is very delayed. Children with developmental dysphasia belong to this group, as do many children with Down syndrome (cf. Launonen, this volume; von Tetzchner, 1984). This subgroup is similar to the alternative language group except for the fact that they tend to have less pervasive disorders and do not need alternative communication as a permanent tool. The alternative communication form is intended as a 'scaffold' to the development of a normal mastery of speech. Adults often solve the problem of not understanding a child by giving more commands and asking fewer questions, as well as giving non-committal answers like *yes, no* or *mm* in response to its communicative efforts (Bondurant, Romeo and Kretschmer, 1983; Schjølberg, 1984; von Tetzchner and Smith, 1986). The alternative communication form is not intended to replace speech – either for the children concerned or for those who communicate with them. Its chief objectives are to facilitate and encourage participation in conversations and other social situations where speech is used, and make available effective means for participating in such situations in the period before expressive speech is acquired. The general focus of the intervention for this subgroup is to make clear the relationship between speech and the alternative language form as well as solving social problems related to lack of speech. Comprehension of spoken language will vary within this group and thus the extent to which comprehension training will be included in the intervention.

Children in the other subgroup of the support group may be paralysed or have spasms that make it difficult for them to control their articulation properly and make it difficult for people to understand what they are saying. They resemble the expressive language group but the alternative communication is not their main form of communication. The degree to which they are able to make themselves understood through speech varies with how well people know them, the topic of the situation, and noise conditions. For example, discussing experiences shared with the listener, the child may easily make itself understood while descriptions of a film the listener does not know may not be understood. A child who is well understood in a small classroom may be nearly unintelligible in a train or on a street with normal traffic. In such situations and with unfamiliar people, children in the second subgroup may need to produce manual signs or letters, or point at graphic signs, written words, or graphemes corresponding to the speech sounds that the communication partner has not understood. For this group, intervention should focus on conditions that help the child learn when it needs supplements to speech, how to monitor the comprehension of the communication partner, and how to use appropriate means and strategies in different situations.

The situational constraints on the use of speech described for the latter subgroup may also to some degree apply to children with severe developmental language disorders. Although they gradually learn to speak, and thus belong to the first subgroup, their speech will generally be poorly articulated throughout the pre-school period (Fundudis, Kolvin and Garside, 1979). This means that for several years it may be difficult for people other than those who know the child well to understand what it says.

## Alternative language group

Children belonging to the alternative language group are characterised by little or no use of speech as a means of communication. The alternative communication is both their main form of expressive communication and the language form they comprehend best. It is likely to be the language form they will depend on permanently. Autistic and severely intellectually impaired children may belong to this group, as well as children with auditory agnosia or 'language deafness' who appear to have special problems in interpreting sounds as meaningful linguistic elements (Luchsinger and Arnold, 1965). Intervention will comprise both comprehension and production, and a principal goal will be to establish conditions where the child may learn to understand and use the alternative language form without needing a reference to spoken language, and an environment where the alternative language form is truly functional.

## Distinguishing between the groups

The division into three groups does not imply that it is always easy to determine the group in which a given child belongs. The same categories are often represented in more than one intervention group. The group of Down syndrome, for example, includes children who develop intelligible speech, children who develop speech that is difficult to understand, and children who acquire little or no speech (cf. Launonen, this volume). Some children with cerebral palsy need a communication aid in order to be able to express themselves at all; others need it to support speech that is difficult to understand, some only for a limited period of time.

It is particularly difficult to distinguish between people who belong to the supportive language group and the alternative language group. This is illustrated by the experience gained from manual and graphic sign intervention for intellectually impaired and autistic people. People who had not learned to speak despite years of speech training, and who therefore were expected to belong to the alternative group, subsequently began to speak. For some of these people, speech has gradually become their main form of communication. Before this it was reasonable to assume that they were incapable of learning to speak.

# Some dimensions of intervention

The conditions needed for developing optimal intervention for the three main groups differ along several dimensions, notably: implicit versus explicit learning conditions and first versus second language teaching; and requirements of the language environment and situation-restricted versus situation-rich intervention.

## Teaching strategies

The distinction between implicit and explicit learning is fundamental in augmentative and alternative communication intervention. Implicit learning means 'that a person typically learns about the structure of a fairly complex stimulus environment, without intending to do so, in such a way that the resulting knowledge is difficult to express' (Berry and Dienes, 1993a, p.2). Thus, implicit teaching does not seek to make the individual aware of its own learning strategies. Explicit learning, on the other hand, means that the individual is aware of and able to verbalise the strategies used to acquire knowledge or skills. Explicit learning conditions imply taking a metaperspective.

The distinction between explicit and implicit learning conditions seems to parallel differences between strategies typically used in first and second language learning. First language learning is mainly implicit, while explicit teaching strategies seems best suited for second language learning (Berry and Dienes, 1993b; Dienes, 1993).

For the expressive group, conditions often resemble second language teaching: the main focus of the intervention is the relationship between the spoken language used by communication partners and the environment in general, and the expressive means of the disabled child. Because there is a large gap between comprehension and expression, spoken instructions may be used to explain the use of the alternative communication forms. Strategies will mainly be explicit although they may result in implicit knowledge of language. These strategies attempt to utilise the asymmetry in knowledge of both speech and the alternative language form that exists between the child and the interventionist.

At the other end of this dimension, the aim of the intervention for the alternative communication group is to develop a first language, a mother tongue. This demands implicit strategies. It is not clear how explicit teaching could be done or how a child with poor language comprehension would utilise such knowledge. A child belonging to the expressive group may be asked to point to the graphic sign corresponding to a particular spoken word, a strategy typical of second language teaching. However, although this instruction is constantly used also in intervention for people belonging to the alternative group, the possibility of following it may be based on skills they do not have. The task will have little meaning for people who do not understand the spoken instruction (cf. Møller and von Tetzchner, this volume).

Metaphorically, implicit language learning may be described as exploration of new territories without knowing where one is going. Implicit teaching implies the use of strategies that develop skills that may increase in functional value and – for children with some comprehension of speech – make the relationships between language forms (speech and manual or graphic signs) and their use apparent to the child. For children who belong to the language supportive group, emphasis may be on explicit or implicit teaching strategies depending on their comprehension of spoken language and the communicative functions to be taught.

## Environment

In order to ensure optimal conditions for the acquisition of an alternative language form, learning must be situated in an appropriate context, that is, an environment that supports the child's narrow or extended possibilities of learning language use and comprehension in social interaction with people in the environment. These people may adapt to users of alternative communication in three main ways. Firstly, they may adopt the alternative mode and use this in all communication with the child, thus creating an enclave of alternative communication use within an environment of natural speakers. Such enclaves may consist of the school, home, institution and similarly restricted environments. Although this would be an optimal learning condition for people with little or no comprehension of spoken language, even in restricted environments this kind of overall adaptation probably hardly exists.

Secondly, people in the environment may speak normally when responding to a child using an alternative communication form. In these interchanges, both the communication impaired child and the communication partners use different modes of communication for comprehension and production. This is the typical environment of people belonging to the expressive group, but it is also common among people belonging to the other two groups. Learning will depend on both the child's speech comprehension and on how the connections between the alternative communication form and speech are made apparent by people in the environment.

Thirdly, people in the environment may speak normally and support their speech with manual or graphic signs. This is probably the most common environment of people belonging to the supportive or alternative language groups. However, for communication impaired children the possibilities of utilising the environment will to a large degree depend on their understanding of spoken language, and such adaptations are probably insufficient for people with comprehension problems (cf. Grove, Dockrell and Woll, this volume).

The ultimate, although not always attainable, goal is that the child be able to communicate freely in all ordinary communication situations and a range of less ordinary ones. For people belonging to the expressive group, intervention tends to be situation-rich. Teaching is often directed at using the alternative language form for active communication in diverse settings, and varying between communicative roles is often a major objective of the intervention. Teaching tends to be explicit and concerned with metaknowledge and general situation-independent language strategies. This is the case even if prototypical examples and exemplary utterances, that is, utterances that may serve as models for a wider range of linguistic constructions, play an important role.

Intervention for children belonging to the alternative language group tends to be situation-restricted. Because teaching has to be both structured and implicit, it is usually necessary to give priority to a limited number of situations. However, since the long-term goal is situation-rich communication, care should be taken not to restrict situations to only one communication function, for example teaching only one type of request. Attempts should be made to select situations that are prototypical and which together may form a scaffold of vocal, manual and graphic signs and communication functions. In this way acquisition of a network of vocabulary and communicative functions can be facilitated, as well as active participation in a wider range of social contexts. For the alternative language group, a selective situation-restricted strategy may be initially applied, but the long-term goal is to gradually reduce restrictions and increase variety.

For the two subgroups of the support group, intervention is typically situation-restrictive. For the early development subgroup, the focus is usually participation in social activities and conflicts. For the other subgroup, whose speech is insufficient in certain contexts only, intervention should aim to identify these situations, and design strategies for coping with them by augmenting speech with an alternative form of language.

## Conclusions

Several changes in perspective have been suggested regarding assessment and intervention for language and communication impaired people. The success of a particular language form in intervention, including speech, may depend not only on the characteristics of the child but also on the potential for creating ample conditions for teaching the child. Teaching conditions are highlighted by the division of candidates for augmentative and alternative communication into three groups. The motivation for using an alternative form of communication and various dimensions of the intervention distinguish the three groups. For people with good comprehension of spoken language, this ability may be utilised in explicit instruction based on metacommunication. For people with little or no comprehension of spoken language, implicit teaching strategies may provide the best results. For the supportive language group, intervention may comprise both explicit and implicit strategies. The language forms applied in the environment should be adapted to support the intervention needs of the individual child.

# Chapter 3
# Joint attention and alternative language intervention in autism: Implications of theory for practice

ENCARNACIÓN SARRIÁ, JUAN CARLOS GÓMEZ AND JAVIER TAMARIT

The aim of this chapter is to discuss the importance of joint attention behaviours for improving and expanding intervention with alternative communication systems in children with autism. First, we offer a theoretical discussion of the relevance of joint attention in the development of normal communication, emphasising its role in so-called 'prelinguistic communication'. We then briefly review the characteristic deficits of joint attention behaviours in autism and, finally, we propose some guidelines for assessment and intervention based upon our theoretical discussion.

## Joint attention and prelinguistic communication

Joint attention behaviours are those that involve the coordination of the attention of two or more people around a common focus of interest. Typically, joint attention refers to the coordination of visual attention, because the visual mode is a privileged way of engaging in shared attention. However, joint attention may be achieved through other sensory modalities, such as vocalisations or physical contact.

Within the visual domain, the two fundamental patterns of joint attention are, firstly, to follow the gaze of other persons towards their focus of interest, and, secondly, to make eye contact with other people. The combination of these patterns may give rise to more complex sequences, such as a child looking into the eyes of someone, then looking at an interesting object, and then checking back to the eyes of the other person to see whether he or she has followed its gaze.

49

The intricacy and meaning of eye gaze in social interactions between adults have been extensively studied by social psychologists (Argyle and Cook, 1976; Fehr and Exline, 1987; Kleinke, 1986). However, this chapter will focus upon the role of joint visual attention in the emergence of intentional communication in infants and young children.

Developmentally, intentional communication about objects precedes the appearance of language. At around 9–12 months of age, human infants are capable of using communicative gestures, such as pointing or reaching, to request or show objects and events to other people. Typically, this happens before infants start using vocal language. This is why this kind of communication is commonly known as 'prelinguistic' or 'preverbal', and has been considered to play some role in facilitating the acquisition of language (Bruner, 1983).

However, prelinguistic gestures are remarkable in themselves in that they seem to be the first genuine manifestation of intentional communication. The term 'intentional communication' implies that the child wants to provoke the communicative effect its gestures have upon the receiver. The distinction between intentional and unintentional communication is illustrated in the following example:

> A girl leans and reaches towards an object that is out of reach; in doing so she vocalises as a result of her effort and perhaps of frustration. A nearby adult, upon hearing the noise, looks at her and sees her behaviour. The adult understands that she wants the object, approaches and consequently gives it to her.

In a sense, the girl 'communicated' her desire to the adult. However, this communicative effect was accidental, not intentional. Indeed, it would be more accurate to say that the girl's behaviour has accidentally informed the adult of her desire. However, since there is no agreement as to the proper use of the term 'communication', this distinction will be made with the qualifiers 'intentional' and 'unintentional'.

For communication to be intentional, it is necessary that a child wants to inform the adult of its desire, that is, that it purposefully shows or directs its behaviour to the adult. This is what happens in the following example:

> A girl first tries to reach the object. When she does not succeed, she leans back, looks at the adult and vocalises until the adult looks at her; then she points to the object while looking back again at the adult.

Why should this be more readily accepted as a case of genuine intentional communication? Bates and her associates (e.g. Bates, 1979; Bates, Camaioni and Volterra, 1976; Bates, O'Connell and Shore, 1987) and

Sarriá and Riviére (1991) suggest that several factors contribute to such an identification: the schematised nature of the gesture (it is no longer a real attempt at taking the object), the goal-directed way in which children orchestrate the whole sequence, and the fact that they usually seek the gaze of the other person, that is, the fact that the gesture is embedded in a joint attention situation.

We have argued elsewhere (Gómez, 1991; Gómez, Sarriá and Tamarit, 1993) that this third factor – establishing joint attention – is the crucial component of preverbal communicative intentionality. If intentional communication happens when one purposefully wants to inform someone of something, and one is using gestures to communicate, the only way to fulfil this goal is to make sure that the other person sees the gesture. No signal can function as communication if it is not perceived by the addressee. Hence, the ability to call the attention of other people upon oneself and redirect this attention towards the communicative target is an essential part of intentional communication. Within the realm of vision, these two attentional goals are commonly achieved by means of eye contact and gaze following.

Genuine intentional communication can only happen when one is capable of understanding the role of achieving joint attention in the communicative process. (Sometimes this understanding may be used to avoid communication, for example, waiting to do something until a person is not looking at one). The reason one-year-old children look like intentional communicators is that they are already showing the rudiments of this ability: they call the attention of other people when producing their gestures, and the gestures function to redirect the attention of others to the targets of the children's interest.

### Protoimperative and protodeclarative communication

One feature of infant preverbal communication that has had a major impact in the field of autism is the distinction between 'protoimperative' and 'protodeclarative' gestures (Bates et al., 1976). Protoimperatives are requests, that is, gestures intended to make another person do something for one's benefit. The above example with the girl pointing to the object she wanted is an instance of a protoimperative gesture. Protodeclaratives are gestures intended to make other persons look at something apparently for the sake of doing so. A typical example is a child pointing to a train or a plane passing by while checking the mother's gaze.

From the point of view of joint attention, protoimperatives involve the use of joint attention behaviours as a means subordinate to a final goal (e.g. getting an object), whereas protodeclaratives consist of using joint-attention behaviours for the sake of sharing the experience of an interesting object or event.

Described in this way, it would seem that protoimperatives are more complex than protodeclaratives, since they must always be subordinated to a further goal, and this would involve a more complex behavioural sequence. However, in the literature, exactly the opposite has been argued: that protodeclaratives are more complex communicative acts than protoimperatives. According to some authors (Baron-Cohen, 1989, 1991; Leslie and Happé, 1989; Riviére, 1990), in order to have the goal of sharing one's attention on a target with someone else, one must be able to understand the effect of gestures upon the minds of other people. That is to say, children who use protodeclaratives are interested in directing other people's attention to objects because they somehow understand that, by doing so, they make people 'know' things about the world. Otherwise, there would be no point in establishing joint attention for its own sake.

The distinction between protoimperatives and protodeclaratives, and its theoretical explanations, has had an important bearing upon practice, both for diagnosis and intervention reasons. This point will be addressed in the next section, devoted to joint attention deficits in autism. Then, an alternative interpretation of the distinction between protoimperatives and protodeclaratives will be presented.

To summarise, prior to acquiring language, normal infants use a range of gestures and vocalisations to communicate with other people. This preverbal communication is said to be 'intentional' because it involves the strategic use of joint attention behaviours, such as making eye contact, following the gaze of others, making others follow one's gaze, etc. Such behaviours can serve different communicative intentions – protoimperative or protodeclarative – which, according to some interpretations, might involve different cognitive abilities.

## Joint attention deficits of children with autism

Children with autism seem to be uniquely affected in their communicative abilities, and one of the most important consequences of their impairments seems to be a lack or severe deficit of joint attention behaviours. The most characteristic deficit in the non-verbal communication of children with autism is the lack or severe impoverishment of protodeclarative gestures (Baron-Cohen, 1989; Curcio, 1978; Loveland and Landry, 1986; Mundy, Sigman and Kasari, 1993; Mundy, Sigman, Ungerer and Sherman, 1986; Riviére et al., 1988). In comparison, protoimperative gestures have been reported in several studies (e.g. Baron-Cohen, 1989). This finding led some authors to consider that the autistic deficit might affect only the declarative function of prelinguistic communication. Moreover, this purported selective deficit played an important role in developing the hypothesis that protoimperative and protodeclarative communication may have different underlying cognitive mechanisms (see above). Since it is known that children with autism are deficient in their capacity to represent the mental states of other people (the so-called 'theory of mind'; cf. Baron-Cohen, 1993; Baron-Cohen, Leslie and Frith, 1985; Frith, 1989), this would explain their inability to produce protodeclaratives, if these really have the goal of affecting other people's 'knowledge', (Baron-Cohen, 1989, 1991). Protoimperatives, however, requiring only the ability to predict other people's actions, would pose no special problem to children with autism.

However, the assumption that children with autism do produce protoimperatives is based upon a 'gestural' definition of communication which does not take into account whether the gestures are or are not accompanied by joint attention. According to the above discussion, genuine communication occurs only when children demonstrate that they understand the joint attention components of communication. Simply making a movement towards an object because one has learned the contingency between this movement and a desirable effect – getting the object – is not communication, strictly speaking.

There is evidence that the joint attention deficit in autism is a general one affecting not only protodeclarative communication but any behaviour requiring an active coordination of attention with other people, hence including protoimperatives.

A recent study (Phillips et al., 1995), comparing normal, intellectually impaired and autistic children in a simple request task, shows a significant difference in the tendency of children with autism to perform requests without taking joint attention into account. As many as 60 per cent of the children with autism would never look even once at the eyes of the other person when producing a gesture. This was the case in spite of a lack of initial response by the adult, a condition that usually prompts eye contact in both normal and intellectually impaired children. This suggests that autism may imply a deficit in joint attention behaviours in general, not specifically in protodeclaratives. Further evidence for this comes from several other studies. There is evidence of a deficit in spontaneous gaze-following in young autistic children in comparison with developmentally matched controls with intellectual impairment and normal development (Sarriá and Riviére, 1986), and in simple referential looking (Loveland and Landry, 1986) even when the direction of gaze is emphasised with pointing (Mundy et al., 1986).

Although some studies have found no differences in the frequency of eye contact (Riviére et al., 1988) and in the time that autistic children spend looking at other people (Dawson and Adams, 1984; Sigman and Mundy, 1989), there is evidence that they have problems in the coordination of looking at others and performing an activity (Lord and Magill, 1989; Mirenda, Donnellan and Yoder, 1983), or even in the simple alternation of gaze between a person and an object when it is the other person who is manipulating the object (Mundy et al., 1993). In relation to requests, Canal and Riviére (1993) found that children with autism did not use eye contact initiated by the adult as an opportunity to carry out a request, in contrast to their developmentally delayed and normal matched controls who seemed to seize this opportunity as if they understood eye contact as a signal of communicative availability. (A more detailed review of studies about joint attention can be found in Mundy et al., 1993; although these authors sometimes restrict 'joint attention' to protodeclarative-like behaviours; see also the review in Gómez et al., 1995).

Burack (1994) and Ciesielski, Courchesne and Elmasian (1990) suggest that these difficulties in social attention might stem from a more basic deficit, on a primitive level of information processing, such as rapid attention shifting, which would be especially evident in social situations. Whatever the ultimate explanation, the available evidence shows that young children with autism have a general deficit in joint attention skills, which might explain their problems with preverbal intentional communication, irrespective of whether it is protodeclarative or protoimperative.

## Alternative interpretations of joint attention

Returning briefly to the theoretical interpretations of prelinguistic communicative behaviours, the apparent selective impairment of protodeclarative gesturing in children with autism has been taken as strong support of the 'theory of mind' hypothesis about protodeclaratives (i.e. the hypothesis that to make protodeclaratives children have to understand the effects of their gestures upon the minds of other people). However, if the interpretation that the available data show a general impairment of joint attention in autism, affecting both protodeclaratives and 'true' protoimperatives (i.e. requests making use of joint attention), is correct, then this hypothesis should be changed. It should either be extended to all preverbal communication (thereby attributing to one-year-old infants the ability to understand how their gestures change other people's minds), or be abandoned in favour of a different interpretation.

We have explored elsewhere (Gómez et al., 1993; Gómez et al., 1995) an 'expressive' interpretation of early joint attention understanding. Essentially we hold that what infants and young children understand about the attention of others is precisely its external manifestations – changes in gaze direction, eye contact, body orientations – which usually are accompanied by expressive behaviours such as smiling, laughing, speaking, shouting, etc. (Interestingly, these expressive behaviours tend to appear in the same area in which attention is manifest – the region of the face). Early communicative behaviours, both protoimperative and protodeclarative, would be based upon an understanding of such attentional and expressive behaviours as explicit causal links mediating the child's gestures and the adults' reactions. Initially, children would not understand the difference between the external manifestations of attention and attention as a mental state. (See also Baron-Cohen, 1989, 1993; for another 'expressive' interpretation within a broader theoretical framework).

This interpretation could be taken to imply that there is no difference between protoimperatives and protodeclaratives. However, there is a relevant source of evidence that suggests an important difference between both types of communicative functions. Non-human primates, such as gorillas and chimpanzees, are reported to engage in quite complex protoimperative behaviours, involving the use of joint attention (Gómez, 1991), but they seldom, if at any time, engage in protodeclarative communication (Gómez et al., 1993; Gómez et al., 1995).

This suggests that being able to use joint attention as a means to affect the behaviour of other people does not guarantee that one will also be able to use joint attention for its own sake. It is as if protodeclaratives involve the addition of intrinsic 'motives for interaction' (to use the terminology of Trevarthen, 1986) that allow the use of the attentional/expressive machinery involved in protoimperative communication as a goal in itself. Indeed, much of early protodeclarative communication in infants presents an appearance of playful, exploratory interactions, rather than serious information transmission. If anything, it could be said that in protodeclaratives, infants use joint attention with the goal of provoking expressive reactions about objects in others (Gómez et al., 1993).

The theoretical reinterpretation of joint attention and its role in early intentional communication is an open question that will raise further debate and controversy (for more detailed discussions of different positions, see Baron-Cohen, 1995; Gómez et al., 1995; Hobson, 1993). However, what is of interest in this chapter is the practical implications of the debate.

To summarise, although when adults use joint attention behaviours (e.g. calling the attention of somebody before pointing to an object), they understand their mental implications (e.g. making the other *know* that one *wants* to *inform* him of something), infants' and young children's use of joint attention might involve only a 'shallow' understanding of it. Nonetheless, this understanding allows them to be more effective both as senders and receivers of communication (for example, adapting their signals to the attention and inattention of other people). Joint attention is thus an important component of communication even before there is a 'deep' understanding of its mental implications. This means that joint attention should be considered as an important area of alternative communication teaching, an area that is closely related to the issue of the intentionality of communication. In the next section, some implications of our theoretical views for augmentative and alternative communication intervention for children with autism are presented.

## Implications for intervention

Intervention for children with autism using alternative communication systems began in the early seventies (Bonvillian, Nelson and Rhyne, 1981; Howlin and Yates, 1989; Kiernan, 1983). Currently, the use of these systems is largely recommended by experts in the field (e.g. Baron-Cohen and Bolton, 1993; Jordan and Powell, 1995). For example, in Spain, the use of alternative communication systems has significantly increased in the last years. Specifically, the programme of Schaeffer and his colleagues (Schaeffer, Musil and Kollinzas, 1980) is used by more than 64 per cent of Spanish special schools using alternative communication systems (Tamarit, 1993). There is now a variety of texts about the use of augmentative and alternative communication systems well suited for practical intervention in autism and related disorders (e.g. Baumgart, Johnson and Helmstetter, 1990; von Tetzchner and Martinsen, 1992). In addition, there is an increased interest in naturalistic approaches for communication teaching programmes (Koegel, O'Dell and Koegel, 1987; Koegel and Johnson, 1989).

However, it is still rare to find instruction-oriented papers focused upon deficits in joint attention behaviours, despite the fact that, as Lewy and Dawson (1992) suggest, this is a 'promising therapeutic strategy' (p. 564). On the other hand, in the last years, there has been a generalised feeling that many of the methods used to teach communication to children with autism do not always teach real communication, but rather ritual behaviours linked to particular contexts that have to be performed on the requirement of the therapist (Jordan and Powell, 1995). Furthermore, these ritual behaviours nearly always 'simulate' an imperative function, whereas declarative communication remains extremely difficult to teach even at the most rudimentary level.

In this section we are going to argue that if the role of joint attention in communication is taken into consideration, one might be able to start dealing with some of these problems. An important part of teaching alternative communication systems must involve teaching how to engage in and take advantage of joint attention. Among the aims of teaching it is necessary to include how to call, keep or manipulate other people's attention in relation to the signals used by the child. It is also important to teach the difference between failing to reach a communicative goal because the signals do not reach the receiver (a failure in joint attention), and failing because the receiver is not ready, willing and able to respond. In the latter case, where there is a temporary inability to respond by the receiver, an important skill to be taught is how to recognise indications that the message has reached its destination (i.e. signals other than the desired answer, such as *Wait a minute!* or some non-vocal equivalent). Including joint attention in alternative communication programmes may render these systems more versatile and functional. These considerations are valid both for intervention and assessment.

## Assessing joint attention for alternative communication

An important part of any evaluation of the communicative skills of disabled people should involve their understanding of the role of joint attention in communication. For this, it is not enough to record whether, for example, a child's gestures are accompanied by eye contact. This does not guarantee that the child understands joint attention. It is necessary to design situations where the individual is confronted with varying degrees of inattention in his or her audience. An example of such a situation has been developed by us according to an experimental paradigm originally designed to study the understanding of visual attention in chimpanzees (Gómez, 1995).

This task allows assessment of different levels of attention understanding in terms of the cues to which the subject is sensitive. These cues may range from very gross (e.g. the adult's back is turned to the communicator) to more subtle ones (e.g. the adult is facing the communicator, but looking somewhere else). In a preliminary study with young children with autism, we used the following arrangement.

In a small room, an adult was sitting behind a table. At his side, there was a tray on which desirable objects could be placed. Since the table blocked direct access to the tray, children had to ask the adult for the items on the tray. A few preliminary trials were conducted in which the adult would pay full attention to the children's actions, responding as soon as a request (verbal, gestural, manipulative, etc.) had been recognised. This part of the task is similar to situations used in other studies on preverbal communication, in both children with autism (Curcio, 1978) and normal children (Martinsen and von Tetzchner, 1988). However, in the present study, when the child proved capable of engaging in requesting behaviours, 'inattentive' trials were intermingled with the normal, 'attentive' ones. These experimental trials included:

- adult oriented towards the child but with eyes closed;
- adult with head turned sideways;
- adult with body turned sideways;
- adult with back turned to the child;
- adult looking at the desirable object;
- adult looking at subject but not responding for a few seconds.

Of course, this situation would allow other variations in the signs of inattention shown by the adult (for example, the face could be oriented towards the child, but the eyes could be turned sideways), depending upon how detailed one wants the assessment to be.

The point of the situation is that it allows assessment of which signs of inattention, if any, a child is sensitive to. For example, in our preliminary study, most of the children with autism were sensitive to the 'back turned' situation. However, only some of them showed skills for overcoming the situation, for example approaching the person and touching his back or pulling his clothes. The other children would simply stop making requests when the adult was in such a position. However, these latter children would persist in making a request when the inattention of the adult was less clearly expressed (e.g. head turned sideways or eyes closed).

Many of the children used manipulative gestures as their means of making requests. For example, they would take the hand of the adult and lead it towards the target (a typical procedure for children with autism). Of course, if the hands of the adult were resting on the table, the children had no need to call the attention of the adult – their requesting gesture functioned as an attention-getter as well. This led us to introduce an additional type of experimental condition, where the hands of the adult would be unavailable. Many of the children using manipulative gestures were unable to deal with this situation, except for stretching and trying to reach the hand of the adult. They did not seem to notice the attentional behaviours of their 'communicative' partner.

Procedures like this allow assessment of both an individual's sensitivity to different cues of inattention and the means available to draw the attention of inattentive people.

It is important to emphasise that, even if from a theoretical point of view, many of the gestures and signals used by children with autism might not qualify as genuine intentional communication because they are not accompanied by proper joint attention, this does not mean they are worthless. Indeed, it is much better to have limited means of controlling your environment than to have none at all. The first step in communication intervention may often consist of establishing a simple grasp of the contingency between the child's behaviour and a particular consequence in the environment. This contingency grasp may be further enhanced by establishing some sensitivity to discriminative cues, such as having somebody present when making the signal or establishing eye contact with the addressee. (Cf. the notion of 'precommunicative intentions' developed by von Tetzchner, in preparation).

This does not involve a genuine understanding of joint attention and, therefore, is not 'genuine' communication; but it is a useful means of interaction and should be treated as such. It is important to keep in mind the possible beneficial effects of permanently attributing social intentionality (including, of course, communicative intentionality) to any acts of the children, independently of their 'real' level of intentionality. For example, if a child reaches for objects without ever checking the adults' attention, it could be helpful to react to these 'requests' even if one doubts that they are genuine communicative acts. Indeed, authors like Bruner (1975) and Lock (1980) have defended the idea that overattribution of intentionality could play some role in the development of intentional communication in normal children. But whatever role the strategy of overattribution might play, both for normal and atypical children, it is important, first, that the professional is aware of the actual level of communicative proficiency achieved by the persons he or she is teaching, and second, that overattribution is likely at best to be only a complement to other teaching strategies.

According to this, a goal of intervention programmes must be to build up the joint attention components absent in the interactive patterns of children, such as checking the adult's gaze or calling the attention of inattentive people before making gestures to them. For this it is important to develop means to assess the understanding of attention and inattention, such as the procedure outlined above.

## Joint attention in alternative communication intervention

The theoretical distinction between protoimperatives and protodeclaratives has important practical implications. Whereas gestures with some protoimperative function seem to be relatively easy to establish in most individuals (not so their corresponding joint attention behaviours), even the most rudimentary protodeclarative functions seem to be highly elusive to teaching when one is working with persons with autism and severe developmental impairments. The reason seems to lie in the intrinsically motivating nature of these gestures: as mentioned before, whereas protoimperatives use joint attention to make others do something, protodeclaratives involve using joint attention for its own sake. As Schaeffer (1978) points out: '...the handicapped child's first sign may be viewed as a highly conventionalised protoimperative' (p. 326). As to the protodeclarative function, Schaeffer, Raphael and Kollinzas (1994) state that it is not likely that children with autism will master it 'even with extensive instruction and encouragement' (p. 131).

Teaching abilities like gaze-following could be relatively easy (of course, depending upon the student's impairments). It is enough to find out which objects the students are interested in and then arrange situations where an adult's attention is the cue that directs them to the objects. However, in the case of protodeclaratives, it is the students who have to figure out what the adult might be interested in; furthermore they have to find the adult's interest interesting (be it an inner 'mental' interest or outer expressions of interest). This is the difficulty with teaching protodeclarative communication.

As to protoimperative communication, it has already been pointed out how difficult it is to teach 'genuine' intentional requests in which the student takes the other person's attention into account.

In the remainder of this chapter, intervention strategies will be explored which might facilitate the use of joint attention behaviours in both protoimperative and protodeclarative communication.

### Interrupting behaviour chains

As Hunt and Goetz (1988) proposed, one may elicit, and enhance, a variety of joint attention behaviours if, in a previously well-known routine or behavioural chain, a different, unexpected step or item which suddenly interrupts it is introduced, as in these examples:

> Carlos was a 10-year-old non-verbal boy with autism and moderate intellectual impairment. He received manual sign intervention following the *Signed Speech Programme* (Schaeffer et al., 1994). He spontaneously used a lot of manual signs to ask for things to satisfy his desires and needs. Every day, after lunch, along with his peers and teacher, he had to go to the bath room and brush his teeth. It was always the same routine: getting the tooth brush, spreading the tooth paste, brushing the teeth, turning on the tap, etc. The things he needed were always in their usual place. But one day the teacher – obviously, without Carlos seeing her doing it – hid his tooth brush and put a colourful pencil in its place. When seeing a pencil instead of a tooth brush, Carlos was likely to look at his teacher, and, since she was waiting for this reaction, she showed off as if Carlos had said 'Look, the tooth brush has disappeared'. The adult 'shared' the problem with her student, imitated his facial expression of surprise, and immediately helped him to solve the problem by looking for a solution 'together' with him.

> Laura was an 8-year-old non-verbal girl with autism who followed the same manual signing programme as Carlos. At snack times, she usually drank a glass of milk with some sugar. But occasionally, the sugar bowl was carefully emptied by her teacher. The moment Laura discovered that it was empty, whatever she did was interpreted by her teacher as if Laura had said 'There is no sugar' or 'I want some sugar, please'.

Note that this technique of routine interruption can be designed to emphasise the 'protodeclarative' aspects of communication (enhancing the surprise component of the interruption), as in the case of the pencil appearing instead of the tooth brush; or its 'protoimperative' dimension, as in the case of the simple absence of sugar. In the latter case, instead of an empty bowl being shown, some surprising and unexpected object could be placed in the bowl, thereby making the situation similar to the tooth brush example. The teacher's task was to capitalise upon the expressive signs of surprise, interest or whatever, shown by the student upon finding the unexpected object. After that, the request of the appropriate object and the search for it could be orchestrated.

## Do I know that you cannot do anything?

An important aspect of requesting is that the thing one is asking for can or cannot be provided. Unlike a machine that always responds in the same way when a button is pushed, a human being may react in quite different ways to exactly the same request at different moments. Sometimes, the addressee cannot fulfil the request because he or she is not in a condition to do so. It is the responsibility of the sender to appreciate when people are or are not in a condition to do something, and it is the addressee's responsibility to offer an explanation of the failure to respond.

Concerning the relevance of the schema 'I know/do not know that you can/cannot do something' in teaching social and communicative behaviour, it is our belief that programming and planning events in naturalistic environments for teaching this strategy is a way to develop joint attention behaviours. For example, imagine that there is a person physically available to reach something (for example, a person who has nothing in his hands and is close to a shelf with desired objects), whereas another person is not physically available (for example, a person who is behind a table with both hands busy typing on a keyboard). A child enters into the room: To whom should the child address its request?

A similar situation might be designed for introducing emotional cues. In the room there are two familiar persons. One of them seems to be tired and angry. The other one looks calm and is smiling: To whom should the child address its request?

One could work with these issues in real life situations or by means of pictures or video-recordings. We have just started our firsts attempts at teaching children with autism in such situations. Preliminary results look promising, but more time and data are necessary to draw conclusions about the usefulness of the strategy.

## Wait a minute!

There is another skill worth teaching in relation to the problem of learning when somebody can or cannot respond to requests. Sometimes, the person's inability to respond is only momentary. It is a matter of waiting a little until the person can answer the request. In everyday situations, this involves two reactions by the addressee: first, she has to recognise that the request has reached her attention and she has understood it;

second, she has to tell the communicator to wait a little. The question is how one can teach children with autism to adapt to a situation like this.

The aim is to teach the student that once the request is performed, although the reward will eventually be obtained, occasionally it will be necessary to wait a little before getting it without having to repeat the request. A step-by-step teaching plan can be established. At the beginning, the time elapsing between the request and its accomplishment will be no more than a few seconds, and during this interval, the adult will offer continuous verbal comments about the request. The comments are intended to function as a signal that the request will be attended to, as the temporal delays are extended before the request is fulfilled. However, the comments themselves should be progressively faded until the student can accept a simple acknowledgement of the request together with a 'promise' that it will be fulfilled a little later.

These situations have a great potential in intervention. They can be used to distinguish different reasons why requests do not always immediately succeed. Sometimes it is because the request has failed to reach the other person's attention. The solution in this case is to call properly on the attention of the addressee. At other times, it is because the person is unable to respond. It will be better to recognise this inability and refrain from repeating the request or using misplaced attention-getting procedures. Still, on other occasions, the problem is the person's unwillingness to respond, and it may be possible to try to persuade, entice or somehow convince the person to act. Finally, the person may have noticed the request and be willing to respond, but may not be sure what the exact request is and requires some clarification. Essentially, all the 'deferred response' situations should be contrasted with 'negative response' situations, where the requested item is not going to be provided at all. In each case, the reason for the request failing is different and, therefore, a distinct strategy is required. Understanding the reasons for the failure is largely a matter of paying attention to the attentive and expressive behaviours of the other person.

Thus, a function that is traditionally considered to be simple and straightforward – requesting things – turns out to be highly complex and sophisticated. Requesting, if properly handled, may offer excellent opportunities for teaching children about the importance of attention and expression in others. One might attempt to capitalise upon the external motivation provided by requests to teach something about the relevance of other people's interest in objects.

For example, when teaching strategies for calling the attention of other people, it is common to do things like shaping the behaviour of tapping onto the adult's shoulders and then making a request. However, an alternative strategy might be to teach the student to get the attention of an 'inattentive' adult by providing her with an object of interest to her. For example, a woman is playing a game (e.g. Tower of Hanoi) while showing a joyful and happy face. After that, she leaves the game and goes into the next room where she sits down with a tired attitude. The student needs to make a request to her, but how can the student get the attention of the 'tired' woman? A second adult could shape the action of taking the Tower of Hanoi and offering it to her. The adult will react with delight at the 'kind' action of the student, telling the student: *Oh, thanks … is there anything I can give you in return?*

The initial goal is not so much that the student shall understand all the intricacies of this complex interaction, as that she shall grasp the idea that other people's attention and availability can be influenced by means of objects – objects of special interest to the other. In this way one may be able to direct the students' attention to relations between other people and objects that may not in themselves be particularly interesting to the students.

## I am trying to get your attention… sometimes in good ways… sometimes in less good ways

So far, acceptable and positive ways of calling the attention of others have been discussed. However, children with autism and related disorders may spontaneously develop inadequate ways of capturing the attention of other people.

> Antonio was a 17-year-old adolescent with autism and severe intellectual impairment. He and his teacher were in the playground of the Centre, resting during a break. Suddenly, Antonio ran to his teacher, biting his own index finger while, at the same time, looking at his teacher's face and smiling. Clearly, Antonio was looking for the teacher's reaction.

Usually, this behaviour would have been interpreted as a 'negative' way of seeking attention. However, it might also be interpreted as a teasing behaviour, similar to those described in young babies (cf. Dunn, 1988; Reddy, 1991). If this interpretation is chosen, Antonio's self-biting behaviour would not be reacted to with anger, but in an exaggerated and fictitious way as if one were frightened by him. This form of interaction might then be transformed, step by step, into a better form of expression (with no fingers bitten).

# Conclusions

Before starting to use language, young children display a variety of communicative expressions in the form of gestures and preverbal vocalisations. An important part of this system is joint attention. Behaviours like gaze-following and eye contact facilitate both reference and intentionality. We have proposed that a consideration of the functions of joint attention in prelinguistic communication may provide important insights for assessment and intervention with alternative systems of communication for disabled populations such as children with autism. Taking into consideration the joint attention conditions in which early prelinguistic communication occurs, may allow one to elaborate apparently simple functions such as requesting, and to approach the traditional complex issue of teaching protodeclarative communication.

## Acknowledgement

Support to write this paper was provided by Direction General de Investigación Cientifica y Tecnica (PB92-0143-C02-02). At the time of writing, Juan Carlos Gómez was enjoying a grant from Ministerio de Educación y Ciencia (Subprograma General en el Extranjero; EX94-01103673).

# Chapter 4
# Words and strategies: Conversations with young children who use aided language

STEPHEN VON TETZCHNER AND HARALD MARTINSEN

Conversations involving young communication aid users and adults differ in significant ways from conversations between normally speaking children and adults. Hence, intervention with communication aid users cannot be based solely on existing knowledge about speech development. In order to be able to create appropriate situations for both learning and practising linguistic and communicative skills, it is necessary to gain insight into the dialogue context of aided speakers. However, within the traditional education-oriented approach to aided language, the nature of the children's participation in dialogues, which is the focus of the present chapter, has not been a central issue. Acquisition of aided language has been approached mainly as a technical skill and a motivational problem (e.g. Cook and Coleman, 1987; Shane and Bashir, 1980; Vanderheiden et al., 1975).

It is the recognition that language is individually 'reconstructed' within a variety of social contexts, through communicative interaction with other people (Garton, 1992; Lock, 1980; Luckman, 1990; Schaffer, 1989), that has directed the focus of aided language to development and dialogues. Within a transactional model of development (Sameroff and Chandler, 1975), dialogues reflect characteristics of the communication aids and the users, and how these, through transactional chains, have contributed to forming the conversational strategies and interactional styles of communication aid users and their communication partners. There is a dearth of knowledge about these dialogues and young aided speakers' development of conversational skills. A pressing issue for research in aided language acquisition is to reveal how transactional characteristics determine the developmental course. Some of these may to a large extent be inherent in the aided language form itself, but it may still be possible to influence acquisition and strategies used through changing other elements of the communicative context.

Early use of aided language usually consists of pointing to, or otherwise indicating, graphic signs, such as Blissymbols, pictograms (PIC, PCS, etc.), drawings and photographs (see Introduction). As children get older, traditional orthography may be used. Several concatenated characteristics of aided communication influence the interaction between the children and their partners. The two most important ones are that:

•    it takes longer to select a graphic sign than to articulate the corresponding word;
•    the expressive vocabulary is restricted to the number of signs made available by the communication aid; e.g. the number of items on a communication board.

These two characteristics are interdependent. Even if traditional orthography is disregarded, it is in principle possible to design a graphic sign system in which the equivalent of any word of the spoken language is available for a communication aid user. The more signs an aid contains, however, the longer it will take for the user to access and select a sign.

In Norway, most children who are taught aided language are unable to speak or use manual signs due to motor impairments. Many have cerebral palsy while others have less clearly defined conditions of motor impairment or dyspraxia (von Tetzchner, 1995). Their ability to understand spoken language varies. Some need mainly a means of expression, due to a significant gap between their ability to speak and their understanding of what other people say to them. This subgroup is termed the *expressive language group*. For another subgroup, the aided language is used as a support system and to facilitate acquisition of spoken language. For a third subgroup, comprehension of spoken language is lacking or clearly limited. The graphic sign system functions as their 'mother tongue' throughout life. Intervention strategies will differ for these three groups, as will their conversational skills. (For a discussion of different groups of alternative language users, see Martinsen and von Tetzchner, this volume).

For children belonging to the expressive language group, the primary focus of this chapter, the main code of the conversation is speech. The aided language may be conceived of as a form of 'translation' where utterances the children are unable to articulate are being replaced by graphic language forms. The words corresponding to the graphic signs indicated by the children are articulated by the communication partner, or, if they use high-technology aids, through synthesised or digitised speech. The parents and other significant persons communicate with the children through speech, it is rare for them even to complement their spoken words by pointing to a graphic sign.

Aided language users tend to get their communication aids at a much later age than that at which children usually start to speak (Joleff et al.,

1992; Light, Collier and Parnes, 1985a; Smith, 1991; Udwin and Yule, 1990; von Tetzchner, in press). Before a graphic system is introduced, conversations between the children and their caregivers are in most cases limited to the child pointing with hand or eye at objects, people and locations in the environment, and, by non-verbal means, expressing the equivalents of 'yes' and 'no'. Children with some motor ability may have learned a few manual signs. A substantial part of the conversations consists of the parents asking the children whether they want something and the children indicating whether this is the case. When somewhat more advanced matters are addressed, the dialogues resemble the game 'Twenty Questions'. In principle, the introduction of graphic sign systems makes it possible for the children to express themselves with greater precision, introduce topics not thought of by the adults, and comment on objects, people and events in a less dependent manner.

The present chapter discusses dialogues involving four children, aged 5;4–8;4, who needed graphic signs mainly as a means for expressing themselves and who were able to understand the spoken language of others. The children participated in a larger study investigating aided language intervention in a representative group of young children considered by their teachers to have graphic language as their main form of communication (cf. von Tetzchner, 1995, in press). The children were representative of those with a large gap between comprehension and production of spoken language. One child had 12 spoken words, the other three had none. Intellectually, they were among the seven highest functioning children in the study. (Two other children in this category in the larger study were not included, because although the educational staff could hardly understand anything they said, their speech was understood by their parents to a considerably greater extent. One child obtained a relatively low language comprehension score). They were all established communication aid users, having used graphic language for an average of 4;8 (range 2;4–5;7). The average size of their graphic vocabularies was 431 items (range 145–845). Intervention at the time of the study focused mainly on expression, speech comprehension being considered appropriate for educational purposes. The assessments made of the children varied. However, all had obtained an age-equivalent score of three years or higher on a computer-based test of language comprehension with small demands on motor skills (von Tetzchner, 1987). Although comparable expressive language ability cannot be taken for granted, the results on the language comprehension test indicate that the children probably would have used complex sentences if physical impairments had not rendered them unable to speak.

The dialogues were drawn from video recordings of conversations between the children and their parents in situations chosen by the parents and considered by them as constituting good communication situations. The examples presented here are typical of these inter-changes. In addition to the video recordings, parents and professionals were interviewed about the intervention process, and the children's language development, communication, and performance in preschool and school.

## Characteristics of the conversations

Dialogues involving children who use communication aids and their parents have several characteristics that set them apart from dialogues involving children, of the same age and younger, who are able to speak. The differences found in the present study relate to the form of the dialogues, the roles of the two communication partners, and characteristics of the children's utterances.

In conversations between speaking children and their parents, both partners use the same mode of communication. The communication aid users and their parents used different communication forms. The adults talked to the children. Only in certain situations did they point to items on the children's communication aids when communicating. The children indicated graphic signs. The parents articulated the words corresponding to the graphic signs and typically expanded the utterances into comments based on situational interpretations. The parents thus spoke both for themselves and on behalf of the children.

The fact that the dialogues were based on a speech code, and that only the parents were able to speak, probably contributed to making the parents dominate in a manner not usually found in dialogues involving speaking children. The double role of being both a communication part-ner and the one who articulates for a disabled communicator typically leads to an asymmetry in the roles of the communication partners (Blau, 1986; Harris, 1982; Light et al., 1985a; Marková, 1995; Sutton, 1982). The parents tended to decide the topic of the conversation, assigning the subordinate role of answering questions to the children. They also openly expressed judgments about the children's conversational perfor-mance.

### Adults' use of questions

Dialogues involving children using communication aids have been shown to contain a high proportion of turns where the communica-tion partners ask questions, mainly *yes/no* questions. As a conse-quence, most of the children's turns are directed towards giving answers (Basil, 1992; Harris, 1982; Light, 1985; Sutton, 1982). The use of questions may be traced to pre-aid communication strategies and fulfils a number of communicative functions. (For notations, see Table 0.1).

(1)     Henry, aged 8;4, used a communication book with 145 PIC signs
        through dependent scanning. His father had just read Henry's
        'message book', in which the teachers and the parents daily
        communicated the most important events and activities in which
        Henry had participated, and had initiated a conversation about
        Henry's school day.
    F:   *Did you learn about any particular animals today or which*
         *animals did you learn about?*
         *It is in your book, so I know about it.*
         *Which animal did you learn about in school today?*
    H:   DOG.
    F:   *Yes. Dog, yes. Did anybody bring a dog to school today? Who*
         *was it? Who brought a dog to school today?*
    H:   Looks at the table and smiles.
    F:   *Was it Mary?*
    H:   'No' (head movement).
    F:   *Was it Joan who brought a dog?*
    H:   'Yes' (head movement).
    F:   *Yes, it was in your book that Joan brought her dog.*
         (Time elapsed, 0:32).

The father phrased the questions so that Henry never had to indicate
more than one graphic sign. A majority of the questions could be
answered with 'yes' or 'no', which Henry indicated with head movements. This is also the most common strategy in conversations of non-
speaking children before they have received communication aids. It
does not usually require the use of a graphic sign. Henry, like most children in the expressive group who use communication aids, was able to
express 'yes' and 'no' by other means.

Dialogue (1) contained two questions that made it necessary for
Henry to refer to the communication aid, the wh-questions *Which*
*animal did you learn about in school today?* and *Who brought a dog to*
*the school today?* Henry answered *DOG* to the first question. The other
was reformulated into a series of *yes/no* questions because the father
could not expect a direct answer from Henry: the communication book
did not contain the name (a pictogram or photograph) of the person in
question. However, the father's use of a rhetorical question may in this
case have been functional, serving to provide Henry with a target for the
following *yes/no* questions, and making it easier for him to answer
correctly.

Reverting to a communication form in which the aided system
becomes irrelevant may to some extent be a result of insufficient vocabulary. However, it may also be done to speed up communication, due to
the long time it takes for the child and its partner to select an intended
graphic sign. Adults may be reluctant to invest the time and the effort

that is necessary for the child to use the communication aid, particularly when they, like Henry's father, already know the answers to the questions they have asked. In fact, in this study, both parents and professionals seemed to prefer to communicate by asking questions that could be answered with 'yes' or 'no'. The communication aid was considered more an educational instrument than a general means for communicating. One of the parents said:

> 'We chose the way of least resistance. We worked with PIC signs but when we communicated, we used a lot of *yes/no* questions'.

Similar opinions were expressed by the teacher of a nine-year-old Irish girl using Blissymbols (Smith, 1991).

It may also be of significance that communication aids tended first to be introduced as 'problem solvers'. Parents were advised to start using them as a means of help when the pre-aid strategies failed and communication broke down. This may initially have been done as an effort to demonstrate the usefulness of communication aids to parents and teachers. However, they may have continued to use the communication aids mainly in this restricted manner, causing them to be infrequently employed. George's mother expressed it like this:

> 'Because he communicates well using his eyes, he can always tell us what he wants to talk about. It is only in emergencies, when he gets stuck, that he asks for the PIC book'.

Similar attitudes were apparent in the school setting, for example as expressed by Eva's preschool assistant:

> 'We bring it out when there is an emergency. When she has eaten, it is used for choosing an activity. We bring it out when she is sad, approximately every second week'.

The conception of aided communication mainly as a means to solve a problem may in fact have been an important determinant of the strategies that were developed (cf. Collins, this volume). The focus of this type of communication is to convey a single item of information – usually in the form of a single graphic sign – whose particular function is interpreted by the partner in accordance with the problem in question. The formulation of a relational meaning in the form of a sentence did not seem to be an important goal. In the comments made by parents and professionals, communication breakdowns were usually related to the child's wants and needs, rather than to ideas or opinions that the child might hold about some event or state.

Dialogue (1) also demonstrates that adults may tend to encourage young aid users to reiterate known events rather than to tell something new. None of the parents in the present study chose situations where the children were expected to present new information or contribute in a substantial way to the dialogue. Henry was not really supposed to communicate anything to his father, at least not in the sense of transferring unknown information. Henry's father even made it clear beforehand that he already knew the answers, and the dialogue ended by the father confirming that Henry got the story right. Although the father did show interest and closeness, the meta-message implicitly communicated to Henry may have been that the point of the communication was to check out that Henry remembered what had happened. In communication involving speaking children and parents, such dialogues are rarely found, except in very early dialogues when a parent is helping the child to tell a story. Even in these instances, speaking children may not only reply to questions, but provide unexpected views and comments, sometimes reflecting a childish misunderstanding of the facts (cf. Aukrust, 1992; McTear, 1985). Similar dialogues may also be found when speaking children undergo oral examinations in a school setting. This similarity may be a result of teacher influence and encouragement to praise 'correct' communication (cf. Scollon and Scollon, 1994). The parents' choice of frames for the dialogues may be linked with their use of a guessing strategy, and the fact that it is difficult to guess outside one's own communicative frame (cf. Goffman, 1974; van Dijk and Kintsch, 1983).

The limitations of the guessing strategy were illustrated in a communication task where the children were asked to relay the content of pictures to their teachers who were ignorant of the contents of the pictures. The communication aid of the boy in (2) was not used much in the classroom, and although the teacher had been made aware of the nature of the task and explicitly told that all forms of communication were allowed as long as the picture remained face down, she still failed to bring along his communication aid, a book containing 447 items.

(2)    Helmer, aged 8;3, communicated with direct selection. He had been shown a picture of a red flower. This was the second picture, the first one depicted a chair.

    T:  *A new picture. Do you remember what it is?*

    H:  'Yes' (vocalises).

    T:  *Is this an object as well? Could it be a chair?*

    H:  'No' (head movement).

    T:  *It was not a chair on the picture. Can you tell me about the picture, what you saw on the picture. What did you see?*

    H:  Smiles.

    T:  *Did you see something funny? Was it a table or a chair or something?*

H: Looks out of the window.
T: *I think you are looking at the children.*
*Are you going to tell me what is on the table? Could you point*
*at something?*
*Is there anything in the room looking like it?*
*Nothing in the room?*
H: Looks towards a shelf.
T: *Is on at the shelf up there? Maybe it is a toy? Is it something*
*you can play with?*
(Time elapsed, 1:50).

The teacher did not manage to guess the content of the picture within the time limit of eight minutes. Helmer lacked the means to communicate this to her. His communication aid was not available to him, and there were no flowers present in the room that he could point to. There is no doubt that he would have been able to relay the information in a few seconds if his communication aid had been present. On a later occasion, he had no problems telling his parents by the use of graphic signs that a live cat had visited him in the classroom earlier in the day (another communication task). In fact, in the following lesson he was writing on a computer together with another teacher who did not know the content of the task, and on his own initiative, he managed to write rose.

The fact that adults have to revert to a guessing strategy when they believe that the children are trying to express something they lack the means to convey, suggests that the children may need signs especially selected to direct the adults' guessing, such as *ALMOST-YES, ALMOST-NO, GETTING-HOT, FURTHER-AWAY*, etc. (von Tetzchner, 1993c).

### The adult as a helper

Parents are their children's communication partners. However, in order for children who use aided communication to express themselves, unless they use a high-technology aid, parents must also assist in articulating their messages. In some situations the parents' behaviour resembles the act of a ventriloquist. Part of the reason why parents become the dominating partner in the communication to such a degree may be the difficulties embedded in taking on such a double role. In addition, the parents have to be their children's helpers in most everyday activities; washing, putting on clothes, moving about, eating, etc., at an age when most other children have become independent. Avoiding confounding the roles of being a communication partner and a communication helper may be made even more difficult if strategies are transferred from activities where the helper role is more clearly defined. This is the case in situations where a parent does something on behalf of the child, and in which neither the parent, nor the child, is the object of the activity.

(3)     George, aged 7;4, communicated with eye pointing and depen-
        dent scanning. His communication aid was a book containing 845
        PIC signs, drawings and photographs. He and his father were
        building a house on a square.
        F: *We should start with the living room.*
        G: 'Yes' (eye movement).
        F: *Yes. And a sofa there. Sofa.*
            *Did you want the living room there?*
        G: Looks at the square and the house.
        F: *Or?* (turns the house around).
            *Here?* (turns it again, looks at George).
            *Here?* (points to another room).
            *There?* (points to the last room).
            *Here? Where do you want the living room?* (Tries to follow
            Henry's gaze).
        G: Looks at the roof of the house they are building.
        F: *Hello.*
        G: 'Yes' (eye movement).
        F: *Here?* (points).
            *Is it so difficult to make up your mind? Hm?*
            *Should we rebuild the house, or what are you thinking of?*
        G: Looks at the father and quickly up.
        F: *Hm. The roof. Should we move the roof? The wall?*
        G: 'Yes' (eye movements).
        F: *Hm. Should we move the wall?*
        G: 'Yes' (eye movement).
        F: *This?* (points). *Should we move it?*
        G: 'Yes' (eye movement).
        F: *Yes* (takes George's hand and moves the wall).
            *Where should we move it? Just take it away?* (Points at the
            square) *Over here?*
            (Puts down the wall) *Like this?*
        G: Looks at the father.
        F: *Did you think it was too small?*
        G: 'Yes' (eye movement).
        F: *All the way?* (moves the wall).
        G: 'Yes' (eye movement).
        F: *Yes.*
            (Time elapsed, 1:55).

In order to be a successful helper, the adult must be able to help without
changing the intentions of the child. In (3), the father placed the bricks
according to George's wishes without imposing his own standards or
interest into the boy's construction. He used a guessing strategy, waiting
patiently for George's confirmations of the guesses and suggesting other

possibilities when guesses were not acknowledged. However, all that
was achieved in (3) was moving a wall, the meaning negotiated during
the two minutes of 'conversation' may be expressed as 'Please, make the
room bigger by moving the wall to the edge of the square'. George did
not communicate any story which, for other children of the same age,
would have been the main focus.

(4)    Ann, a normally speaking three-year-old girl, and her mother were
       playing with dolls and talking about somewhere they would be
       going the next day.
       A:  *Drive the car home.*
       M:  *Yes, we will drive the car home tomorrow.*
       A:  *Don't bring the doll. The doll must stay inside.*
       M:  *Yes, the doll has to stay in when you are going to see all the
            children tomorrow.*
       A:  *Yes.*
       M:  *Hm* (affirmative).
       A:  *The doll must be in the chair.*
       M:  *Yes, the doll may be in its chair.*
       A:  *When the girl comes home, the doll must stand up.*
       M:  *Yes.*

In dialogue (3), the structure of the building movements made guessing
a functional strategy. If George or his father had introduced a story-
making activity during the construction, unless it was a routine story
with a known course, George would have needed graphic signs in addition to answering *yes/no* questions. The communication form would
have forced the communication partners to shift focus between the
activity and the communication aid, stopping the activity while communicating. The fact that the communication was very time-consuming
made it difficult to transcend the directions and communicate about
what was going on.

## The role of the child

Although several factors may predispose parents towards taking the
dominant role, parents' communicative behaviour may not be a sufficient explanation of the way the children act in the communication situations. In some sense of the word, the children must allow the parents to
take the control. Thus, it becomes important to consider to what extent
children who use aided communication are forced into a passive role by
problems imposed by their disability, characteristics inherent in the
communication system, or the parental behaviour. In order to approach
this question, it is necessary to focus on the children's contributions to
the dialogues.

In conversations between speaking children and their parents, the parents will follow the lead of the children. This happens at all ages, starting when children begin to speak (Snow, 1986). Dialogues between children who use aided language and their parents tend to be initiated by the parent (Light et al., 1985a). As a consequence, in most cases the topic of the conversation is also introduced by the parent. This may partly be explained by the fact that the children control few means of directing the parents' attention towards matters other than ongoing activities and cues in the immediate situation. Furthermore, even communication about the immediate situation may depend on the partner somehow 'reading' non-verbal expressions, as an indication that the child may want to say something that is not part of the activity frame introduced by the partner.

(5)   George and his father were going to start playing, but the father saw from George's expression that something was wrong.

F:   *Here?* (Turning pages, asking for each page).
G:   *BODY.*
F:   *Body. Body?* (Turns pages).
G:   Vocalises and gets tense in the body.
F:   *Hm? Was it not the body? What was it? Was it this one?*
G:   'No' (eye movements).
F:   *This one?* (Points at *CLOTHES*).
G:   'Yes' (eye movements).
F:   *Clothes.* (Indicates domain. The father turns the pages to the clothes pages). *And here?*
G:   'Yes' (eye movement).
F:   *What?*
G:   *SWEATER* (gaze).
F:   *Is it something with the sweater?*
G:   'Yes' (eye movement).
F:   *What?*
G:   'Yes' (eye movement, probably prompts guessing).
F:   *Are the sleeves too long?*
G:   'Yes' (eye movement).
F:   *Oh, they are. Yes.*
     (Time elapsed, 2:0).

However, most dialogues were related to activities and themes that were introduced by parents.

(6)   Eva, aged 5;4, was using direct selection and a communication book with 285 PIC signs and photographs. She and her mother were communicating about a trip to an aunt, a frame introduced by the mother.

E:  *DOLL.*
M:  *Did you bring this along to Aunt Kari? The doll?*
E:  'Yes' (nods)
    *READ.*
M:  *The doll went along to Aunt Kari. Hm?*
E:  *DUPLO.*
M:  *And you like to play with Duplo.*
E:  'No' (shakes head).
M:  *No.*
E:  *TRAIN.*
M:  *What can you do at Aunt Kari's?*
E:  *READ.*
M:  *Can you read there?*
E:  'Yes' (nods)
M:  *Hm. What else can you do?*
    (Time elapsed, 0:33).

The dialogue was typical in the sense that the frame of the conversation was chosen by the mother. *READ* was used by Eva to relay an intention that was not acknowledged at first by the mother. *READ* may have been an attempt to change the topic of the conversation, or suggest that they should read. However, the attempt to change the direction of the conversation or the activity was not successful. Eva repeated it once later and the mother interpreted *READ* in accordance with the topic she herself had chosen for the conversation, and continued to talk about the trip. (A similar pattern may be seen in dialogue (8) below.)

Eva and the other aid users could, in principle, have insisted on communicating about something else and actively sought to change the topic during the conversation. Even in the first stages towards the acquisition of speech, children usually persist until they succeed in directing the attention of the partner in comparable child-adult dialogues, as in this example from Martinsen and von Tetzchner (1989, p. 64):

(7)  A normally developing child, aged 13 months, is talking with its
     mother
     M:  *Åh, der er en pus.*           *Oh, there is a cat.*
         *Pusekatt.*                     *Pussycat.*
     C:  *Tju.*
         *Tchju.*
         *Pu.*
         *Ekche.*
         *Esjekatt.*
     M:  *Pusekatt.*                     *Pussycat.*
     C:  *Pusche.*
         *Tej.*

Comparing (6) and (8) with (7) and (11), it may seem that children who use aided language are less insistent than speaking children on adult partners shifting their attention towards the topic of the child, and thereby are also less insistent on their attempting to understand what the children want to communicate.

(8)     Eva and her mother were sitting on the sofa with a doll's house and several Duplo figures on the table in front of them.
        M: (Points to a Duplo figure). {*Look, Eva, the mother is hungry HUNGRY*}.
        K: 'Yes' (nods).
        M: {*CRY Yes, I will cry if you don't go to the shop and buy food for me*}.
        K: 'Yes' (nods).
        M: *Hm.*
        K: (Turns the pages of the communication book).
        M: (Helps to turn the pages).
        K: *BICYCLE.*
        M: *Oh, you are going to use the bicycle.*
        K: (Stretches towards the Duplo figures)
        M: *When are you going to shop?*
            (Time elapsed, 0:25).

In dialogues with aided speakers, partners have rarely been reported to point at graphic signs (Bruno and Bryen, 1986) like the keyword point-ing of Eva's mother in (8). The reason for pointing at the pictograms, however, may not have been to provide language models but rather that the mother had sat down with Eva to have a 'conversation' and use the communication aid. She used it like a traditional picture book. The graphic signs were used as cues for comments, rather than for express-ing something in particular. Both she and other parents sometimes went slowly through the book, making comments and entertaining the child by conversing about matters relating to some of the graphic signs.

(9)     Eva's mother was going through the communication aid, turning pages and asking questions.
        M: *And Tom?*
        E: 'No' (shakes the head).
        M: *What does he have on? Does he use glasses?*
        E: 'Yes' (nods).
        M: *Who else uses glasses?* (Turns page). *Is it Mary?*
        E: 'Yes' (nods).
        M: *Hm.* (Turns page). *Which colour is your car?*
        E: *ORANGE.*
        M: *Which colour is your car? Do you remember?*

E:   'Yes' (nods).
M:   *Which colour is your car?*
E:   *RED.*
M:   *Yes, that one. Your car is red. Hm.*
     (Time elapsed, 0:37).

The communication resulted in a fragmented conversation, in which various topics were presented in relation to particular pictograms and photographs, but in which the topics were unrelated in meaning. Sometimes the parents first found a pictogram or photograph in the communication book and then posed a question, to which pointing to that graphic sign would be an appropriate answer.

(10)   Henry and his father were having a conversation using the communication aid.
     F:   *Is there anything more you want to tell about this page?*
     H:   *BALL.*
     F:   *Yes, ball, yes. What do you do with the ball, Henry? Let's see if we can find something here that we use it for* (turns pages). *Do we use the ball for anything here? What can we use the ball for?*
     H:   *FOOT.*
     (Time elapsed, 0:25).

In the dialogue below, and probably also in (7), the child seemed to add a comment to the topic, after the adult confirmed the topic (from Martinsen and von Tetzchner, 1989, p. 64).

(11)   A normally developing child, aged 11 months, was talking with its mother.
     C: *Se.*                    *Look.*
        *Se.*                    *Look.*
     M: *Ja, se der.*         *Yes, look there.*
     C: *Åi.*                   *Oy* (expression of excitement).

In most of the examples where the young aided language users succeeded in choosing the topic by the use of a pictogram, they only contributed to the conversation by pointing to a single sign, letting the adult provide the comment. The adult typically started to guess on the basis of the indicated sign, and the child ended up either by confirming the adult's comment, or by answering a *wh*-question which the adult had used to elicit a comment from the child. This was true in (6) and (8), and even in (5), where the comment guessed by the father was related to discomfort experienced by the child. It is part of the pattern observed, however, that examples such as (5) seldom occurred. Usually, the children failed even to choose the topic. Furthermore, there were hardly any examples found of dialogues in which the parents questioned the child in such a way that it was encouraged to comment independently upon the topic.

The lack of insistence on determining the topic of the conversation may thus be related to the adult partners' preoccupation with providing topics that create successful interactions, and the children's lack of means to make the adults change their direction of attention. The result, however, may be that repeated failures to express themselves and make the adults understand what they want to talk about discourage the children from trying to do so at a later stage.

## Expressive vocabulary

The crucial role of vocabulary for expressive communication has made selection of words and design of standard vocabularies for various groups the most central issue in aided language intervention (Fried-Oken and More, 1992; Fristoe and Lloyd, 1980; Karlan and Lloyd, 1983). The expressive vocabulary of children who use a graphic sign system will always be limited. This implies that the children lack graphic signs corresponding to words which are necessary for expressing particular meanings. In clinical work one has attempted to compensate for this by selecting the signs that are most likely to be useful for the child in various situations throughout the day; for example food items at meals, and animal names in biology lessons (e.g. Musselwhite and St. Louis, 1988). Accordingly, a child's communication aid may contain different vocabularies in different situations. A consequence of this strategy is that the topics that can be introduced by the child are limited by the situational board arranged by the adult. Moreover, the lack of appropriate signs may force the communication partner to attempt to guess what the child wants to communicate in the situation.

The limited expressive vocabulary and lack of relevant signs available in a communicative situation are not a necessary attribute of communication aids. In principle, it is possible for the child to insist on a particular sign being made available in a situation – for instance, by repeatedly pointing to the communication board making distress sounds or an unhappy face. However, this would imply not only that the child knew the spoken word the parents needed, in order to express what it wanted to say, and was able to make them guess it, but also that the parents had a graphic sign present, equivalent of that word, to include in the child's communication aid.

Alternatively, the children could combine two or more graphic signs to create the intended meanings, using them in a somewhat metaphorical way. However, the parents and professionals interviewed were hardly able to provide examples of such combinations or metaphorical use.

One parent mentioned *MEATBALL* for 'hamburger', another that *BEDROOM* had been used to indicate that the child's leg was 'asleep' (a Norwegian idiom). *CHEESE+SANDWICH* was also mentioned. One parent thought the use of *ACCIDENT* for falling down stairs was metaphoric because the PIC sign displayed two cars colliding. The scarcity of examples indicates that interpretations of messages expressed with pictograms may tend to be literal and more related to the pictorial content of the pictograms than the gloss written on them (cf. Basil, 1992; Raanaas, 1993).

Both of the strategies mentioned above require well-developed metalinguistic skills (cf. Hjelmquist and Sandberg, this volume). None of the parents of the children included here had been explicitly taught to use such strategies. Neither did the professionals seem aware of this as a possible strategy for pictograms. (With Blissymbols, the use of combination and analogy is an inherent strategy of the system). In addition, except for photographs denoting people, neither parents nor professionals seemed to utilise non-system vocabulary items to any large extent, thereby limiting the vocabulary by their choice of system. None of the children in the present group used Blissymbols, or had advanced beyond PIC before they started reading instruction at 6–7 years of age (cf. von Tetzchner, 1995).

The dearth of combinations and metaphors, as well as information provided in the interviews, indicate that the children had not been taught these strategies. Moreover, if the children had attempted to use combinations and metaphors for conveying new meanings to their communication partners, because of the literal interpretations leading the adults in other directions, they may well have learned that these strategies would not lead to communicative success. It is possible that such learning experiences may reinforce an existing tendency to become passive, common among children using communication aids, and thereby partly explain why adults become the dominant partners of the conversations. Inclusion of strategies utilising combinations and metaphors might have contributed to allocating greater responsibility to the children for producing elements of the message, thereby reducing their dependence on guessing.

## Creative pointing

Pointing and other ways of indicating objects, persons and locations outside the communication board may be part of an aided language strategy. When a child lacks a useful sign, indicating an object or person may be a way to overcome this. It may also save time if such items are more readily available than the graphic sign which may take more time to select. For example, Henry, sitting next to the door of his room, looked at this door to express 'I'. This strategy, which is a kind of trope, was faster than going through the pages of his communication aid, provided that he was understood by his communication partner. In (3), George looked up and this was (mistakenly) taken to indicate 'roof' (see also Chapter 5.)

In many communicative interactions, there may be little functional difference between pointing to an object and pointing to à graphic sign, except for the fact that objects may tend to be taken as an indication of that particular object, rather than an object category, and that this type of 'utterance' is unlikely to be understood metaphorically. Pointing to an object may even be considered symbolic communication, if the object is used to name or represent a category, an activity, or a larger context.

In national manual sign languages pointing is part of the formal grammar. A location may be used as a pronoun or have an adverbial function (Loew, 1980; Meier, 1990). No such formal use of pointing has been reported for children who use graphic sign systems. In the dialogues observed here, except when used to indicate a graphic sign, pointing was mainly limited to the same communicative function as is usually found in the speaking community (cf. McNeill, 1992). This suggests that spoken language conventions also determine whether the pointing gesture should be part of the language system, or merely used in a non-verbal manner. It is not, however, obvious that this has to be the case. It might be taken as evidence that not all means of communication have been developed to their full potential, and that conventions of the spoken language may restrict the functionality of aided communication.

## Making the adult talk about a topic

The children's contributions to the conversations indicate that they may have developed communication strategies that are very different from strategies found among naturally speaking children. The function of their utterances often seemed to be to make the communication partner say something about a particular topic. Helmer's mother expressed it in this way:

'He turned the pages and pointed. I had to say 'music', 'piano', 'record player' or whatever it was. He has very consciously used us to speak for him, or to talk about something he wanted talked about. This was the way we used it (the communication book)'.

The children typically used a few graphic signs to prompt the adult partner to tell a story connected with the topic suggested by the graphic signs. To paraphrase, they seem to say something like: 'Tell me something that is connected with the following topic'.

(12)  Eva was sitting in the living room together with her mother, communicating about a visit to an aunt.

M: *When we went to Aunt Kari, what did you bring?*
E: *BICYCLE.*
M: *You brought that bicycle when we went to Aunt Kari.*
E: *BICYCLE.* (TO) BICYCLE (lifts the arm up and down, which is a manual home sign for 'to bicycle').
M: *Yes, you did bicycle there.*
M: *Hm?*
E: *SANDBOX.*
M: *Were you also in the sandbox?*
E: 'Yes' (nods).
M: *Hm.*
E: *SWING.*
M: *And then you used the swing.*
E: 'Yes' (nods).
M: *Hm.*
E: *SWITCHBACK.*
M: *And the switchback was there. Eva was in a playground when we visited Aunt Kari.*
(Time elapsed, 0:35).

At the start of the dialogue, the mother had prompted Eva to indicate *BICYCLE* with the request: What did you bring? Thereafter, however, Eva took control of the dialogue, directing the mother to create a narrative where (TO) BICYCLE, *SANDBOX, SWING* and *SWITCHBACK* were parts. Although the frame of the conversation was provided by the mother, Eva introduced new topics to the conversation by using manual and graphic signs. However, unless (TO) BICYCLE is regarded as a comment to *BICYCLE,* she did not attempt to add comments. This was left to the mother. Eva made exophoric references to events that were known beforehand to both herself and the mother, and the dialogue became a retelling of what she did at that specific time. The mother went easily along with Eva's change of content during the dialogue. Indeed, the dialogue seems typical in that it demonstrates that such pragmatic use of graphic signs was common and accepted by both partners. The mother articulated Eva's utterances but did not ask her to comment or expand them, taking that role upon herself. Eva did not herself attempt to make a comment.

This particular pragmatic use of signs in dialogues may be coined *directive*, since the signs are used to direct the attention of the speaking partner towards a topic, on which the user wants the partner to comment on his or her own behalf. The use of single-sign utterances to direct the questions of the adult and make him or her talk about something, seems to be a natural developmental complement to the guessing strategy applied by adults, and a continuation of the pre-aid interactions.

### Single-sign utterances

As implied several times in the discussions of the dialogues above, the children used primarily single graphic signs, not signs strung together in a sentence structure. As a consequence, they rarely put words together with predicates and arguments, and their utterances had no syntactic structures. The interviews with parents and professionals confirmed that this was a general feature of the children's communication. Helmer's parents expressed it in this way:

> 'When he marked that there was something he wanted to do, he would bring the communication aid. He would then point at *OUT* or *COMPUTER*. Or he would indicate that he wanted to play with the train by pointing at *BASEMENT*. It was that kind of a train. He pointed at *FIRE* to indicate that he wanted us to light the fire.

George's teacher:

> 'He uses sentences when prompted, but when things are in a hurry, he uses single signs'.

The children's use of single-sign utterances as directives and for answering questions may be regarded as a compensatory strategy, utilising basic language skills typically found among speaking children at the single-word stage in their development. The lack of multi-sign structures, with the concomitant lack of communication of relational meanings, was underlined by a lack of independent vertical structures.

Even among children in the first half of the second year of life, the relational use of words interspersed with pauses is commonly found. These structures are called 'vertical' to underline that it is mainly the presence of pauses and lack of sentence-like intonational contours that distinguish them from ordinary sentences. They link words together in a way that conveys relational meaning (Scollon, 1976).

(13)  Brenda, a normally developing girl aged 1;7, was interacting with her father. She held up her mother's shoe and stared directly at it.
      B: *Mama*
         *Mama*
         *Mama*
         *Mam*
         *S*
         *Si*
         *S*
         *Sls*

> *Su*
> *Su?*
> *Sus*
> F:  *Shoes!*
> B:  *Si*
> *Si*
> *Su?*

Scollon argues that vertical structures precede and seem to be precursors to later adult-like use of sentences, that is, 'horizontal' structures. The relative lack of vertical structures in the dialogues between children who use graphic signs and their parents may partly be explained by the parents' communicative behaviour. It may be argued that parents, by dominating the communication and being more concerned about maintaining interaction than about fostering formal language skills, make it difficult for the children to string graphic signs together in sentence-like structures. Thus, the single-sign utterances may reflect the fact that the children presented here rarely participated in conversations where they were expected to make sentences. The adults' strategies required single-sign utterances only. The children, adapting to this, have acquired a general single-sign strategy.

Another contributing factor may have been a focus on activities in conversations with young aided speakers. Even utterances which were vertically related in the conversations were seldom true vertical structures, that is, utterances which expressed both topic and comment. If the children expressed related successive single-sign utterances, these tended to contain events, often represented by an object sign, rather than graphic signs with different linguistic functions; that is, sentences expressing relational meaning.

(14)  Henry and his father were communicating about Henry's school day.
> F:  *Is there something you want to tell here?*
> H:  *DRAW.*
> F:  *Draw, yes. It is a long time since you did that at home. You do it at school, I think. What else did you do in school? Do you see what...?* (stops).
> H:  *READ.*
> F:  *Read, yes. Did you do more? What?*
> (Time elapsed, 0:25).

In this dialogue and (12), the graphic signs that the children used were linked together, as events of the school day. Henry's father commented *DRAW* but only acknowledged *READ*. He did not ask Henry what he drew or read or in any other way made him comment upon the activities he had participated in at school. It is the adults who make sentences 'redundant' by filling in the rest, and it is not known to what extent the children learn to express themselves from this (cf. Clark, 1982; Smith, this volume). Although parents typically may expand utterances made by their young children (Snow and Ferguson, 1977), the above kind of vertical dialogue has not been described for speaking children. This suggests that the communication strategies developed by children who use aided language and their adult communication partners, may lead to a specific kind of sentence structure not usually found among speaking children and adults. Helmer's teacher said:

> 'It is not a long sentence he tells in the PIC book, it is stories he has told. Sequences of signs that comprise the same topic. For example, if he had been to hospital he might have pointed at *DADDY, CAR, EAR, HOSPITAL* and *PAIN*. It wouldn't be a sentence, but a narrative. He writes the same way'.

The fact that it often takes a long time before children begin to use sentence-like structures, even when they obtain a text-based communication system and communicative partners that allow such communication, as indicated by Helmer's teacher, suggests that the narrative connection between graphic signs used by young aided speakers may be qualitatively different from ordinary sentence-like structures.

## Discussion and implications for intervention

Several issues arise when the characteristics of the conversations between children who use graphic signs and their adult communication partners are considered. The issues are intertwined. The study shows how the children's impairments and mode of communication contribute to forming the parents' communicative strategies, as well as how the parents' adaptations to the children's impairments contribute to forming the children's strategies. The children's contributions reflect the strategies used by the adults, which again are influenced by the children's communicative behaviour, and so on, in a transactional chain. In some sense, both partners have to allow for the dialogical asymmetry. For practical purposes, however, one may still distinguish three factors: effects of the communication form, the adults' communicative behaviour as a limiting factor, and consequences of developmental problems among children using graphic signs.

Any spoken word may have its correspondence in graphic language. There is nothing in the language modality itself that precludes a particular sign or type of signs. This is evident from the fact that the role of script is to mirror speech (de Saussure, 1977), and that anything spoken may be expressed in alphabetic or non-alphabetic writing. It is further demonstrated in full in the sign language literature of the last 20 years (e.g. Friedman, 1977; Klima and Bellugi, 1979; Kyle and Woll, 1983; Siple and Fischer, 1991). Thus, in principle, there is no difference between learning to speak or sign manually, and learning to write or point at graphic signs for face-to-face interaction. In practice, the vocabulary will be limited for children who have not learned to write. The major effect of the system may be a combination of the time it takes to select a graphic sign and the impracticality of accessing large vocabularies, limiting the number of vocabulary items for children relying on pictograms. The time factor is also at least partly responsible for the adult's tendency to target the child's utterance as a single sign or non-verbal equivalents of 'yes' and 'no'. In the present dialogues, poor vocabulary organisation in books with up to 100 pages probably amplified this effect.

Moreover, with small vocabularies it may be difficult to construct meaningful utterances. With large vocabularies, the time it takes to get from one graphic sign to another may ruin the coherence that is basic to a feeling of 'sentence intonation' (cf. Collins, this volume). This calls for better access strategies and more use of high-technology aids also in the 'dependent' mode; that is, operated by adults under the direction of the children. The time it takes for the adults to get to a particular page and item may determine how much an aid is used. Anything that can reduce this time will increase the independence of the child.

Several, partly concatenated, factors may have acted together to make the adult take a dominating part in the communication. Firstly, the fact that only the adult mastered all aspects of the speech-based dialogue form made it difficult for the children to become equal partners. Secondly, the impracticality of aided language compared with speech encouraged the adult to circumvent the restrictions of the aided language system by reverting to a register of simplification strategies, usually ways of communicating that were used before the graphic sign system was introduced. The result of this was guessing, often including rhetorical questions, possibly in order to inform the child of the target of the sequence of *yes/no* questions that followed, and to reduce the cognitive effort needed. It is also easier to create an impression of true dialogue if the answers to be guessed are known beforehand. Rhetorical questions thus contributed to maintaining the dialogue, even if the answers were provided by the parent. Moreover, even answers that came from the children and were unknown to the adults, were articulated by the adults. Hence, the difference between rhetoric and true questions became blurred.

Parents of normally speaking children also sometimes apply similar strategies when their children are at the initial stages of language development. However, for these children, such 'scaffolding' functions to foster independent contributions, because the children have the means to transcend the actual situations (Bruner, 1975). For motor-impaired children, it may become a straightjacket, hiding their real communication problems and potentials, and hindering the provision of appropriate means and ways of communicating.

The dominance of adults may also be related to the fact that children in need of aided communication constitute a high-risk group for the development of passivity problems (cf. Basil, 1992; von Tetzchner and Martinsen, 1992). The adults' strategies may represent attempts to compensate for such problems, paradoxically thereby enhancing a passive communicative style in their children. The children's need for help from adult caregivers in most of their daily activities may foster a generalised dependency and lack of initiative, which also influences the way that they communicate with their parents and other adults. A generalised helper role may make the adults more dominant in the communication situation than they actually need to be.

The strategies used by parents and other adults may be linked with the kind of attentional focus and attitudes with which the adults enter into the communication situation. The adult-child conversations indicate that parents may be more concerned with establishing social interplay and mutually shared and comforting social situations, than with what the children might tell about events which are unknown to the adults (cf. Light, 1985). The parents' typical way of framing the conversations may be paraphrased as: 'Yes, we are here together now. I am informed about, and interested in, what you have done while we have been apart'. However, in spite of the fact that the parents seemed to succeed in establishing a comforting and safe haven for their children, they may at the same time unintentionally have signalled a lack of interest in what the children may have wanted to communicate to them.

Given the background that the children included here had fairly good comprehension of spoken language, one might have expected that the dialogues would reflect that parents were constantly mindful of this fact. The dialogues did not, however, demonstrate such an attitude. On the contrary, the dialogues somewhat resembled the ways that very ill, infirm, and elderly people are talked to. This apparent gap between the parents' stated beliefs about their children's language comprehension and the way that they talked to their children may also be indirectly caused by the parents' diverse roles in relation to the children. The parents talk to their children as if they understand everything that is said, but reply to them as if the children have little to say. The necessity of being a helper both in the children's daily activities and in the communication process might focus the parents' attention on their own helping behaviour, diverting attention from the children's efforts towards being agents in their own lives.

Nevertheless, it seems important to realise that the decisive factor governing parents' dialogue behaviour is probably a yearning for success in the situation in which social interaction takes place. This may have been more prominent in sessions being video recorded by a researcher than in other situations, but it is probably a general characteristic of all parent-child interactions. Awareness of the difficulties their children were facing daily may have made success even more important for this particular group of parents. For motor-impaired children, mastery of language is the key, not only to successful communicative interactions, but to most self-motivated activities. Many of the strategies the parents used seemed to provide immediate satisfaction in the sense that interaction was maintained. However, these strategies may have failed to sustain development of gradually more functional and complex linguistic and communicative skills. The major implication for intervention is a need to create an awareness of both the possibilities and limitations of graphic sign systems and aided communication, so that the use of strategies related to long-term developmental goals can be balanced against immediate needs for fast communication and successful interactions of limited scope. Helping parents and other significant people to achieve this awareness, and guiding them in the process, is also the major challenge for professionals who are responsible for aided language intervention.

**Acknowledgement**

The present project was funded by the Norwegian Research Council.

# Chapter 5
# Referring expressions in conversations between aided and natural speakers

SARAH COLLINS

This chapter is based on an ongoing study of referring expressions in the context of conversational interactions between aided speakers and natural speakers. Some uses of referring expressions in these interactions will be detailed, drawing on video recordings of communication tasks and conversations.

The first aim is to demonstrate how referring expressions are used in conversational interaction by aided speakers using some form of graphic communication system. This will be done by describing referring expressions in two kinds of communicative situations: communication tasks and conversations. In this respect, this chapter aims to contribute new insights to the study of referential communication, which (as far as I know) has only dealt either with communication tasks or with conversations. A second aim is to identify ways in which communication for aided speakers may be made more effective.

In interactions between aided speakers and natural speakers, establishing understanding of what the aided speaker is referring to is often problematic. Long and elaborate sequences of conversation often ensue, in which the referent has to be physically constructed, piece by piece, by both participants (see, for example, Collins and Marková, 1995; Higginbotham, Mathy-Laikko and Yoder, 1988; Kraat, 1985; Linell, 1991).

The present approach is based on the assumption that arriving at a mutual understanding of a referent is a collaborative process. Thus, the focus is on referring expressions as they occur in conversational interaction. They are considered as part of the turn-taking process: they elicit collaboration, and are collaboratively constructed themselves. That is to say, the concern is with how the referring expression, as it is produced by the aided speaker, may be recognised for what it is by the natural speaker, and then built on in ensuing talk. This is in accordance with the principles of conversation analysis (cf. Heritage, 1984).

The following extract, taken from the conversations in the present study, exemplifies how a referent may be collaboratively constructed by both participants. In this extract, Fiona and Arnold were talking about Arnold's brother's forthcoming wedding, and Fiona had asked Arnold what he would be wearing. (For notations, see Table 0.1).

(1)    Arnold had no useful speech, and used a communication book with 400 Blissymbols. Fiona held the book, and Arnold guided her to the Blissymbols he wanted by eye-pointing to coloured and numbered stickers on his wheelchair corresponding to the colours and numbers of the pages and grids in his communication book.

F:    *Are you wearing a kilt?*
A:    'No'(screwing up his eyes).
F:    *No.*
A:    Indicates sticker by looking at it, but stops as Fiona continues to speak.
F:    *Dinner suit* (Waits for 2 seconds). *Dinner suit* (quietly).
A:    Indicates sticker by looking at it.
F:    *You don't know you're not sure.*
F:    (Following Arnold's gaze to stickers) *Purple.*
A:    Indicates sticker by looking at it.
F:    *Yellow.*
A:    Indicates sticker by looking at it.
F:    *Five.*
A:    Smiling.
F:    (Turning pages of communication book) *Purple, yellow, five I must see this.*
A:    Stops smiling.
F:    *Trou.. Oh, yeah ... I should think you're wearing trousers yes. Is it going to be a fancy sort of dinner suit thing...?*
F:    *Oh, so it's trews.*
      (Time elapsed, 2:00).

In the context of Fiona's guess that Arnold might be wearing a dinner suit, Arnold provided the clue *TROUSERS*. He did not explicitly reject her guess of *dinner suit,* but used it to build on. He was going to be wearing a suit of some kind, but it was not a <u>dinner</u> suit. He began to communicate to Fiona what he would be wearing: Fiona's suggestion had not been exactly correct. As it eventually turned out, it was *trews* (tartan trousers), but *dinner suit* was on the right track and could be employed by Arnold as a clue, by following on from it with the clue *TROUSERS*. Fiona thus recognised that *TROUSERS* was a clue; that it was linked with her guess *dinner suit*; and that what Arnold was attempting to describe was *a fancy sort of dinner suit thing*. Through the subsequent talk it emerged that Arnold would be wearing trews. In this example, the collaborative nature of the talk is clearly illustrated by the fact that the guess provided by the natural speaker *(dinner suit)* was worked into a sequence of clues by the aided speaker.

Constructing referents often involves prolonged sequences such as the one above, with strings of referring expressions. Therefore, the referent construction may become the focus of the conversation: that is, it may become a topic in its own right. To put it another way, pursuing understanding of an aided speaker's referent may become the central activity in the conversation, within which the original topic becomes subsumed. Similar observations have also been made by Linell and Korolija (1995) in their study of aphasic discourse.

## Method

The aided speakers in this study had cerebral palsy. They comprised two sub-groups: those who relied mainly on low-technology communication aids with Blissymbols; and those who relied mainly on high-technology communication aids with Minspeak icons. The natural speakers in this study comprised carers, friends and family of the aided speakers.

Two different sets of observations were made: conversations and communication tasks. For the conversations, the aided speaker was asked to select a natural speaker of their choice. The two participants were then instructed to talk on any topics they wished, for as long as they wished. The video camera was switched on, and the participants were left to talk. Once they had finished, they were asked whether they felt the conversation had been natural; if they did not, the video recording was not used in the analysis.

The communication task consisted of a drawing activity adapted from language teaching (Ur, 1981). The aided speaker was given a picture of a kitchen (containing cupboards, a sink, a cooker, a table, a window, a cuckoo clock on the wall, and a dog standing on a stool making coffee). This picture was hidden from the natural speaker's view. The aided speaker had to describe this picture to the natural speaker in such a way that the natural speaker could reconstruct the picture in a drawing. The natural speaker could ask questions about the picture while drawing. This task was designed to allow the aided speaker access to information that the natural speaker did not already have, and could not readily assume. For successful completion of the task, the information available to the aided speaker had to be communicated to the natural speaker. The participants were in full view of one another. As for the conversations, the video camera was switched on, and the researcher left the room for the duration of the activity.

## Constructing a referent

In both sets of dialogues, referring expressions were used as clues to the thing that was being referred to and were presented in a sequence of turns. Dialogue (1) provides an example of this. In the following extract, taken from the communication tasks, Tom used his communication board to present a sequence of words *(SOFT, FURNITURE and CHAIR)* when referring to an object in the kitchen on the picture.

(2)    Tom had no useful speech. He used a communication board with 400 Blissymbols on a wheelchair tray, which he accessed directly by pointing with his finger. His partner was Doris.

       T:   *SOFT* (vocalises).
       D:   (Looking down at communication board) *Soft.*
       T:   *FURNITURE.*
       D:   *Furniture.*
       T:   Looking down at the communication board.
       D:   Looks up at Tom, then down at the communication board.
       T:   *CHAIR.*
       D:   *Chair.*
       T:   Looks up at Doris.
       D:   (Looks up at Tom and then down at drawing) *Where am I gonna ... on here ... on the ... on the cabinet.*
       D:   (Looking at her drawing) *I've done my window too big, haven't I?*
       D:   (Looking up at Tom) *Couch kind of thing.*
       T:   *YES.*
       D:   *So where should I put the couch?*
            (Time elapsed, 0:36).

Tom presented *SOFT, FURNITURE* and *CHAIR* in sequence. By juxtaposing these words, with no break between them (he did not look up, but on receipt of one Blissymbol by Doris, simply moved to the next), he conveyed that each word was a clue to some whole. After some deliberation over her drawing, Doris then presented the candidate interpretation *couch kind of thing*, leaving the reference fairly unspecific. Her presentation of this interpretation left Tom in a position either to agree with it, or to develop it further. She thus displayed her understanding that Tom had presented her with a string of clues to some whole, the exact nature of which he himself had not specified. Once he had acknowledged that her interpretation was correct, Doris used the definite referent *the couch,* and displayed that her understanding was complete by asking him where she should put it.

Dialogues (1) and (2) illustrate the use of referring expressions to construct referents. In these examples, noun phrases played a pivotal role. A sequence of noun phrases were presented as clues to the referent: as a way of delivering the referent in instalments. In this respect, their use was commensurate with the findings of others who have looked at referent construction using communication tasks (e.g. Clark and Wilkes-Gibbs, 1986; Wilkes-Gibbs and Clark, 1992).

Clark and Wilkes-Gibbs (1986) report that referring expressions (commonly in the form of noun phrases) play a central role in initiating the process of construction of mutual understanding of a referent. These authors observed that, commonly, a noun phrase was presented by one participant to another, and then worked on by both participants, until they came up with an understanding of the referent that was mutually accepted. The following example, taken from their data, serves to illustrate this. The task in their study was based on the description of a set of Chinese puzzles called tangram figures, each one a different shape. Two participants sat divided by a screen. One participant had the tangram figures set up in a particular order. The other participant had the same figures. The object of the exercise was for them to arrange the figures in the same order (Clark and Wilkes-Gibbs 1986, p. 22).

(3)    A: *Uh, person putting a shoe on.*
       B: *Putting a shoe on?*
       A: *Uh huh. Facing left. Looks like he's sitting down.*
       B: *Okay.*

In his receipt of A's description, B identified the part he was not sure about *(putting a shoe on)*, and A then expanded on her original description, giving more information about the figure. B then conveyed that he had understood A's description (and could thus identify the figure) by saying *Okay*.

This study focused on tasks in which the main purpose of the interaction was to arrive at a shared understanding of a referent (the tangram figure). Describing such figures necessitated the use of noun phrases, and did not require any elaboration on these noun phrases. The predominant use of noun phrases and referring expressions to initiate the process of referent construction may therefore have been a function of the particular task, as Clark (1992) himself has implied. Thus, it may not be possible to extrapolate from these findings to interaction in other settings. In a subsequent study (Clark and Schaefer, 1989), collaborative processes in conversational interaction were explored in the context of conversations, thus moving away from the consideration of noun phrases in referential communication, to looking at utterances as a whole.

In the dialogues from the communication tasks, referring expressions were used by aided speakers not only to describe the objects in the room, but also to describe their location in relation to one another. That is to say, where natural speakers would use prepositional phrases to describe locations of objects, aided speakers, in this communication task, used referring expressions in the form of noun phrases. The aided speakers attempted to convey information about the location of objects through the sequential placement of the noun phrase in the interaction. The following extract provides an example of this.

(4) Donald had no useful speech of his own. He used a LightTalker with synthetic speech which he accessed by means of a chin switch. He had the 'Language, Living and Learning' application package, which contains some 2500 words. He had been using this system for a number of years and was quite familiar with it. His partner was Mary.

   M: *Cupboard at the top ... cupboard at the bottom ... the cooker with the pot ... and the cup ... the window ...*
   D: Starts operating his chin switch.
   M: *... with a blind and that's it.*
   D: (Looks up at Mary, smiling) *'Sun'.*
   M: *Sun. What through the window?*
   D: 'Yes' (nods).
   M: (Starts drawing) *Draw the sun.*
      (Time elapsed 2:30).

At the beginning of this extract, Mary began to present Donald with a summary of her picture. When she said *window,* Donald started operating his chin switch. As she completed her summary, saying *and that's it,* Donald said *'Sun'* and looked up at Mary and smiled. Mary repeated *Sun,* and then presented her interpretation of what Donald was intending by saying *'Sun',* by asking *What through the window?* Donald then nodded, displaying acceptance of this interpretation, and Mary then proceeded to draw the sun coming through the window.

By starting to talk as Mary said *window* in the middle of her summary, Donald displayed that the drawing was not yet complete, and that there was something to add. More than this, by saying *'Sun'* immediately after Mary had said *window,* he conveyed that the sun and the window were related in terms of their location in the picture. And Mary understood this to mean that the sun was coming through the window, on the basis of which she proceeded to draw it.

In certain respects, there was a closer fit between the communication tasks and the conversations in the present study than, perhaps, one might assume there to be in these two types of interactions between natural speakers. While the task-based interactions were activity specific, involving the construction of a series of referring expressions relating to objects in the picture, it is clear that these interactions closely resembled what regularly happens in conversation for aided speakers in attempting to reach a mutual understanding of a referent. In both sets of observations, referents might need to be constructed through clues, or presented in instalments.

## Referring expressions and activity types

Dialogue (4) illustrates that referring expressions were not used merely to communicate an object in the picture (e.g. *'Sun'*). They also, in how they were presented by the aided speaker, were used to communicate something else about that object, for example, its location ('the sun is coming through the window'). In the conversations, similarly, referring expressions, as used by aided speakers, often were intended to convey to natural speakers more than a referent.

Therefore, in order to understand what the aided speaker is saying, the natural speaker has to do some inferring, on the basis of the referring expressions with which they are presented. In the conversations from the present study, referring expressions were used in various other contexts. The following example illustrates that determining the relationship between a series of referring expressions may be problematic. In this extract from the conversations, the issue arose of determining whether the noun that had been initially presented was a subject or an object. This caused problems for the participants in constructing the whole utterance, in terms of how the topic of the conversation was being developed. Conrad, the natural speaker, and Fay, the aided speaker, had been talking about Fay's recent holiday.

(5)    Fay had no useful speech. She used a communication board with 200 Blissymbols, which she accessed directly by pointing with her finger. The board also contained a few names of places and people.

    F: {*FATHER Mmm mmm*}.
    C: *Wanna tell your father.*
    F: *HOLIDAY.*
    C: Looks up at Fay, then down at communication board.
    F: (continues pointing) {*HOLIDAY Mm mm mm*}.
    C: *Oh you're going ...* (Looks down at communication board)
    F: Shakes head and vocalises.
    C: *... on holiday with your father.*
    F: Leans forward over communication board.
    C: *Right.* (Leans back a little and says something inaudible).
    F: *LIKE.*
    C: *You like.*
    F: {*FATHER Mmm mmm*}.
    C: *Your father.*
    F: Moving finger to point to another Blissymbol.
    C: *To go on holiday.*
    F: {'Yes' (looks up at Conrad, nods) *Mm*}.
    C: Right.
    C: (Sits back) *You'd like that to happen.*
    F: Mmm. 'Yes' (nods).
       (Time elapsed, 0:40).

Fay pointed to *FATHER*. Rather than just acknowledging this initial Blis-symbol and waiting for the next, Conrad attempted to guess the whole of what Fay was beginning to say. In this guess, Conrad treated Fay as the subject and her father as the object *(You want to tell your father)*, thus assuming that this was something about Fay in relation to her father, rather than simply something about her father. When this understanding was rejected (implicitly through continuing on to point to *HOLIDAY* and providing no confirmation of Conrad's guess), Conrad proffered a second guess, again of the whole of what Fay was trying to say. This time Conrad understood Fay to be continuing the prior talk by saying some-thing about what she would like to do for her next holiday. However, it ensued that Fay was trying to talk about something new: not connected to herself, or her holidays, but saying that she would like her father to go on holiday.

In (5) there was some difficulty for Fay in indicating, and for Conrad in discerning, whether Fay was developing the prior talk or whether what she was saying was not topically related to it. Fay presented nouns that had already been referred to (for they had been talking about holi-days), and so it was not clear whether these related back to the prior topic, or began a new one. The natural speaker had to work this out. Fay indicated *FATHER* at a possible topic closure (immediately prior to the extract given above, they completed some arrangements for her next holiday). However, Fay had no way of indicating that she was starting up a new topic. Therefore, in the first instance, the natural speaker assumed that Fay was continuing with what they had previously been talking about.

The difficulties of determining the relationship between referring expressions raise the question of what kind of activity types (Levinson, 1979) are being carried out through the talk. Activity types in the present study comprise constructing a referent in conversation, reconstructing the picture in the drawing activity, talking about holidays, or pursuing an answer to a question (see dialogue (6) below). The particular activity that was currently being pursued through the talk placed constraints on the contributions made by the participants. In dialogue (5), some confu-sion arose over the activity of the talk, because the aided speaker attempted to start up a new line of talk solely by the reference to her father. It was not clear to Conrad what activity Fay was intending to carry out: that is, whether she was still engaged in reviewing her holiday, in making arrangements for a future holiday, or, as turned out to be the case, was expressing a wish that her father should go on holiday. In these dialogues, understanding <u>what</u> was being referred to might depend on the ability to understand <u>why</u> it was being referred to in that particular sequence of interaction. This did not present such difficulties in the communication task, in which the range of activities that a noun phrase might be projected to do was relatively constrained by the nature of the task: it would either refer directly to a thing in the picture, or describe some feature of that thing. So the natural speaker only had to work out which of these activities the referring expression was intended to carry out. However, in the context of ongoing conversational interaction, there were many possible activities that a referring expression might be used to project. The following question–answer sequence, taken from the conversations, may serve to exemplify this further.

In this extract, the natural speaker, Mona, asked the aided speaker, George, what he had been doing at college that day. By saying his address and pointing at a pile of papers on the table, he tried to tell her that he had been writing letters. He thus began to present his answer by giving two referring expressions as 'clues' to what he had been doing. Mona did not initially recognise his references (to his address and to the papers on the table) as an answer to her question.

(6)    George had no useful speech of his own. He used a TouchTalker with synthetic speech output which he accessed directly by pressing the keys with his finger. He had the 'Language, Living and Learning' application package, containing approximately 2500 words, and was in the process of learning to use it. He also had some of his own messages programmed in the TouchTalker, such as his address.

M: (Looking down at the communication aid, then up at George) *Well ... what are you doing (here) today ... hmm.*

G: Starts pressing keys on TouchTalker, then points at, and looks over at, some papers lying on the table beside them.

M: Follows George's point and gaze, looks over at papers.

G: Withdraws point.

M: (Looks up at George) *What is it?* (Looks down at the communication aid) *What's going on today? ... Hmm?*

G: *'I live at 65 ...'* (Gazes at papers, points at papers) *'... Longbenton Avenue York'.*

M: *Yes, I know you do but wha... Mm, what are you telling me that for? Oh ...*(looks down at papers) *because of this address here* (points at papers, holds gaze on papers... tuts) *Hhh, at's you being nosey, isn't it?*

G: Looking round over his right shoulder, across the room.

M: *Are these strange surroundings?*
....

G: *'Dinner'.*

M: *Dinner. Hh ... are they writing letters about you going out for your dinner?*
(Time elapsed, 8:04).

Eventually it evolved that George was trying to tell Mona that they had been writing letters that morning. At the outset of the sequence, Mona found explanation of George's actions (i.e pointing to the pile of papers and saying his address) in George *being nosey,* and put his behaviour down to the *strange surroundings* in which their conversation was taking place. Through the simultaneous production of these two actions, and their reiteration in the ensuing talk, in response to Mona's reformulations of her initial question *What are you doing here today?,* and, finally, by saying *dinner* as well, George got his answer understood as such. The difficulties here lay in George using these two referring expressions as an answer to a question which demanded a verb *(What have you been doing)*, and Mona being able to infer, on the basis of his actions, that this was what he was trying to communicate. Mona realised that these two actions were connected when she surmised that he was telling her his address to draw attention to the papers on the table, but a lengthy sequence ensued before she realised that the two combined to give 'writing letters' in answer to her question.

## Conclusions

On the basis of the above discussion, the use of referring expressions in this study can be summarised as follows. Firstly, referring expressions may be used as clues in the construction of a referent. This is the case not only in the communication task, but also in the conversations.

Secondly, referring expressions may be used by aided speakers to do more than referent construction. In the communication task employed in the present study, it seemed that referring expressions played a more extensive role than has previously been acknowledged. They were not only used by the aided speaker to communicate objects in the picture (see dialogue (2) about a couch kind of thing); they were also used to describe the location of these objects (see dialogue (4) about the sun through the window). In the conversations, aided speakers made use of referring expressions to carry out various activities. They used them to elaborate on current references in order to perform activities other than referent construction, such as changing topic (see dialogue (5) about the holiday), or answering a question (see dialogue (6) about writing letters).

The aided speaker's use of referring expressions to carry out activities other than referent construction presents certain difficulties for both participants in the interaction. From the point of view of the natural speaker, the difficulties relate not only to understanding each referring expression in a sequence, but also to working out the relationship between them. Clark and Brennan (1991, p. 137) state that 'until the referent has been properly identified, the rest of the utterance will be difficult, if not impossible, to understand'. However, it appears from the present study that it is not only the difficulty of understanding what is being referred to that has to be overcome, but why it is being referred to at a particular time and place within the talk. It seems, then, that for the natural speaker it is not, as stated by Clark and Brennan, simply a question of first identifying the referent, and then proceeding to understand the rest of the utterance. It is more a question of establishing understanding of the particular activity that the referring expression is designed to project. For example, in dialogue (6) about writing letters, the natural speaker presumed the aided speaker was being nosey when he referred to his address and the pile of paper on the table. Once the natural speaker had understood these referring expressions to be interactionally significant, she then had to work out how they were being employed by the aided speaker. That is to say, she had to work out whether they were intended to connect to the prior activity in the conversation, or were intended to start up a new activity. The natural speaker did not initially recognise that the aided speaker's actions constituted an answer to her question, and (mistakenly) assumed that the aided speaker was starting on a new line of talk.

The difficulties for the aided speaker may be stated as follows. The aided speaker not only has to construct the referring expression, but also may be using the referring expression as a vehicle to convey other talk. For example, where natural speakers might use initiatory talk such as *well, by the way* and *what about* to start a new topic and project the activity the talk is performing, referring expressions may provide an alternative resource for aided speakers.

In how aided speakers position their contributions in relation to those of the natural speakers, they have a way of demonstrating the activity their talk is carrying out. They may display relationships between referring expressions through their sequential placement of words or contributions, in which they build on or make use of the natural speakers' talk. In dialogue (4) about the sun through the window, the aided speaker conveyed that the sun was coming <u>through</u> the window by saying '*Sun*' immediately after the natural speaker has said window. In dialogue (5), the aided speaker seemed to be trying to convey that she was introducing a new topic by placing the previously unmentioned word *FATHER* first in her utterance. In dialogue (6) about writing letters, the aided speaker attempted to convey that his utterance of his address, followed by his gesture to the papers, constituted an answer to the natural speaker's question by producing them immediately after her question.

There are certain ways in which these difficulties may be resolved. Many graphic communication systems do not appear to give aided speakers the opportunities to convey pragmatic aspects of interaction. However, it seems that they could be adapted to include words or symbols that indicate the activity that is currently being pursued by the aided speaker, such as 'new topic', 'question', or 'answer'. Such 'activity indicators' might be employed by the aided speakers as a preface to their contribution. As aided speakers may not be aware of how to employ pragmatic markers, specific training may need to be provided in this area.

It may not always be realistic or useful to expect aided speakers to be able to manage interaction in the same way as natural speakers. Natural speakers may also need to adapt their communication. At present, at least, natural speakers need to be able to infer to a large extent, and so it may be helpful if they are made aware of the various ways in which aided speakers may draw on referring expressions in the absence of other ways of communicating. It may then be necessary for the natural speaker to consciously employ understanding checks that are designed to clarify the activity the aided speaker is trying to carry out. For example, they might ask whether the aided speaker is starting a new topic; or, whether the aided speaker is formulating an answer to a preceding question.

## Acknowledgement

The study reported here forms part of the research project *The joint construction of referent in conversations involving non-speakers,* funded by the Economic and Social Research Council of Great Britain.

# Chapter 6
# The two-word stage in manual signs: Language development in signers with intellectual impairments

NICOLA GROVE, JULIE DOCKRELL AND BENCIE WOLL

It is more than twenty years since manual signs were first used with people with intellectual impairments who had failed to develop intelligible speech (cf. Kiernan, Reid and Jones, 1982). However, although a wealth of experimental research has been undertaken to explore the factors affecting the learning of manual signs, and the relationship between sign and speech development, there are relatively few detailed descriptions of the communication of children who rely on this modality to express themselves. This makes it difficult for teachers and speech and language therapists to assess development, and plan appropriate intervention. Experimental studies carried out into the use of manual signs by people with intellectual impairments need to be complemented by studies of how they use their language in meaningful and creative interactions.

The research described in this chapter focused on a group of relatively advanced users – children who communicate primarily through manual signs, and who spontaneously combine signs to convey different meanings. Multi-sign utterances are interesting, because the ability to produce creative combinations is regarded as something of a watershed in language development (Atkinson, 1992; Bloom and Capatides, 1991; Brown, 1973; Caselli and Volterra, 1990). Once two words are produced within a single unit, it is possible to analyse the relationships between the words, that is, the emerging grammar. Children generally begin to combine words when they have a productive vocabulary of about 50 words, towards the end of their second year. From then on, progress is very rapid in the areas of syntax and morphology; by the age of three, children are using well-formed grammatical sentences (Ingram, 1989).

# Typical patterns of language development in the two-word stage

Language development is commonly related to stages of mean length of utterance (MLU), following Brown (1973). As utterances increase in length from 1 to 4 constituents, so does grammatical complexity. At Stage I (MLU 1.0 – 2.0), children's word combinations appear to be pre-syntactic (Bates, Bretherton and Snyder, 1988; Brown, 1973; Radford, 1992), reflecting consistent patterns of semantic relations, such as Agent + Action, and Locative + Entity (Bloom, Lightbown and Hood, 1975; Lahey, 1988). These have been found across different spoken languages (Bates and McWhinney, 1982), and are also robust with regard to modality differences, since they are produced by children acquiring manual signs as a first language (Meier and Newport, 1990).

It is comparatively rare for children's output to show errors in word order (Brown, 1973; Ramer, 1976). Those that do occur typically involve pre-position of Objects in relation to Verbs (Patient before Action), as in *Balloon throw* (Bloom, 1970) and *Paper find* (Brown, 1973). Subjects (Agents or Actors), however, tend to be placed before verbs (e.g. Byrne and Davidson, 1985). This contrastive distribution led Bates and associates (1988) to propose that children have an established notion of 'agency' at the point where they begin to combine words in utterances. Again, the pattern appears to go across modalities, as it has been replicated in a recent study of young children acquiring manual signing as a first language (Coerts and Mills, 1994).

Consistency in ordering patterns does not necessarily imply that children have grasped the syntactic function of word order. A series of studies which have investigated children's receptive performance have concluded that at first, children use semantic and pragmatic cues to determine meaning. Sensitivity to the linguistic significance of word order develops gradually between the ages of about three and four. At the point where they are beginning to combine words, children do not seem to use word order to distinguish between sentences such as *The boy kisses the girl* and *The girl kisses the boy* (Bates and McWhinney, 1982; Bridges, 1984; de Villiers and de Villiers, 1973; Wetstone and Friedlander, 1973).

A second feature of multi-word utterances which is relevant to the study of multi-sign utterances, is that they are produced in sequences, linked through repetition to preceding utterances – either their own, or those of another person (Anisfield, 1984; Bloom, 1973; Martinsen and von Tetzchner, 1989). A common pattern involves the repetition of the first word as the final element in a three-word utterance – as in the ABA constructions reported by Fenn and Rowe (1975). Veneziano, Sinclair and Berthoud (1990) view this as the first signs of formal patterning in expressive language – and once again, the same phenomenon is observed in deaf signing children (Kyle, Woll and Ackerman, 1989; Woll and Kyle, 1989). The pattern seems likely to be a feature of typical language development, rather than purely an imitation of a teaching strategy.

The first evidence of a developing morphological system appears once children are consistently using two words at a time. They begin to make productive use of inflections and 'closed class' lexical items such as determiners, questions, prepositions and pronouns (Fowler, Gelman and Gleitman, 1994). When speaking children with moderate and severe intellectual impairments are compared to typically developing children, research suggests that they follow a similar pattern, although they may not progress beyond the level of simple clause and phrase structure (Fowler et al., 1994; Rosenberg and Abbeduto, 1993). Although a substantial proportion of people with intellectual impairments never achieve more than a lexicon of single words, many do develop grammatical structures (Fowler et al., 1994; Rutter and Buckley, 1994). In theory, children who have difficulties producing speech might have the linguistic potential to develop a grammar in manual sign. The question is what form it would take.

## Options for grammatical development in manual signs

Logically, there are two possibilities. Provided that they hear and understand spoken language, children could use the structure of the spoken input as a basis for organising their output, through a process of translation. The alternative option is to organise the output in ways that are independent of spoken language.

### Translating from spoken words

At a lexical level, signs may be regarded as corresponding to words. At its simplest, the non-speaking child who recognises a furry animal with whiskers and a tail which says miaow, may be able to produce the manual sign CAT and use it in the same contexts as the spoken word *cat*. However, at a grammatical level, the picture is more complicated. The child must induce the grammatical rules of the spoken input, and apply them to its output in manual signs. In the discussion which follows, the examples will refer to spoken English.

To express syntactic contrasts the child can use word order. It can translate the words it hears into manual signs, and thus produce sentences such as CUP ON BOOK; BOOK ON CUP; BOY KISS GIRL; and GIRL KISS BOY. This is the principle underlying the 'keyword signing' approach which is prevalent in the input (Kiernan et al., 1982). The assumption is that the child will operate in the same way as the teacher. This option is not available for the inflectional morphology of English – it is difficult to imagine a child spontaneously developing inflected endings for manual signs which correspond to possessives, past participles and copulas. In Signed English systems, of course, educators have attempted to do just this. However, such systems are rarely taught to children with moderate or severe intellectual impairments. The main evidence that a child is developing an expressive language system which is based on the structure of the spoken input is therefore most likely to be found in patterns of word order.

## Creativity within the modality

The alternative to the translation option is that children who have to rely on manual signs could exploit the potential of the modality to produce systematic contrasts in meaning. Recent studies by McNeill, Singleton and Goldin-Meadow demonstrate that the gestures produced by hearing people undergo structural changes when they are produced in the absence of speech (McNeill, 1992; Singleton, Goldin-Meadow and McNeill, 1995). Specifically, gestures which accompany spoken narratives are produced singly (average of one per clause) and are global and synthetic. By contrast, when the narrative has to be conveyed without speech, gestures are produced in temporally integrated sequences, and show systematic patterning. There is evidence of segmentation (e.g. a 'crown' gesture is used in combination with other gestures to signify king or queen), and the incorporation of transitive objects into action gestures, with the hand shape denoting the object, and the movement denoting the action. These researchers have concluded that language properties can emerge in gesture once the modality becomes the principal vehicle for the intentional communication of meaning. The process may be regarded as an example of *representational reconstruction* (Karmiloff-Smith, 1979). The system becomes self-contained and self-referential, and the units which compose it are treated as functioning in their own right.

Other examples are provided by research with deaf children who grow up in predominantly oral environments, with limited exposure to sign language. Analysis of their signs and gestures shows a capacity to transcend the input, and introduce creative modifications to the form of signs which are consistent with meaning (Knoors, 1991; Loncke, Quertinmont, Ferreyra and Counet, 1986; Volterra, Beronesi and Massoni, 1990). In the most detailed of these studies, Goldin-Meadow and her colleagues have provided evidence which suggests that gestures are systematically organised over time by such children in ways that are typical of early child language. Specifically, they expressed the same semantic relations, showed developing predicate structure, and expressed consistent orders. Typically, in their two-gesture sequences, Patients preceded Actions and Recipients (e.g. CHEESE EAT and HAT HEAD), and Actions preceded Recipients (e.g. MOVE-TO TABLE) (Goldin-Meadow and Mylander, 1990). Note that the precedence of Patients in the sentence differs from the order of spoken English – it is necessary to look for internal consistencies within the child's system, as well as looking for matches between input and output in language.

The researchers looked for evidence of morphological structure as well as syntax in the children's manual signs. Only one boy's production has been analysed in depth. His gestures involved a restricted set of hand shapes and movements, and showed consistent form-meaning correspondence. The morphology was idiosyncratic, and not the same as that of a sign language, although subsequent investigations have shown several areas of overlap (Morford, Singleton and Goldin-Meadow, 1994). However, its development over time is strongly suggestive of a conventional linguistic path, moving from unanalysed wholes to a system of component morphemes. For example, at first the C (curved) hand shape combined with circular movement was only used to refer to opening a jar. Later, the C hand shape was used to refer to a class of objects, and the circular movement to a class of rotating actions.

There are, of course, crucial differences between Goldin-Meadow's subjects and hearing signers with intellectual impairments. Nevertheless, it is possible that a child's linguistic potential could find expression in the alternative manual modality, when access to speech is blocked. The child who is treating this modality independently from speech might show evidence of general organising principles (such as segmentation and combination) as well as modality-specific features (such changes to the movement of a manual sign to indicate manner or direction of an action, or the systematic use of spatial locations).

This option has not been explored to date by researchers in the field of augmentative and alternative communication. The assumption has been that the receptive modality will form the basis of the expressive system (Light, Remington, Clarke and Watson, 1989; Lloyd, Quist and Windsor, 1990; Romski and Ruder, 1984).

## Studies of manual sign production by people with intellectual impairments

Research suggests that relatively few hearing people with intellectual impairments spontaneously produce multi-sign utterances. Kiernan and associates (1982) carried out a survey of schools for children with severe learning difficulties in England and Wales. In a sample of over 400 pupils, 72 per cent used only one sign per message. Bryen, Goldman and Quinlisk-Gill (1988) carried out a survey of the communication abilities of 118 adults with severe and profound learning disabilities. An average of only one in five sign combinations per person is quoted in this study. The findings from case studies of small groups and individuals are consistent with the survey data, with multi-sign combinations reported for only 19 out of a total of 104 subjects, taken across five studies (Daniloff and Shafer, 1981; Hodges and Schwethelm, 1984; Hoffmeister and Farmer, 1972; Kahn, 1981; Kopchick, Rombach and Smilovitz, 1975). Children who reach this stage of development therefore seem to be exceptional, so it is of interest to consider the structure of the utterances they produce.

Three descriptive studies provide data on a total of 70 children with moderate and severe learning disabilities who had learned some system of manual signs. Fenn and Rowe (1975) studied seven children with cerebral palsy and multiple impairments. Udwin and Yule (1990) studied 14 children aged 3;6–9;8, also with cerebral palsy, and Grove and McDougall (1991) observed 49 children aged 4;7–12;11. Some general conclusions can be drawn from these studies.

Firstly, use of multi-sign combinations is relatively rare. In Udwin and Yule's study, MLU was 1.06, and on average, only 12 per cent of utterances were 'multi-term'. In Grove and McDougall's study, MLU was 1.17, and the majority of children used only single signs.

Secondly, children do not seem to progress beyond the earliest stages of sentence construction. In Udwin and Yule's study, most sign combinations were two-term, with a few three-term utterances. The children were said to use no clause expansion, and the range of structures employed was limited, with very few examples of questions, commands, negatives, adjectives and auxiliary verbs. Grove and McDougall found that many sign combinations consisted of a lexical sign and an index finger point, to express meanings such as 'that's a cupboard' or 'there's a cupboard'.

Thirdly, it is questionable whether children develop rules to generate word order in sign. Fenn and Rowe found no syntactic regularities in the children's combination of signs.

> 'Word order appeared to be chaotic and there was an excessive amount of repetition. ... On the other hand, there was no doubt whatever that the children were producing signs in meaningful sequences and that genuine communication between child and interviewer was taking place' (1975, p. 9).

Although word order was flexible, it was not bizarre. Adjectives preceded or followed nouns, but noun phrases remained units, and were not split by verbs. One pattern which did seem to be common and consistent was an ABA sequence such as TELEVISION BROKEN TELEVISION. Fenn and Rowe conclude that this was an artefact of a teaching style which repeated, and then expanded upon a child's contribution –

thus the child might sign CAR to which the adult would reply CAR. WASH CAR.

These studies suggest that there may be a plateau in development for manual signers who have intellectual impairments. They are complemented by experimental studies specifically concerned with the teaching of generative sign combinations in the context of 'matrix training' (Karlan et al., 1982; Light et al., 1989; Romski and Ruder, 1984). This approach uses X and Y axes to represent each element of a two-term combination (e.g. colour + object, action + object, object + location). The child is taught certain sets of combinations directly, whereas other sets represent generalisations of the ordering rule. For example, the child might be taught RED + CAR, RED + BOAT, BLUE + BOAT, and BLUE + HAT, and then be asked to generalise to RED + HAT and BLUE + CAR.

In general, the conclusions from these studies suggest that although children may learn to sequence two signs by this method, they have not learned the rules which determine word order. For example, in the most detailed of these reports, Remington and his colleagues describe how they sought to teach contrasts in locative ordering. To succeed on the receptive and expressive post-tests, the children had to realise that the first mentioned item was the object, and the second was the location. None of the subjects were successful in this task. The authors conclude that the linguistic status of achievements in manual signing for the population of children with severe learning difficulties is highly questionable, given the significance of word order in the development of syntax in English. The authors imply that the lack of sensitivity to word order is both atypical and specific to the modality of sign.

Viewed from a developmental perspective, however, certain caveats are in order. It is unclear from these studies whether the problem was confined to the experimental task, or was a general feature of their language development. If analysis of their spontaneous communication were to show that they consistently used the word order of the input, and could produce contrasts in meaning through word order, it might be concluded that the problem was an artefact of the teaching method.

Another question is whether the problems experienced by the children in expressing consistent word order were modality specific. Four of the children in these studies are said to combine spoken words as well as manual signs (Watson, 1986), but it is not clear if they spoke as well as signed in the experimental task – and, if so, whether they exhibited the same problems in speech as they did in sign.

A final question relates to the children's level of cognitive and linguistic development. Since five of the six children in the study had mental ages and receptive language levels of four years and below, it is possible that they had not reached a stage of development where they could be expected to learn rules in a relatively artificial context.

It is clear from these studies that although word order may be problematic for signers with intellectual impairments, it is necessary to know more about their patterns of language in order to determine whether the underlying difficulty represents a delay, or a fundamental difference in the children's development.

## Clinical observations

The questions which motivated the research described in this chapter were prompted by the first author's experiences in a special school for children with moderate and severe intellectual impairments. A number of pupils used manual signs as their main means of communication. Observations of their signing revealed features which did not appear to have been modelled on the teachers' sign production. Specifically, sign order sometimes deviated from that of the spoken language input and individual signs were occasionally elaborated in ways that seemed to convey additional meanings.

*Sign order.* Students sometimes placed objects before verbs (as in CAKE EAT), or started with a location (as in TABLE, CUP ON). One very striking pattern was the ABA sequence, reminiscent of Fenn and Rowe's findings.

| | |
|---|---|
| DUCK EAT DUCK | 'The duck is eating' |
| BUS RED BUS | 'The bus is red' |
| CHAIR MUMMY CHAIR | 'Mummy is on the chair.' |

The children seemed to be generating this pattern spontaneously, rather than copying their teachers, as Fenn and Rowe had thought.

*Sign modifications.* Manual signs, like spoken words, are composed of bundles of discrete features. Each sign can be analysed as a unique combination of hand shape, movement, location, and orientation of the palm and fingers (Stokoe, Casterline and Croneberg, 1965). The children used signs from British Sign Language, within the context of the Makaton Vocabulary programme (Grove and Walker, 1990; Walker, 1977). They had been taught the basic 'dictionary' form of the signs. However, it was noticeable that they sometimes introduced changes to the way the signs were made, as the following examples illustrate:

Robbie was presented with a picture of three men standing at a bus stop. He produced the manual sign MAN three times in succession. He seemed to be using repetition to pluralise the meaning.

Brendan was describing how he had told his mother to stop talking to her friends and come home. He used the manual sign SHUT-UP, displaced from himself towards her, out of the normal signing space (a change in location). This seemed to carry the meaning 'I told you to shut up'.

Michael was in the swimming pool, and wanted people to notice a new achievement. He used the manual sign LOOK, which in the Makaton Vocabulary is an index finger moving outwards from the eye. Michael used two hands, and reversed the movement towards himself, effectively conveying 'All of you look at me!' by 'doubling' the sign and changing its orientation.

In each of these cases, the children were changing the sign to add meaning, rather than using additional lexical signs, such as THREE-MEN and YOU-LOOK-(at)-ME. Teachers did not show the same features in their signing. Such observations suggested that signers with intellectual impairments could show potential for modality-specific development of morphology.

The aim of the present study was to explore the evidence for linguistic structure in the multi-sign utterances produced by a group of ten intellectually impaired children who were dependent on manual signs for communication.

## Method

### Subjects

The children attended day schools for pupils with severe learning difficulties (moderate to severe intellectual impairments). They were identified on the basis of a survey of 126 schools in the South East of England (Grove, 1993). The survey data were used to rank children on the basis of reported length of sign utterance, and a potential group of subjects was identified and visited in school. Children were selected who spontaneously used signs in conversation with their teachers, and whose speech was rated as difficult to understand, even by familiar adults. Table 6.1 provides summary statistics on the chronological age, mental age and sign vocabularies of the subjects. Mental age scores were obtained on the *Snijders-Oomen Test of Non-Verbal Intelligence*, using the norms for hearing children (Snijders and Snijders-Oomen, 1976). Vocabulary estimates were completed on the basis of checklists filled in by the teacher.

Table 6.1: Subject descriptions

|  | Mean | Standard deviation | Range |
| --- | --- | --- | --- |
| Chronological age | 13;8 | 1;9 | 10;5–16;10 |
| Mental age | 4;0 | 0;6 | 2;9–5;3 |
|  |  |  |  |
| Manual signs known |  |  |  |
| Receptive | 221 | 54.1 | 114–313 |
| Expressive | 16 | 68.6 | 35–243 |

Four of these children had no functional speech, and six children had spoken vocabularies of between 10 and 50 words. Intelligibility of speech was very poor, measured both by teacher ratings and on the *Edinburgh Articulation Test* (Anthony, Bogle, Ingram and McIsaac, 1971). Diagnoses were only available for seven children. The group included two children with Down syndrome, one with cerebral palsy, one with brain damage following a febrile convulsion, and two with chromosomal abnormalities (one suspected Fragile X, one unspecified). All the children could hear and respond appropriately to spoken language in conversation. On an adapted version of the *British Ability Scales Verbal Comprehension Test* (Harris and Beech, 1995) they achieved raw scores of 13–23, corresponding approximately to the level of a typically developing child of 3 years of age.

## Procedures

Samples of spontaneous language (signed and spoken) were collected and transcribed in three contexts: picture description, story recall and conversation with the class teacher. The pictures and the story, which was shown to the children on videotape, were designed to elicit particular contrasts in sign production, such as directionality, hand shape incorporation, and contrastive movements. Samples were of 20–30 minutes duration. Inter- and intra-reliability measures were collected on 20 per cent of the data. Agreement ranged from 81 to 100 per cent across all categories used in the analysis.

# Results

The results describe some general characteristics of the children's signed output and the teachers' input, then focus on issues of word order and morphology.

## Children's sign production

The data consisted of all intelligible communication produced by the children in the three contexts, excluding those which were purely imitations of a preceding adult turn. For each child, the number of utterances, MLU and upper bound of utterance length were calculated. The mean number of utterances produced was 64.3 (sd. 16.38, range 27–86). Utterance length was calculated as the number of signs and points (to people, objects and locations) produced per communication turn. The Mean Length of Sign Turn (MLST) across the group was 1.84 (sd. 0.45, range 1.31–2.58). Six children had an MLST below 2.0, and upper bounds between 3 and 6. Four children had MLST's above 2.0, and upper bounds between 7 and 9. The two groups appeared comparable to Brown's Stages I (MLU 1.0–2.0) and II (MLU 2.0–2.5), in terms of the number of signs they produced in sequence (Brown, 1973). Table 6.2 shows the number of single and multi-sign utterances produced by the children in the two groups.

Table 6.2: Number of utterances of various length produced by individual children

| Name | 1 | 2 | 3 | 4 | 5 | 6 | 7 | 8 | 9 | Total |
|------|---|---|---|---|---|---|---|---|---|-------|
| Bina | 33 | 17 | 10 | 2 | 0 | 0 | 0 | 0 | 0 | 62 |
| Louise | 52 | 19 | 0 | 2 | 0 | 0 | 0 | 0 | 0 | 73 |
| Jon | 35 | 12 | 7 | 5 | 2 | 1 | 0 | 0 | 0 | 62 |
| Mark | 30 | 23 | 6 | 1 | 0 | 0 | 0 | 0 | 0 | 60 |
| Ana | 35 | 12 | 6 | 2 | 1 | 1 | 0 | 0 | 0 | 57 |
| Matthew | 19 | 7 | 1 | 0 | 0 | 0 | 0 | 0 | 0 | 27 |
| Adam | 40 | 23 | 6 | 5 | 3 | 0 | 1 | 0 | 1 | 79 |
| Amita | 30 | 21 | 17 | 1 | 5 | 2 | 1 | 0 | 0 | 77 |
| Pardeep | 33 | 8 | 6 | 7 | 2 | 2 | 0 | 1 | 0 | 60 |
| Jayesh | 27 | 31 | 17 | 5 | 4 | 1 | 0 | 0 | 1 | 86 |
| Total | 334 | 173 | 76 | 30 | 17 | 7 | 2 | 1 | 3 | 643 |

## Teacher input

Manual sign input to the children consisted of the full model of the spoken language, paired with lexical signs (key-word signing). Two measures of teacher signing were collected in the conversation context, which lasted five minutes: total number of signs used, and the mean number of signs per clause (i.e. a sentence with a main verb). The mean number of signs used was 57.1 (sd. 51.44, range 15–160). On average, the teachers used signs in 58 per cent of the main clauses they produced. The mean number of signs per clause was 1.45 (sd. 0.48, range 1.00–2.52). Only two teachers regularly produced multi-signed clauses with a manual sign density of over 2.0.

Where teachers did produce signs in sequence, the order of signs followed the order of speech. Thus although children were provided with a very limited model of language in sign, they were not presented with ordering patterns which differed from those of speech.

## Word order patterns

The children's multi-sign utterances were categorised into three patterns: conforming to English word order; deviating from English word order and ambiguous, where word order could not be determined (as in lists of items). On average, 22 per cent of sign utterances conformed to English (e.g. EAT CAKE); 11 per cent violated the rules of English (e.g. CAKE EAT), and word order could not be determined for 67 per cent of utterances. The range of word order violations was between 7 and 23 per cent for seven of the children, which is high compared to the figure of three per cent quoted in the child language literature (e.g. Ingram, 1989; Ramer, 1976).

It is not clear whether the underlying problem is one of delay, or difference. If the children's language is delayed, features of early Stage I word order patterns might be expected, such as the contrastive distribution of Subjects/Agents and Objects/Patients referred to above. At the two-word stage, children tend to express the subjects of intransitive and state verbs (such as *baby sleep; mummy ill)* but drop subjects in favour of objects when the verb is transitive (*wash dolly; eat cake)* (Lahey, 1988). Word order errors, although uncommon, typically involve the placement of objects before the verb, rather than subjects after the verb. On the other hand, if development is atypical, there might be random distribution of subjects and objects in relation to verbs.

The patterns of word order observed in the children in the study suggested that the children were following a typical path. They were more likely to include the subject of an intransitive or state verb than the subject of a transitive verb. Eight children produced a total of 26 intransitive or state verbs (ranging from one to ten tokens per child), all with a Subject. Nine children expressed a total of 48 transitive verbs (ranging from three to nine tokens per child). The Subject was expressed in only 34 per cent, whereas the Object was expressed in 88 per cent of these manual sign utterances. This suggests that there is a systematic deletion of Subjects by the children in the context of transitive verbs, similar to that observed in typically developing children.

Analysis of the distribution of verb position showed that Subjects were more likely to precede the verb, whereas Objects both preceded and followed verbs. Only one child produced utterances (2) where the Subject followed the verb. Nine children produced a total of 37 combinations of Objects and verbs. Of these, 16 were Verb-Object and 21 were Object-Verb. Eight of the nine children produced both patterns. Again, this suggests some sensitivity to the category of Subject or Agency – and that a common error involves pre-positioning of Objects in relation to verbs.

Another aspect of the analysis was concerned with patterns involving the repetition of items in an ABA sequence, such as BOOK ME BOOK ('put my name in the book') or SHOP MORE SHOP ('I will get some more glasses at the shop'). If the children in this study are following a typical path, one would expect that ABA repetitions would be found in sequences across dialogues. However, if Fenn and Rowe (1975) are correct that ABA patterns are produced in imitation of a teaching strategy, one might expect that teacher use would exceed child use.

A total of 41 ABA combinations were produced by nine children, The majority (28) were produced across sequences of dialogue. By contrast, teacher use of this construction was very infrequent, amounting to one or two per teacher. One teacher was exceptional in producing 6 instances – however, this was in response to the child, functioning to clarify his utterances (e.g. {GLASSES BROKE GLASSES *Who broke your glasses?*}). The children's productions of ABA utterances therefore look very similar to those of typically developing children at Stage I, and do not appear to be modelled on teacher input.

A final point about the children's multi-sign utterances is that the patterns of semantic relations they expressed were typical of MLU Stage I, primarily involving Actions, States, Locations and Attributes (Bloom et al., 1975; Lahey, 1988). These results are consistent with the hypothesis that the children's multi-sign combinations are pre-syntactic, but very typical of early language development.

### The relationship between speech and manual signs

A further question which might be asked is whether the children's speech was any more advanced than their signing. The six speaking children all used some multi-word utterances, sometimes in parallel with signing, and sometimes in isolation. The semantic content of utterances that were simultaneously signed and spoken was the same. The mean number of word combinations was 24, ranging from 5 to 32. All six produced multi-word utterances which both conformed to English word order (average 33%), and violated English word order (average 13%), with a high frequency of the ambiguous category (average 54%). There were no significant differences between modalities in the proportionate frequency of each category. As with manual signs, the most frequent errors (71%) involved the pre-position of objects in relation to the verb. ABA repetition patterns were also observed in speech. When production in the two modalities is compared, development looks very similar. If the children were experiencing problems in developing word order rules, these did not appear to be specific to the sign modality.

### Developmental word order patterns

The findings suggest that children who are reliant on manual signs are following a typical path, but reaching a plateau at a very early stage – about equivalent to Brown's Stage I. It is not clear why this should be so. If the children can understand spoken language, they should in principle be able to induce the rules of word order, and reflect these in their signed (and spoken) output. Two possible explanations are suggested by the data.

Firstly, there may be an underlying syntactic problem which is not modality-specific. Since word order errors are not unknown in typically developing children, maybe there is a transient stage of language acquisition which is experimental before the rules governing word order are established. This is hardly perceptible in typical development, but may be extended and prolonged in children with learning disabilities, as has been found in other areas such as morphology (Hodapp and Burack, 1990; Kamhi and Masterson, 1989). One problem with this explanation is that word order errors do not feature in the literature on reports of spoken language development by children with intellectual impairments who have not been exposed to bimodal input (e.g. Harris, 1983; Rosenberg and Abbeduto, 1993).

A second possibility is that the problem lies with the input. The children are seeing fewer signs per clause than they would need to perceive word order contrasts in sentences like:

> *Mary kissed John,* and *John kissed Mary.*
> *The paper is on the book,* and *The book is on the paper.*

The teacher signing showed that most of the children were presented with very incomplete models of language in manual sign. The 'density value' of sign-word pairing in clauses may simply not be great enough to allow the children to induce word order rules that they can apply to their own sign production. This explanation needs to account for word order errors in the children's speech, since the spoken input <u>does</u> provide the full model of the sentence. There are two possibilities. The children might have problems with uptake of the spoken input, and hence rely on signs for comprehension as well as expression. Alternatively, they may understand the spoken input, but be unable to transfer their knowledge from the receptive to the expressive modality (cf. Remington and Clarke, 1993).

## Morphology

The term morphology is traditionally applied to the structural analysis of words (e.g. Crystal, 1991). In sign language, some morphology is linear (e.g. affixation), but most commonly, morphological marking takes place through changes to the forms of hand shape, location, movement or orientation, which result in changes to meaning. In the present study, the question was whether children with intellectual impairments would display any creativity at the level of morphology, by modifying the form of their signs.

Sign modifications were defined as changes to the citation form of lexical signs which were consistent with meaning. The three anecdotal examples provided above would all meet this criterion. If only the 'dictionary' meanings of MAN, LOOK and SHUT-UP are assigned to these utterances, it can be argued that there is under-representation of the information conveyed. To do justice to their communicative skills, it is necessary to provide extended glosses, such as THREE-MAN, ALL-OF-YOU-LOOK-AT-ME and I-TELL-YOU-TO-SHUT-UP.

The results showed that a total of 24 signs were modified in a way which added meaning, by six of the children. The majority of changes were associated with hand shapes (10) or locations (12). Relatively few changes were made to movement (4). These changes reflected an associated dimension of meaning. Thus changes to hand shape indicated something about the type of object which was the referent of the sign; changes to location indicated something about where an object or action was located; and changes to movement indicated something about how an action was carried out. Figure 6.1 describes some of these in more detail. No such modifications were evident in the signing of teachers.

It is therefore clear that some children were able to vary their sign production to convey specific meanings. However, the morphological status of these meaning-based changes may be questioned. It was important to try to establish whether they formed part of a contrastive and consistent system, and were linked to grammatical or semantic development.

As before, predictions were based on what is known about typical development. Traditionally, language researchers look for contrastivity and consistency in morphological production (Bates et al., 1988). That is, the manual sign (or spoken word) should be produced in two different ways to produce two different meanings (e.g. *walk-ed* and *walk-ing*; and GIVE-ME and GIVE-YOU). The same type of modification should be seen across a class of manual signs (or words) to convey similar meanings (*walk-ing* and *eat-ing*; and GIVE-ME and ASK-ME). Also, consistency would be expected across time and contexts – the modification should be produced more than once. Analysis showed that 18 out of the 24 modifications were contrastive. On two or more occasions when a sign was produced, two or three parameters would be held constant, and one would be varied (see Figure 6.1).

Secondly, in the development of both signed and spoken grammar, it is the verb which is central to the structure of a sentence (Bloom and Capatides, 1991; Brien, 1992; Radford, 1992). If children are to develop a language through sign and gesture, they must discover how to manipulate verbs to provide contrasts in meaning. Meaningful sign modifications associated with verbs might therefore be expected. Results from the four children who produced more than one meaningful modification were analysed. Twenty-one out of the 22 meaningful modifications they produced were associated with verbs rather than nouns. The difference was statistically significant ($\chi^2 = 42.6$, df $= 1$, p$< .001$).

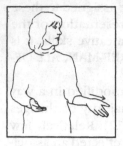
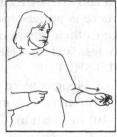

Hand shape
a. GIVE. Flat hand shape, location in neutral space, and outward movement.
b. GIVE-SMALL-OBJECT. Hand shape changes to fingertip contact, indicating that the object given is something small (it was in fact a sweet).

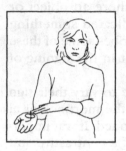
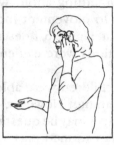

Location
c. CREAM (performed on wrist)
d. CREAM (performed on cheek). A flat hand and circular movement is kept constant, but location is changed to indicate where the cream should go.

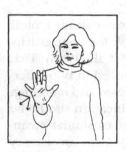
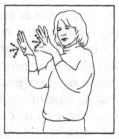

Doubling and movement
e. LIGHT. Performed with one hand, a spread hand shape with a single opening and closing movement.
f. LIGHTS-FLASHING. Pluralised by the use of both hands. The palms oriented to show that the lights face outward. The movement is repeated which conveys the impression of the lights flashing on and off.

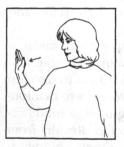
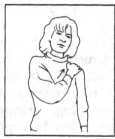

Orientation
g. HIT. Flat hand shape, directed away from self.
h. HIT-ME. Flat hand shape, directed inward toward self to describe how he was slapped on the shoulder. This has the effect of suggesting a distinction between active and passive.

**Figure 6.1:** Examples of meaning-based modifications to signs

Finally, if the modifications are morphological, they should be associated with other linguistic achievements by the children, such as stability of word order, an increased range of semantic relations (Lahey, 1988), and the growth of a 'closed class' lexicon (prepositions, questions, modals and pronouns) (Fowler et al., 1994). Analysis showed that production of modifications was not associated with any other linguistic developments in the children. The children who produced these modifications were not more advanced than other children in their lexical, syntactic or semantic development. The fact that the achievement was relatively isolated suggests that it may be gestural and iconic – a product of the general cognitive system, rather than the linguistic system. On the other hand, this situation may reflect the limitations of the children's input in manual signs.

## Conclusions

At the beginning of this chapter, a question was raised about the expectations speech and language therapists and teachers should have of the hearing child with intellectual impairments who is introduced to manual signs as a means of expression. The results of this study of multi-sign utterances suggest some starting points for both current practice and future research.

Children who are dependent on manual signing seem to plateau at an early stage in their expressive language development. As previous researchers have found, they develop a lexicon of signs (and in some cases, words) which they can combine productively, sometimes in relatively long utterances – but they do not seem to be developing a grammar. This is not to say that this population is necessarily *incapable* of developing a grammar through manual sign. It is entirely possible that if they were provided with linguistic input in sign, hearing children with intellectual impairments might develop certain features of the language. A study in progress on the language development of hearing twins with Down syndrome who have deaf parents, and are bilingual in speech and manual sign, will provide insights relevant to this question (Woll and Grove, 1995).

Even if the children in this study are not developing a grammar, they showed some remarkable evidence of creativity in the way they conveyed meaning in sign. For children with intellectual impairments, their ability to go beyond the sign input, and transcend the limitations in environmental 'scaffolding' represents a significant achievement. This means that researchers and practitioners need to be prepared to look for modality-specific behaviours, rather than necessarily expecting to see an influence from spoken language in sign. We feel strongly that in order to recognise and document these developments, it is necessary to have some understanding of the structure of sign language, the role of gesture in typical development and the relationship between manual sign and gesture (Caselli and Volterra, 1990; McNeill, 1992).

There may also be some individuals who, despite their disabilities, have the linguistic capacity to develop rules for representing meaning in gestural forms. Again, this means that researchers and practitioners must look for evidence of contrastivity and consistency which are internal to the child's system. The studies by Goldin-Meadow, which determined consistency of ordering patterns in gestures and points, provide some guidelines.

Alternatively, it is possible that under certain circumstances, children will develop an understanding of the syntactic rules governing speech, and apply these to their expressive sign output. It is necessary to explore the relationship between comprehension and production, and the contribution of sign input by teachers when considering this question.

Clearly what is needed are research studies which consider the relationship between input, reception and expression in the two modalities of sign and speech. Smith (this volume) found that children's expressive output in PCS was more related to their comprehension of messages presented through PCS than to their comprehension of spoken language. This suggests that processing of some graphic material may be modality specific. It raises a more general question of cross-modal transfer in language between input and output (Bishop, 1982). Additionally, more information about the early process of syntactic development in the speech of children with intellectual impairments would help to clarify whether the level of word order errors observed in this study is unique to this population of signing children.

# Chapter 7
# The medium or the message: A study of speaking children using communication boards

MARTINE M. SMITH

Over the past four decades, aided communication has been highlighted as a means of circumventing the speech production difficulties of many individuals with combined severe speech and physical impairments (for an historical review of developments in this area, see Zangari, Lloyd and Vicker, 1994). Early research in aided communication focused primarily on interaction (e.g. Kraat, 1985; Light, Collier and Parnes, 1985a,b). More recently, attention has turned to language development and language functioning in individuals using aided communication, with discussion of appropriate models of development (Gerber and Kraat, 1992; Kraat, 1991; Nelson, 1992; von Tetzchner, 1991a), and initial research explorations (Iacono, 1992; Soto and Toro-Zambrana, 1995; Sutton and Gallagher, 1993).

One of the key milestones in the language development of speaking children is the breakthrough into grammar – the ability to manipulate the structure of language to convey an infinite range of meanings. Typically, this emerges productively during the third year of life (Ingram, 1989; Radford, 1992) and continues to adolescence (Crain, 1993; Nippold 1988). Some would argue that this is a discontinuous process (e.g. Radford, 1992), with a change from a lexical-thematic to a functional-nonthematic grammar. Others (e.g. Bates, Bretherton and Snyder, 1988; Bowerman, 1994) propose that, from the earliest stage, form and meaning are analysed together. All researchers, however, would agree that this breakthrough is an important milestone in development, and one which is achieved apparently effortlessly by the vast majority of children.

Clinical experience suggests that the same transition from single-word to multi-word utterances is much more difficult for children using communication boards, even where receptive language is well beyond the stage at which expressive syntax is typically firmly established. Bruno (1989) reports on H.J., aged 4;6, whose receptive language was age appropriate. H.J. used a 60-item picture/word board, with a variety of word classes, for a wide range of communicative functions, but despite her age-appropriate language scores 'her language board messages were telegraphic (i.e. 2–3 words) in form' (p. 90). Udwin and Yule (1990) followed a group of 20 children using Blissymbols (as well as 20 using British Sign Language), over a period of 18 months. The Blissymbol users were assessed as functioning receptively between 3 and 4 years and, at the start of the study, were using communication boards containing a mean of 68.6 Blissymbols (range 9–180). When first seen, more than 65 per cent of their utterances consisted of only one Blissymbol. Eighteen months later, over half of their utterances still consisted of only one Blissymbol. Similarly, Spiegel, Benjamin and Spiegel (1993) report on a 19-year-old adult who scored a receptive vocabulary age equivalent of 9;5, but whose output consisted essentially of 'successive single word sentences with no syntactic organisation' (p. 112).

Such restricted output patterns have been noted even where aided communicators have the ability to use more complex structures. Kraat (1991) describes two children, aged four and seven, who rapidly acquired spoken language, having used a communication board for an extended period of time. Kraat comments on the differences between the spoken output and communication board utterances of the two children:

> 'The 4-year-old, for example, typically produced 'object' or 'actor' utterances when using his board, even though the lexicon for more complete or grammatically complex utterances was known and available. In speaking, this child immediately produced a variety of complete and relatively complex grammatical structures. His board utterances remained unchanged during that transition time' (1991, p. 120).

The persistence and consistency of such findings beg the question: why should the transition to multi-word utterances be so difficult for individuals using communication boards? Given that this is a step which many two-year-olds take in their stride, why is it so difficult for children whose receptive language is far more advanced? Three possible explanations present themselves:

> Output reflects an *underlying linguistic deficit*. Asymmetric receptive-expressive language profiles are commonly reported in the literature on childhood language impairment (e.g. Adams, 1990; Camarata, Nelson and Camarata, 1994; Fey, Cleave, Long and Hughes, 1993). Bishop and Edmundson (1987) proposed that the components of language are differentially vulnerable to impairment, with an increasing vulnerability across receptive language, semantics, syntax/morphology and phonology, a pattern borne out by their study of 55 children.

Board output is a function of the *communication process* in aided communication. Generating output is a slow, effortful process for many aided communicators, particularly those using indirect access techniques. Use of telegrammatic constructions may reflect a choice of effective language style, thus suggesting communicative competence, rather than deficits.

Board output reflects *modality-specific influences*, as yet largely unexplored in graphic communication, though the focus of considerable research attention in relation to manual signing (cf. Supalla, 1991).

Natural sign languages (such as Irish Sign Language, American Sign Language and British Sign Language) have a grammar and structure that exploits the spatial context of signing, and that is quite different from the temporally organised structure of spoken language. Considerable research over the past two decades has been devoted to demonstrating that such natural sign languages are 'full' languages, sharing equal linguistic status with spoken languages (e.g. Klima and Bellugi, 1979; Kyle and Woll, 1983; Wilbur, 1976). In addition to natural sign languages, several manual signing systems have been devised, with the aim of coding a spoken language into a manual mode, like the *Paget Gorman Sign System* (Paget, Gorman and Paget, 1976; see also Introduction). Such signing systems are not regarded as full languages. Unlike natural sign languages, they do not exploit spatial context, but rather, map the linear order sequence of spoken language in a manual medium. Even where instruction is exclusively in a manual signing system, with extremely limited exposure to natural sign language, children developing language using sign tend to exploit the spatial medium, as seen in natural sign languages, in preference to conforming to the linear ordering of signing systems (Supalla, 1991). Supalla refers to this process as 'modalitisation' and concludes that, while language is clearly modality-independent, 'the role of modality in signed language development can no longer be overlooked' (p. 109).

It is possible that similar modality influences operate where graphic signs are being used. If pictograms exert modality-specific influences on communication, these effects must be separated from both the linguistic ability and the physical and lexical access limitations of those using them. In order to address this issue, a project was undertaken using communication boards with speaking preschool children without disabilities.

# Method

Five children, aged 3;5-4;7, participated in the project. All were attending a preschool, and none presented with any reported disabilities. On the *Renfrew Action Picture Test* (Renfrew, 1989) all scored up to age level on both information and grammar measures (Table 7.1).

Table 7.1: Chronological age and age-equivalent scores on the *Renfrew Action Picture Test*

| Subject | Chronological age | Information score: age-equivalent | Grammar score: age-equivalent |
| --- | --- | --- | --- |
| Una | 3;5 | 3;6–3;11 | 3;6–3;11 |
| Oisín | 3;7 | 3;6–3;11 | 4;6–4;11 |
| Natalie | 4;2 | 8;0–8;5 | 8;0–8;5 |
| Olwen | 4;3 | 5;6–5;11 | 5;6–5;11 |
| James | 4;7 | 6;0–6;5 | 6;0–6;5 |

The children were seen in a group once weekly, over a ten-week period, for sessions ranging from 60 to 90 minutes. The author and a research assistant, a final year student in speech and language therapy, led each session. In the first session, a bird puppet was introduced. The bird had large eyes, but no ears, and it was explained that he could see very well, but was unable to hear. For this reason, in order to communicate with the bird, it was necessary to explain messages using picture boards. Each participating child was presented with their own identical picture board, containing 53 PCS signs (Table 7.2), covering a range of grammatical classes: nouns, verbs, modifiers and prepositions, in addition to six 'colour' attributes. It should be noted that the classification of lexical items according to grammatical class relies heavily on context in the early stages of language development, particularly where output typically consists of single words or signs.

A variety of activities was used during each session, introducing the vocabulary on the boards, modelling and encouraging the use of single-word utterances, progressing to combinations of two, three and four words over the ten-week period. Activities were selected to encourage use of a range of syntactic structures to fulfil varying communicative functions, in relation to real objects, miniature objects and pictures. The bird puppet was in charge of each activity, and in order to take part, it was necessary to communicate with him. For example, in a shopping game, the bird was the shopkeeper, and the children were required to use their boards to indicate what they wanted to buy; in the 'action song', the children sang songs, showing PCS signs for actions like *SIT*, *WASH* and *DANCE*, and miming the actions; and in 'Who has what?' PCS signs were used to name objects in the children's bags. All target structures were modelled and demonstrated, and all sessions were video recorded.

Table 7.2: PCS signs on communication boards

**Actions**

| | | | |
|---|---|---|---|
| GO | SIT | DRIVE | EAT |
| BUY | KISS | HAVE | SLEEP |
| WASH | WANT | LOOK | SEE |
| DRINK | STOP | HELP | READ |
| PUSH | DANCE | | |

**Nouns**

| | | | |
|---|---|---|---|
| HOUSE | BED | CHAIR | TABLE |
| TABLE | DOOR | SHOP | CHEESE |
| HAMBURGER | CUP | WATER | SPOON |
| DRINK | DRESS | JUMPER | PANTS |
| SOCKS | SHOES | SOAP | MOUSE |
| DOG | HORSE | CAT | CAR |
| AIRPLANE | TEDDY | DOLL | BOOK |
| BALL | PUZZLE | TRAIN | |

| Colours | People | Descriptors | Prepositions |
|---|---|---|---|
| BLUE | MOTHER | HOT | ON |
| GREEN | FATHER | LITTLE | IN, INSIDE |
| ORANGE | GIRL | BIG | UNDER |
| RED | BOY | DIRTY | OUT |
| YELLOW | BABY | BROKEN | |
| BLACK | | | |

At the end of the ten-week period, the children were seen individually for assessment of their communication board use. A picture test was devised for the evaluation, consisting of a total of 35 plates. Each plate presented either three or four contrasting pictures, only one of which was the target picture. Pictures were selected to elicit sentences covering a range of semantic probability and structural expansion possibilities. Within each test plate, such contrasts formed the basis of the picture selection, to ensure a minimum of two and a maximum of four 'Information Carrying Words'. For example, on plate 10, three pictures were presented: a pencil in a blue shoe (target); a blue pencil in a shoe; and a pencil in a blue box. None of the target sentences had been specifically taught, but the structures required had all been targeted in intervention.

The method of presentation of the test stimuli varied, across three contexts. In presentation A, the target picture was described verbally by the researcher (R), addressing verbal comprehension. In presentation B, a description of the target picture, formulated in PCS signs, was taped to the test plate (addressing PCS comprehension). In presentation C, (the results presented here), each child was asked to describe one of the pictures in the array, (indicated for the child by a star), so that the bird could find a matching picture in his array, and affix a star on the correct picture. The latter presentation resembled the referential communication task described by Glucksberg, Krauss and Weisberg (1966). The bird puppet was placed behind a barrier, and so could not see which picture had a star. However, the aim was not to assess the ability to convey appropriate information, but rather to use PCS signs for multi-term utterances, in a relatively spontaneous, but semi-controlled format. Therefore, help was given in identifying the key features of the target picture, and where it was considered necessary, utterances were rehearsed verbally.

All of the children were verbally able to describe the target pictures. The varying formats (A, B, C) were devised to allow a comparison of verbal comprehension and PCS comprehension, and of PCS comprehension and PCS expression (manuscript in preparation). The necessary vocabulary was available on the communication boards and had been targeted in previous intervention activities.

## Results and discussion

### A transparent task?

Una was the youngest of the participants, and the least advanced linguistically. She had great difficulty understanding the communicative status of PCS signs. Pictures exist in many different forms in everyday life, from indicators for bathrooms, to traffic information signs, illustrations in books, and instructional materials for assembling appliances. There is little specific about PCS signs that distinguishes them from other drawings occurring in the environment. PCS signs may be used to talk about a picture in a book, but a child engaged in such a task may have no way of knowing that the 'role' assigned to PCS signs is very different to that of the illustrations in the book.

This is obviously a very different situation to that pertaining for speech. Although non-linguistic vocalisation may occur in the environment, it can be identified as such, because of the formational constraints that govern the make-up of spoken words, both at the phonological and morphological levels. Indeed, it is these very constraints that allow creative use of language, such as puns, to exist. Because PCS signs are not reducible to a finite set of components, no such formational constraints operate, and thus identifying 'true' PCS signs from other line drawings is much more difficult. This may be compounded by colouring in PCS signs (as opposed to colour-coding grammatical categories of signs). This might seem a trivial point. However, as von Tetzchner and Martinsen (1992) point out, confusion may arise for an individual using a communication board in distinguishing their communication signs from ambient environmental pictures. This blurring of boundaries may have implications at least for the development of metalinguistic aware-ness, in relation to the graphic communication system.

It was clear that, after ten weeks, Una still had difficulty with the concept of using the picture board to communicate with the bird puppet. Instead, she liked to label the PCS signs on her board, even where this had no relevance to the task. An example of this is given below. (For notation, see Table 0.1).

(1)  Una was looking at a test plate with pictures of a big book on a cup; a book on a big cup (target); and a small book on a small cup. Target PCS vocabulary was *BOOK, ON, BIG* and *CUP*. (R = researcher).

    U:  *Look, {PUSH Push}*.
    R:  *You've got push, you have.*
    U:  *{DANCE Dance}*.
    R:  *Dance. Is there anyone dancing in the picture?*
    U:  'No' (shakes head.).

Certainly, part of Una's difficulty arose from the nature of the task. Refer-ential communication tasks such as this continue to pose some difficulty for children up to eight years of age (Bowman, 1984). Although consid-erable help was provided in identifying key features of the target picture, throughout the task, Una confused the two types of pictures visible to her: the PCS signs on her board, and the stimulus pictures on the test array. Four times during comprehension testing, she searched her board for a picture which had been described for her, rather than looking at the test array. She needed considerable prompting to produce any PCS descriptions of the pictures, preferring instead to point to the test picture, or, as in transcript (1), label 'irrelevant' PCS signs. The following transcript is typical:

(2)  Una had a test plate with pictures of a boy in a dirty car; a dirty boy in a car (target): and a clean boy in a clean car. Target PCS vocabu-lary was *DIRTY, BOY, IN* and *CAR*.

    R:  *What's the secret going to be?*
    U:  *A boy in a car* (looking at test plate).
    R:  *Quick, tell the bird what you saw.*
    U:  *A boy in a car.*
    R:  *He can't hear you, he has no ears.*
        *You'll have to show him on the board.*
        *You saw a ... where's the boy?*
    U:  *BOY.*
    R:  *Boy.... where's in?*
    U:  *CAR.*
    R:  *Car. A boy in a car.*

There is little doubt that, had more time been available and more experience provided, Una would eventually have mastered the task of communicating with PCS signs. As children show interest in pictures from a very young age, and can typically point to pictured objects by the age of 18 months (Zimmerman, Steiner and Pond, 1992), it is tempting to assume that using a picture based communication board is also 'easy'. However, de Loache and Burns (1994) caution the need to distinguish between recognition and comprehension or understanding of pictures. They report a dramatic developmental change in the ability to interpret pictures as representations of reality between the age of 24 and 30 months. Using pictures to communicate about reality is yet more difficult.

Una was successful in interpreting messages presented to her in PCS, correctly identifying nine out of twelve pictures. This included PCS messages containing three 'Information Carrying Words, such as *BUY ORANGE DRINK* to select the correct picture from an array of pictures with a boy drinking orange; a boy eating an orange; a boy buying an orange; and a boy buying an orange drink (target). Una did not 'translate' her understanding of PCS signs into productive use of those signs, nor did she translate her expressive spoken language abilities into board-based communication. Similar difficulties have been reported by Raghavendra and Fristoe (1995) with preschool children using Blissymbols.

It is possible that, for a speaking child, such translation requires a level of metalinguistic awareness that Una has not yet reached. Certainly, the high transparency of the PCS signs did not make the task of using those signs transparent for her. This finding may not be generalisable to children whose only option for propositional communication lies with graphic communication, where intervention is typically more intensive and context-based than that presented here. However, it does emphasise the need for such context-based intervention, highlighting the function of graphic signs, in general, as well as the specific signs being targeted.

None of the other children had difficulty with the concept of using their boards to communicate during the evaluation, and their results are presented here.

### Single PCS sign utterances

Much of the reported data on the output of communication board users refers to the persistence of single word utterances (e.g. Spiegel et al., 1993; Udwin and Yule, 1990), a reliance on short utterances and minimal structural expansion. Support for the 'underlying linguistic deficit' hypothesis comes from the structurally similar difficulties evidenced by speaking, language impaired children (e.g. Tyler and Sandoval, 1994). In aided communication, an underlying neuropathology may affect not only speech production and control of voluntary movement, but also language functioning. Proposing underlying linguistic deficits as an explanation does not rule out the possibility that some aided communicators may develop appropriate expressive language. (For example, use of complex morphosyntactic structures is reported by Soto and Toro-Zambrana, 1995). Neither does it preclude a pattern of progress for all aided communicators. It does suggest, however, that such progress will be constrained by the extent of the linguistic impairment, and the related underlying neuropathology.

The PCS output of the four children presented here was also 'reduced', though with individual variation. Of a total of 192 PCS utterances produced, 159 (83%) consisted of a single PCS sign, with a further 33 (17%) accounted for by utterances containing two or more PCS signs. The proportion of single PCS-sign utterances varied across all the children, as Table 7.3 indicates.

Table 7.3: Utterances containing 1, 2 and 3 and more PCS signs

| Subject | 1 | | 2 | | 3 or more | |
|---------|-----|---------|-----|---------|------|--------|
| Oisín   | 32  | (91.4%) | 3   | (8.6%)  | 0    | (0.0%) |
| Natalie | 62  | (93.9%) | 3   | (4.5%)  | 1    | (1.5%) |
| Olwen   | 41  | (71.9%) | 15  | (26.3%) | 1    | (1.8%) |
| James   | 24  | (70.6%) | 8   | (23.5%) | 2    | (5.9%) |
| Total   | 159 | (82.8%) | 29  | (15.1%) | 4    | (2.1%) |

The fact that the children studied here produced very restricted PCS output, despite intact receptive and expressive language abilities, suggests that competence in spoken language is not necessarily reflected in similar patterns of PCS use. Separate 'competencies' may be engaged in both tasks. Here, the question of input may assume considerable importance. Given that users function in a speaking environment, it is unavoidable that input to them is biased in favour of spoken language. Even where attempts are made to provide simultaneous input in graphic signs and speech, it is likely that speech remains the dominant and more structurally complete mode of input, due to a combination of lexical restrictions and time constraints.

Research into bimodal communication in speech and manual sign suggests that, typically, propositional content is maintained across both modes, but there is a bias towards use of speech alone, rather than sign alone, and utterances are grammatically more simple in the manually encoded message (Maxwell, Bernstein and Mear, 1991; Wodlinger-Cohen, 1991). Grove, Dockrell and Woll (this volume), in analysing the consistency of the relationship of sign and speech input of teachers to children with learning disabilities, found that most children received very inconsistent sign input. They queried whether the 'density value' of sign-word pairing was sufficient to allow the children to deduce rules to apply to their sign output. Similar asymmetries in input may have implications for language development in aided communication, but these remain as yet largely unexplored.

Certainly, the input to the children in this study was not substantial, given the time frame of the research. Their reliance on single-term utterances may reflect their lack of experience with PCS signs. This again suggests, however, that a direct translation from spoken language to graphic signs relies on something other than competence in spoken language alone.

Chomsky (1968) points out that, in spoken language, competence is but 'one of many factors that interact to determine performance' (p. 117). Given the effort required, and the slow rate of aided communication (Goossens' and Crain, 1986), limiting output to high-content, key words ('telegraphic output') maximises the amount of information provided in a tight time frame. Such an approach is advocated in therapy with clients with aphasia, for example (Schlenck, Schlenck and Springer, 1995). On communication boards with a fixed number of lexical locations, priority is generally given to content words, as was the case in this study. Board users therefore may not have function words or inflectional morphemes available to them in an easily accessible format. (An exception to this may be boards based on Blissymbols, where typically inflectional Blissymbols are included from an early stage). Yorkston, Honsinger, Dowden and Marriner (1989) reported on G.T., a bright non-literate adult who used a language board and who was actively involved in selecting her own vocabulary. G.T. selected only three function words out of a total of 242 selections to be included on her board. 'G.T. felt that, although some other structure words might be useful, she did not consider them sufficiently important to warrant use of a 'valuable location' when other messages may be more important' (p. 105).

Whilst it is clinically useful to consider that the strategy of producing 'incomplete utterances' may reflect linguistic competence, rather than a further deficit, it is hard to see, in the context of this study, why the children would have chosen to restrict output to telegraphic messages, given that they had no obvious physical or motor difficulties, and could quickly and easily access the necessary vocabulary on their communication boards. This suggests that other factors may have influenced the nature of the output.

Analysis of the single-term PCS utterances suggested four subgroupings. These were labelled as: appropriate elliptical responses, complementary PCS utterances, global PCS utterances, and component PCS utterances.

*Appropriate elliptical responses*

All utterances in this group resulted from appropriate use of ellipsis in response to an immediately preceding question. Beyond noting the appropriate use of ellipsis, these data are not considered further here.

*Complementary utterances*

Fischer, Metz, Brown and Caccamise (1991) cite de Filippo, in using the term 'complementary signals', describing bimodal communication, where one mode provides information that the other does not (cf. Heim and Baker-Mills, this volume). A small number of instances were noted where the PCS output differed from the spoken output in a complementary way, both modes contributing to the picture description.

(3)    Natalie was looking at a test plate with pictures of a big book on a cup, a book on a big cup (target), and a small book on a small cup. Target PCS vocabulary was *BOOK, ON, BIG* and *CUP*.
       N:  {*BOOK On*}.
           *CUP*.

(4)    James was looking at a test array containing pictures of a man standing on a horse (target), a man standing beside a horse, a man sitting on a horse, and a horse standing on a man. Target PCS vocabulary was *MAN, ON* and *HORSE*.
       J:  {*MAN Man*} {*HORSE Stand*}.

(5)    Oisín was looking at a test plate with pictures of a girl kissing a teddybear (target), a teddybear kissing a girl, a girl kissing a boy, and a girl washing a teddybear. Target PCS vocabulary was *GIRL, KISS* and *TEDDY*.
       Oi: {*KISS The girl*}.
       R:  *Kissing*.
       Oi: {*BEAR The teddybear*}.

These instances suggest that both lexical sets (PCS and speech) were accessible simultaneously, and that the process observed was not a simple one-to-one translation across lexical sets, but rather the formulation of a proposition, which was then expressed bimodally. Of course, it could be argued that the examples above simply represent performance limitations, resulting in mistiming of spoken utterances and PCS productions. It is difficult to either prove or disprove this argument. However, even if one accepts 'mistiming' as an explanation, the point then becomes one of a choice of speech for some elements of the message, and PCS for other elements. Both explanations challenge the proposal that communication board users formulate a proposition in 'inner speech', and then simply translate this into PCS output.

## Global PCS utterances

All of the children produced spoken descriptions of pictures that were more structurally complete than their PCS descriptions. At times, they produced single-word utterances in PCS, while at the same time producing complex spoken utterances. Examples of some of these instances are provided in Table 7.4.

Table 7.4: 'Global' PCS utterances

| Stimulus picture | PCS production | Spoken utterance | Target PCS |
|---|---|---|---|
| A girl sitting on a chair | *SIT* | *A girl sitting on a chair* | *GIRL, SIT, ON, CHAIR* |
| A girl sleeping in a bed | *BED* | *Sleeping in the bed* | *GIRL, SLEEP, IN, BED* |
| A dirty boy driving a car | *BOY* | *A dirty boy* | *DIRTY, BOY, DRIVE, CAR* |

This pattern was most typical of Oisín. In many ways, it seemed that for him, all the information required for the picture description task was conveyed in a single PCS sign. This is most obvious in his selection of *SIT*, to describe a girl sitting on a chair, where the test array presented three pictures: a girl sitting on a bed, a girl standing on a chair, and a girl sitting on a chair (target). The PCS sign *SIT* (Figure 7.1) is of a person sitting on a chair. In the same way that a graphic sign for a 'fire-exit' presents all the necessary information in a single event-frame, Oisín chose the PCS sign *SIT*, rather than selecting *GIRL SIT CHAIR*, all of which were available to him. (This meant that the contrast in the array of pictures between a girl sitting on a bed and a girl sitting on a chair was lost. Oisín commented *She's standing on the chair, and she's sitting on the bed* in relation to the other two pictures, but, despite prompting, he did not add any further PCS information to his message).

Soto and Olmstead (1993) proposed that 'languages based on pictographic representations do not necessarily require a particular sequence in order to convey meaning' (p. 139). Clearly, combining PCS signs was not regarded by Oisín as necessary, although he had all the PCS signs available to him, and both knew and used the relevant signs on other occasions during the evaluation. In fact, he almost resisted attempts to encourage him to sequence PCS signs, as seen in the following example:

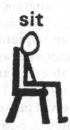

**sit**

**Figure 7.1:** *SIT* in PCS

(6)   Oisín had a test plate containing pictures of a boy in a dirty car, a
      dirty boy in a car (target), and a clean boy in a clean car. Target PCS
      vocabulary was *DIRTY, BOY, IN* and *CAR.*
      Oi: {*CAR The dirty boy in the car*}.
      R:   *Can you show him all the pictures that you need?*
      Oi: *CAR.*
      R:   *Car, yes, and what else..?*
      Oi: {*MAN Man*}.
      R:   *Man, ok ... and what did you say about the man?*
      Oi: {*CAR The man is sitting on the dirty car*}.
      R:   *The dirty car.*
      Oi: {*CAR In the car*}.

Neither underlying linguistic deficits nor physical limitations seem
adequate explanations for this pattern of output.

## Component PCS utterances

Identifying utterance boundaries posed one of the more difficult problems in the research reported here. In spoken discourse, this rarely poses
a problem. Gutfreund, Harrison and Wells (1989) state that a change of
speaker or pause or intonation cues signal utterance boundaries. Where
there is ambiguity, 'utterance boundaries occur where you would naturally use a full stop, question mark, or exclamatory mark in writing' (p. 4).
Eye gaze is also an important indicator of turn changes (Kendon, 1973),
with the speaker looking towards the listener to signal a willingness to
relinquish the floor. However, very often, such cues are not available
where one of the conversational partners is using a communication
board. Furthermore, in aided communication, co-formulation of
messages is a typical feature (Harris, 1982), the speaking partner labelling
graphic signs indicated by the aid user, and clarifying selections. It is not
clear whether this constitutes a change of speaker. Pauses, on the other
hand, may reflect searches for lexical items on a communication board,
rather than a willingness to relinquish the floor. In this context, long

sequences of turns may yield one 'utterance'. The closest analogy in child language is the transitional stage between single-word utterances and multi-word combinations, where sequences of single-word utterances gradually approximate combinations (Bloom, 1973).

The results presented in Table 7.3 are based on speaker-listener changes marking utterance boundaries. However, much of the interaction involving the PCS description of pictures resembled the building up to a single proposition, formulated in PCS, rather than successive single-word comments. The term 'component PCS utterance' was used to refer to such constructions. An example is given below.

(7)  Olwen was looking at a test plate containing a picture of a boy in a dirty car, a dirty boy in a car (target), and a clean boy in a clean car. Target PCS vocabulary was *DIRTY, BOY, IN* and *CAR.*
Ol: *A man in a car.*
R: *Yeah, and he's all dirty, isn't he? Ok, you tell him. Give him the clues and see if can he find it.*
Ol: *{DIRTY Dirty}.*
R: *Dirty.*
Ol: *{CAR Car}.*
R: *Car.*
Ol: *{MAN Man}.*
R: *Man.*
Ol: *{IN In}.*
R: *In.*
Ol: *The {CAR Car}.*

In spoken language development, a rich interpretation of single-word utterances proposes that understanding of semantic relations underlies single-word sequences (Ingram, 1989), and as such the utterances should be treated holistically. Based on Scollon's (1976) work, Martinsen and von Tetzchner (1989) use the term 'vertical construction' where constituents appear in a sequence of utterances. Such vertical constructions may be considered as presenting a single proposition. Given the reservations already expressed in relation to listener-speaker changes or strict timing cues in determining turn boundaries, data from the transcripts were re-analysed in the framework of vertical constructions, ignoring the 'intrusion' of researcher turns and defining turn boundaries using the following criteria:

*  *Pitch:* where speech accompanied PCS indication, a terminal falling pitch was taken as signalling an utterance boundary.
*  *Eye gaze:* where pitch was not sufficient (or if no speech was produced), utterance boundaries were marked where a child looked up at the bird puppet, having indicated a PCS sign.

- *Body movement:* occasionally, the communication board was pushed to one side, or lifted away from the table. This was taken as a clear indication of an utterance completion.

This re-analysis yielded substantially more multi-term PCS utterances, as presented in Table 7.5. However, even using these guidelines, there were many occasions when identifying turn boundaries was difficult. Sometimes, the children did not speak, and continued to look at their communication boards until their attention was directed to the test array. On other occasions, they looked up for clarification of their PCS selection. Given that such difficulties were encountered in dealing with children with no speech impairments, who had no difficulty in directing eye gaze or other physical movements, the argument for a 'vertical construction' interpretation of the output of individuals with multiple impairments is a persuasive one. This seems particularly relevant, in that the 'vertical construction interpretation' changed the balance between single- and multi-term PCS utterances from almost 8 to 1 (83–17%) to an essentially equal balance (48.5–51.5%). In the re-analysis, both James and Olwen produced more multi-term than single-term utterances.

Table 7.5: Number of utterances with 1, 2 and 3 and more PCS signs with a vertical construction interpretation of PCS utterance length

| Subject | 1 | | 2 | | 3 and more | |
|---|---|---|---|---|---|---|
| Oisín | 15 | (57.7%) | 10 | (38.5%) | 1 | (3.8%) |
| Natalie | 25 | (59.5%) | 10 | (23.8%) | 7 | (16.7%) |
| Olwen | 15 | (39.5%) | 17 | (44.7%) | 6 | (15.8%) |
| James | 9 | (34.6%) | 9 | (34.6%) | 8 | (30.8%) |
| | | | | | | |
| Total | 64 | (48.5%) | 46 | (34.8%) | 22 | (16.7%) |

Within these sequenced 'component PCS utterances', contrasts in word order constraints operated across both modes, as illustrated in the following transcript:

(8) James had a test plate containing a picture of a boy in a dirty car, a dirty boy in a car (target), and a clean boy in a clean car. Target PCS vocabulary was *DIRTY, BOY, IN* and *CAR*.
   R:  *Ok, so what will we tell him?*
   J:  *A dirty boy driving a car* (pointing to the test array).
   R:  *Ok, you tell the bird, so he can get the right one.*
   J:  *Bird. {BOY A dirty boy}.*
   R:  *A boy, right.*
   J:  *{CAR Driving a car}* (looks at bird).
   R:  *Well, you just said {BOY Boy} {CAR Car}.*

> J:  *A {BOY Boy} {DRIVING Driving}. Oh, where's dirty?* (looks at board). *Ehm, {DIRTY Dirty}, and a {CAR Car}.*
> R:  *A boy driving, and a dirty car. There's a boy driving a dirty car* (pointing to test array).
> J:  *Not a dirty car.*
> R:  *Oh, a dirty boy driving a car.*

A similar scenario unfolded with Natalie:

(9)    Natalie had a test plate containing a picture of a boy in a dirty car, a dirty boy in a car (target), and a clean boy in a clean car. Target PCS vocabulary was *DIRTY, BOY, IN,* and *CAR.*

> N:  *{CAR Car}.*
> R:  *Car.*
> N:  *DIRTY.*
> R:  *Dirty.*
> N:  *{CAR In}* (looks at researcher).
> R:  *Dirty what?*
> N:  *BOY* (pointing on board).
> R:  *Boy.*

The occurrence of such mode-specific patterns raises questions about the nature of the 'translation' process being observed. The output in PCS is not simply 'reduced', but is different in structure in some important respects. Relying only on the PCS output, an incorrect selection from the test array would have been made in each case above, although the spoken description was both accurate and sufficient.

## Conclusions

The impetus for this research came from clinical experience with children with cerebral palsy using communication boards, where difficulties in producing multi-term utterances seemed disproportionate to receptive language and general communicative abilities. Three candidate explanations were proposed: an expressive language deficit; a communication strategy; and medium-specific influences.

The results presented here are from five children with typically developing language abilities and with no physical impairments. For one, the concept of using a board for communication was still problematic after ten weeks of intervention. This was an unexpected finding, and suggests that transparency studies are needed, not only at the level of signs, but also at the level of the communicative task. For the other four children, it is clear that their output using communication boards was very different to their spoken output. In some instances, complementary information was provided in PCS. In most cases, PCS output was 'reduced', relative to spoken output, essentially consisting of single-PCS utterances, sometimes strung together into a vertical sequence. Within these sequences, linear word order constraints, which were recognised in speech, were frequently violated in PCS output. (Note however that no unacceptable structures, such as *IN BOY CAR*, were produced). In fact, despite their intact linguistic abilities, their easy accessing of their communication boards, and the short messages required, the output of these speaking children is very similar to that of many aided communicators, in the author's clinical experience.

It is unlikely that any one of the three candidate explanations can fully account for the results presented here. The first explanation, that of an underlying linguistic deficit did not apply to these children, although reduced PCS input experience, and as yet incompletely developed metalinguistic skills, may have played a role. The second explanation, that of a language style choice due to physical or lexical access limitations, also has shortcomings. The children presented here did not have any physical or motor impairments, and could access their boards easily and quickly. In many instances they produced all the key information elements, but did not order these elements within the linear order constraints of English. The third explanation, that of modality-specific influences, specifically use of PCS signs as 'wholes' and not as components of an ordered sequence, receives the most support from the data here. This use of PCS signs may be analogous to the modality effects of the spatial medium in natural sign languages referred to by Supalla (1991).

These results may have limited generalisability to aided communicators, given that they are based on a short period of intervention with typically developing children who have intact physical, cognitive, and linguistic abilities. (For discussion of the role of subjects without disabilities in research in augmentative and alternative communication, see Bedrosian, 1995; Higginbotham, 1995).

In introducing augmentative signing with typically developing children, Abrahamsen, Lamb, Brown-Williams and McCarthy (1991) argued 'it is hard to evaluate the results of using atypical input with atypical learners if you do not know what happens when the same atypical input is provided to typical learners' (p. 239). However, cognisance must be taken of the shortcomings of this kind of research. The children in this study have access to a very efficient means of communication. Providing them with a PCS lexical set simply offered another, less efficient option. This is a very different situation to that faced by children with severe speech and motor limitations, for whom picture communication boards may be the only option for propositional communication. In the latter case, the expressive lexicon available may consist entirely of a picture lexicon; there may be overlapping picture and spoken lexicon sets; or there may be separate expressive lexical subsets, with no overlap, so that some lexical items are available in PCS only, while others are available in speech only. Despite these limitations, potentially important clinical implications are suggested.

Inferring a linguistic deficit solely on the basis of telegraphic output constitutes a serious disservice to clients using picture-based communication boards. Assuming that telegraphic output reflects communicative competence may also serve to hide genuine communication difficulties. A rather neglected component in the complex process of aided communication is the graphic medium itself, and its effect on the message generated. The research reported here suggests that, at the very least, the concept of communicating using PCS signs is not completely transparent, even if the signs used are regarded as transparent. It is essential that intervention make explicit the *function* of PCS signs, in general, in addition to targeting specific PCS meanings.

Furthermore, this research suggests that communication in PCS is different to communication in speech. 'Rich' interpretations of PCS output seem justified, in this context, using the framework of vertical constructions. Word order constraints may be more difficult to apply in a graphic medium. Caution should be exercised in using evidence of word order rules as an assessment measure, and it may be necessary to refocus intervention goals. This may involve targeting metalinguistic skills, to facilitate the 'translation' process. For very many individuals using picture-based communication boards, all three candidate explanations may play a role in influencing their output. Attention to date has focused on the first two possibilities, with little consideration of the effect of the graphic medium. The research presented here suggests that one should broaden the framework for evaluating the output of board users. To some extent at least, it seems that for the children presented here, the medium informs the message.

# Chapter 8
# Sounds and silence: Interaction in aided language use

ERLAND HJELMQUIST AND ANNIKA DAHLGREN SANDBERG

In a series of studies of non-speaking adolescents with cerebral palsy, we have focused on basic aspects of communication and language functions. The adolescents' lack of speech puts parents and other people who want to communicate with them in an extremely difficult situation; on the one hand how to know when their own communication, spoken or other, is understood; and on the other hand, to know how to interpret the adolescents' non-speech modes of communication.

The challenges of these kinds of interaction are fundamental since the basis of human communication usually taken for granted is disrupted. A main task for a non-speaking person and a speaking interlocutor is to establish a common ground for communication, to know when the communicated message is understood. Thus one can say that the non-speaking person and the speaking communication partner must put much effort into metacommunication, that is, into discussing the content of the messages of the communication. Metacommunication and metacognition refer to the possibility of making one's own language and thinking the object of reflection (Hjelmquist, Sandberg and Hedelin, 1994). This is an aspect of explicit awareness of the activities of speaking and thinking. These meta-activities are so self-evident that one does not usually think of them as a distinct level of functioning. Normally speaking people tend to take them for granted.

However, it is only through using metacommunication acts that one can successfully take part in interpersonal communication where adjustment, 'audience design' (Clark and Carlson, 1982), clarification and correction of the just expressed message are ubiquitous. Metacommunication implies the use of reformulation, paraphrasing, explanation, etc. when one's own message has not been understood, and one can request such communication acts when one does not understand the interlocutor's message. In conversations with motor impaired persons these aspects of communication exchanges are extremely difficult to handle. Not only is speech lacking. The motor impairments often make non-verbal communication time-consuming and difficult to interpret. The slow pace of the interaction is one of the main obstacles to the communication process.

In general, studies of aided communication have severe methodological limitations. The population of non-speaking communication aid users is small, and the particular groups that have been studied have often been heterogeneous. In the present study, we have taken a dual perspective, analysing the communication and cognitive abilities of the individual, and the characteristics of conversations. We have used special communication tasks and situations with naturally occurring conversations. In the analyses, the language has been categorised in a traditional manner into words and word forms, and combinations of words into utterances and discourse. The development of these aspects of language among naturally speaking children is well known, relatively speaking (Bloom, 1993; Clark, 1993).

'Discourse' refers to a complex of communication acts including formulation of a message, expression of a wish, making a description, and figurative language such as irony, sarcasm, metaphor, understatement and hyperbole. It might be said that figurative language uses the difference between literal meaning and the communicative effect which is created in a particular communication context (Demorest, Silberstein, Gardner and Winner, 1983). People who do not speak but use some kind of alternative mode of communication might have particular difficulties with using this kind of communication. The use of such figurative language may be regarded as an indication of an advanced language ability and of an awareness that one and the same linguistic expression, or form, can convey totally different meanings.

A general topic of studies of aided language interaction and interaction with specific language impaired children is the communication pattern used by the partners (Collins, this volume; Higginbotham, 1989; Light, Collier and Parnes, 1985a; van Balkom, 1991; von Tetzchner and Martinsen, this volume). This includes for instance the way the communication partners start and close interactions, occupy space in the interactions, take initiatives and introduce topics. One major objective of these studies has been to delineate how the strategies of the speaking person influence those of the non-speaking person and vice versa.

Light, Collier and Parnes (1985a,b,c) report great difficulties of communication between parents and their non-speaking children who used Blissymbols. The children were young, 3–5 years of age, and the interaction patterns therefore reflected both the usual features of child-adult interactions and other features due to the disabilities of the children. The adults produced most of the initiative whereas the non-speaking children showed a passive answering role. The children typically answered with one word or asked for specific information. They used various means of communication, and only 18.2 per cent of their turns included the use of Blissymbols. The diverse ways of communicating seemed to correspond to different communication purposes. Blissymbols were used mainly for providing information and explanations while vocalisations and gestures were most effective for expressing 'yes' and 'no'.

Calculator and Luchko (1983) point out the difficulties speaking partners might have in adjusting to the communication exchanges of non-speaking persons. They showed that training of the speaking persons enhanced communication, and that it was more important to change the communication of the speaking partner than to change the communication aid. Light, Dattilo, English and Gutierrez (1992) taught communication partners to give the persons using aided communication more opportunities to communicate and to decrease their own control of the conversation. The results showed a tendency of the persons using aided communication to initiate more topics and that the communication pattern had become more reciprocal.

The present study investigated the communication patterns of motor-impaired, non-speaking adolescents and their parents. We expected to confirm the general features of interaction between speaking and non-speaking persons found in previous research. However, in comparison to previous research, a broader description was included than has usually been the case, in particular by including both structured settings and more natural forms of conversation. It was expected that the communication exchanges between the speaking and the non-speaking individuals would follow the most general principles of conversational exchange. The major question was how such general principles would be instantiated when one of the communication partners was using an aid for communication.

Lindblom (1990) suggests one general conversational feature, namely that speakers as part of the continuous conversational adaptation are just as articulate as is necessary when considering what the listeners can infer from their speech. The adaptive processes shown by a non-speaking person cannot be seen in the speech process, of course, but in the use of the other communication means available. The adaptive processes in situations with free conversation will be compared to those in situations with structured communication. The two conversational situations are very different with respect to the range and specificity of the domain of meaning to be conveyed. Range and specificity are restricted to cards and their features in the structured communication game, while in the free conversations, there are few limitations on what might be suggested as a conversational contribution. These differences made it possible to study whether the non-speaking adolescents acted differently in the two situations, in particular with respect to the explicitness of the messages. If this was the case, it would show adaptation to situational demands, despite the expected generally low level of 'articulation'.

# Method

## Subjects

Seven adolescents participated in the study (characteristics are presented in Table 8.1). All were students at a regional special school for

Table 8.1: Subject characteristics and test results. Scores on Raven based on British norms. ITPA Visual Sequential Memory is based on Swedish norms.

| Subject | Age | Sex | Bliss use in years | Modes of 'yes' and 'no' | Raven Score | Raven Age-equivalent | ITPA-VM Score | ITPA-VM Age-equivalent |
|---|---|---|---|---|---|---|---|---|
| Carl | 11 | M | >6 | Gesture | 10 | <5;6 | 6 | 6;2 |
| Tina | 15 | F | 10 | Vocalisation | 14 | <5;6 | 0 | 5;7 |
| Peter | 13 | M | 10 | Vocalisation | 10 | <5;6 | 2 | 5;9 |
| Tom | 13 | M | 10 | Gesture | 12 | <5;6 | 18 | 7;10 |
| Sven | 17 | M | >10 | Facial expression, Blissymbols | 23 | 8;6 | 22 | 8;10 |
| Olof | 17 | M | 10 | Facial expression, Blissymbols | 10 | <5;6 | 6 | 6;2 |
| Hans | 17 | M | 10 | Facial expression | 17 | 6;6 | 13 | 7;3 |

children and adolescents with motor and communication disabilities, and six of the children were residential, coming from more distant places. They all used wheelchairs. Blissymbols were their primary mode of expression. They all used the standard chart of 462 Blissymbols and all but one had 10–50 additional Blissymbols. They had used the system for 6–10 years. Only two adolescents could express 'yes' and 'no' vocally. The others expressed 'yes' and 'no' with facial expressions, gestures or Blissymbols. All seven participants and their parents were native speakers of Swedish and the parents were all well acquainted with Blissymbols. *The Coloured Progressive Matrices* (Raven, 1965) were used to assess non-verbal intelligence. The subtest Visual Sequential Memory of the *Illinois Test of Psycholinguistic Abilities,* (Holmgren, 1984, Kirk, McCarthy, and Kirk, 1968) was used as a measure of visual memory.

## Procedures

In the structured settings, a traditional 'referential communication' situation was applied (cf. Glucksberg and Krauss, 1967). The adolescent and one of the experimenters sat opposite each other at a table with a screen placed on the table between them. A set of cards was placed in front of each person. The two sets of cards were identical, containing drawings of faces. The faces were small or large, happy or sad, belonged to a boy or a girl, and did or did not have a nose. Thus there were four dimensions, each with two values, making sixteen cards.

One of the persons was instructed to choose one of the pictures and asked to describe it, with the help of Blissymbols in the case of the adolescent, and spoken language in the case of the adult communication partner, in such a way that the other person could pick out the picture that had been described from the set of cards without having seen it. When the describer had made clear that the description was finished, he or she was asked whether the information provided was sufficient for the receiver to pick out the correct card. This was an 'adequacy question'. If the answer was 'no', the describer was prompted to provide more information. If the answer was positive, the communication partner was asked to identify the card, whereupon the describer showed his card and stated if the choice was correct or not. This procedure was repeated three times with the non-speaking adolescents in the role of the describer, and three times with the non-speaking adolescents in the role of the receiver. In this latter role the non-speaking adolescents were also asked an adequacy question, namely whether they had received enough information to pick out the right card. If the answer was 'no', the receiver was prompted to ask for more information. The whole session was video recorded.

In the natural settings, interactions between the non-speaking adolescents and their parents were video recorded. There was one recording for each family, and the sessions lasted 1–1½ hours. The families were instructed to talk about anything they wanted; something that had happened or something on their minds. The recordings were made with two cameras, one directed towards the communication aid, and the other towards the faces and hands of the communication partners.

## Measures

In the referential communication game, a number of mentioned features was counted for both the speaker and the listener role. The transcriptions of the free conversation were segmented into topics, defined as clearly separated parts of the conversation treating a distinct subject and terminated with or without understanding of the message by any of the two participants introducing a new subject. All the topics also had to encompass at least one turn or one turn opportunity, even if left unattended to.

The conversations were coded by two experimenters independently, using a modification of the coding scheme described by Light and her associates (1985a,b,c), indicating function, mode and content of the communication. For each topic, initiations and successful or unsuccessful understanding were coded. The criterion of understanding was an observed confirmation of the interpretation from one or the other of the two persons, whether with spoken words, Blissymbols or non-verbal means.

# Results and discussion

The results will describe and contrast the interactions in the structured referential game and in the natural settings.

## Structured settings

In the referential task, it was a requirement for success that the person describing the picture mentioned all the features that differentiated the picture chosen from the other pictures. Otherwise the description would be ambiguous and the communication might fail. The results show that when the non-speaking adolescents were in the describer position, they succeeded in giving about half of the necessary dimensions (Table 8.2). In the receiver position, they generally asked for very little information. When asked whether they had enough information to pick out the correct card, they answered positively, sometimes even when information about more than one dimension was lacking.

Table 8.2: Number of relevant dimensions in describer and receiver position mentioned and asked for spontaneously or after the adequacy question. (Maximum number of dimensions is 12).

| Subject | Describer position | Receiver position |
|---------|--------------------|--------------------|
| Carl    | 6                  | 1                  |
| Tina    | 6                  | 0                  |
| Peter   | 5                  | 2                  |
| Tom     | 8                  | 2                  |
| Sven    | 8                  | 3                  |
| Olof    | 6                  | 2                  |
| Hans    | 8                  | 4                  |

None of the adolescents described all the relevant variables (12) summarised across the three sender tasks. However, more important, they showed that they had understood the point of the task and worked towards its solution in a systematic manner. The same can be said about their achievements in the listener role. They utilised the Blissymbols effectively, as the dimensions referred to were only indicated by Blissymbols. No other communication means were used for this function.

One important question is to what extent discourse skills can be influenced by instruction and educational arrangements. The participants in this study had all received extensive instruction in the use of Blissymbols. Consequently, they had been taught to distinguish between communication form (the Blissymbol) and what they intended to communicate, that is, to appreciate the distinction between a communicative expression and its content. Such teaching must have taken place at least implicitly. Being able to use a system such as Blissymbolics means that one has acquired the skill to use a referring expression which is not 'natural'. In this sense, the adolescents had been taught to focus attention on communication form. It might be expected that persons whose attention has not been focused on the distinction between form and content, in instructional settings or otherwise, would be less explicit in their language awareness.

It may be concluded from the results that the non-speaking adolescents had acquired a basic ability to manage the discourse of a structured situation with clearly defined goals. They followed the same principles as people without disabilities (cf. Clark and Schaefer, 1989; Hedelin and Hjelmquist, 1991), and understood that the dimensions used by the describer, to distinguish a card from the other cards, also distinguished the cards for the receiver.

## Natural settings

Excerpts will be presented from conversations between Olof (dialogues 1–6), Sven (dialogues 7–8) and Tina (dialogues 9–11), and their parents. In the six dialogues of the first conversation, the content of the conversation was known beforehand by the communication partners, and the interaction was an opportunity for demonstrating this knowledge. Very little, if any, new information was communicated. (For notations, see Table 0.1).

(1)    Olof used a communication board with Blissymbols (for details, see Table 8.1). He was discussing a class excursion with his mother and father. The particular topic was how to travel.

    M:    *You are going on an excursion with your class soon, Olof. How will you travel?*

    O:    *BOAT.*

    M:    *You are going by boat to Keytown, yes.*

    O:    *BUS.*

    M:    *And bus*

    F:    *Where are you going by bus, Olof?*

    O:    *TOWN.*

  M+F: *Town, yes*

    F:    *What town?*

    O:    <u>K.</u>

    F:    *Keytown, yes*

    M:    *Are you starting from Heyborne, I suppose you are?*

    O:    *NO.*

  M+F: *No.*

    F:    *Then you are taking the bus across I suppose.*

    O:    *YES.*

    M:    *Yes.*

       (Time elapsed, 0:40).

(2)    The current topic was where to stay.

    F:    *And then you are going to..*

    O:    *HOUSE.*

    M:    *A house.*

    O:    *STAY.*

    M:    *And see.*

    O:    *STAY.*

    M:    (Puts on her glasses) *You were going to stay in a house.*

    F:    *Where was that? You were going to stay at a nice place, weren't you? What did it say about that?*

    M:    *I don't remember.*

    F:    *Wasn't it hotel Terminus, or?*

    M:    *No.*

    F:    *What?*

    M:    *No, do you remember it yourself?*

    O:    *NO.*

    F:    (Uninterpretable)

    M:    *Are you staying at a hotel?*

    O:    Looks towards the camera and away.

       (Time elapsed, 0:46).

(3)    The current topic was what to do in Keytown.
       M:    *And then you will go to the fun fair? Don't you think so?*
       O:    *YES.*
       M:    *Yes, it is a big place there, believe me, it is much bigger than*
             *Globe fair.*
             (Time elapsed, 0:19).

(4)    The current topic was food.
       F:    (Makes noise with an information leaflet)
       M:    *Can you read it?*
       F:    *Yes, here, you are having lunch at the Valentino restaurant,*
             *menu, what are you going to eat, did you talk about that?*
       O:    *FOOD.*
       M:    *Food, yes*
       F:    *Yes, food, but what kind of food?*
       O:    *DO-NOT-KNOW.*
       M:    *Do not know.*
       F:    *Is it fish or meat?*
       O:    *FISH.*
       M:    *Fish.*
       F:    *Yes, that's right, plaice.*
       M:    *Do you like it? Who does not like it?*
       O:    *MOTHER.*
       M:    *Mother, yes.*
             (Time elapsed, 0:44).

(5)    The current topic was the participants at the excursion.
       M:    *Is Carl coming too?*
       O:    *YES.*
       M:    *Yes, Fanny?*
       O:    *YES.*
       M:    *Yes.*
       O:    *Y*
       M:    *Yvette too, yes.*
             (Time elapsed, 0:11).

(6)    The current topic was the address in Keytown.
       F:    *It's two days, yes.*
       M:    *Hm.*
       O:    (Points at figures)
       F:    *And then it says here that the address is Keytown Hotel*
             *21 Charles Street, Keytown. What address is that? It's the*
             *name of the youth hostel, isn't it?*
       O:    *YES.*
       M:    *Hm.*
             (Time elapsed, 0:22).

Sven had a communication book, and the parent turned the pages in the book. Sven pointed with a head light. The present conversation contained 479 turns and was the longest in the entire material about a single main topic. Sven's interaction with his mother was characterised by laborious work where his messages were brought to the surface and new information was communicated.

(7)    The current topic was choice of topic.
       M: *What are you going to tell now? Tell me first what you are
           going to talk about. Hm, have you decided?*
       S: (Coughs).
       M: *Shall I not turn, shall I turn?*
       S: 'No' (draws down the corners of his mouth).
       M: *No, you are going to be there, yes.*
       S: (Points at the letters).
       M: *Letters?*
       S: 'Yes' (draws up the corners of his mouth). M.
       M: *Mm, shall I turn now?*
       S: 'Yes' (mouth movements).
       M: (Turns the page). *Hm.*
       S: O.
       M: *Y?*
       S: 'No' (mouth movements).
       M: *No, letters?*
       S: 'Yes' (mouth movements) O.
       M: *O?*
       S: 'Yes' (mouth movements, looks to the left).
       M: *Hm, and then back?* (Turns the page).
       S: B.
       M: *Still b?*
       S: 'Yes' (mouth movements).
       M: *Was it that?*
       S: 'Yes' (mouth movements).
       M: *Yes, two?*
       S: 'Yes' (mouth movements).
       M: *Is it about bullying?* ('mobba' in Swedish).
       S: 'Yes' (mouth movements).
       M: (To the experimenter) *We usually to take chances when I
           know a little so that it doesn't take that long.*
           (Time elapsed, 1:06).

The subtopic of the next dialogue had been going on for about 110 turns without Sven having succeeded in conveying his message when the excerpt starts.

8)    The topic was a movie and suicide.
      M: *It must, hm, she tried to take OPPOSITE. No she tried to take*
          *LIVE? I do not understand, have you formulated this wrong or*
          *is it me that..?*
      S: (Bends his head down, searches) *SHE.*
      M: *She.*
      S: *WANT.*
      M: *Want, want, no.*
      S: Looks at mother.
      M: *Yes it was, want.*
      S: *DEAD.*
      M: *She wanted to die, yes, did she want to die?*
      S: 'Yes' (mouth movements).
      M: *She thought it was a hard time, but she didn't die, did she?*
      S: 'Yes' (mouth movements).
      M: *I misunderstood that previously, she thought it was a hard*
          *time so she wanted to die, yes. But what happened, she didn't*
          *die?*
      S: 'No' (mouth movements).
      M: *It was she herself, she wanted to die because she thought the*
          *bullying gave her a hard time, yes, that rings a bell, yes*
          (laughs).
      S: (Smiles) *Mm* (grunts).
      M: *Well, what happened then? Hm, how did it end?*
      S: (Makes a mouth) *Mm.*
      M: *What happened then, at the end, how did the movie end?*
      S: (Looks at mother, smiles).
      M: *It was settled at the end, at the same school, yes. So she stayed*
          *at the school?*
      S: (Looks at mother) *Ha.*
      M: *And the other ones, they changed their minds?*
      S: Continues to smile.
      M: *Yes.*
          (Time elapsed, 1:45).

The main topic of the conversation between Tina and her mother was
museums. In dialogue (9), Tina took several initiatives and successfully
conveyed many of her intentions. However, the most notable feature in
this dialogue is a misunderstanding.

(9)   The particular topic was a building called Fishchurch.
      T: *MUSEUM.*
      M: *Is there something you want to tell about what you have*
          *experienced?*
      T: *FISH.*

M: *About fish.*
T: *HOUSE.*
M: A house.
T: *GOD.*
M: *God, God's house, is that what you want to tell me about?*
T: *FISH.*
M: *Was there fish?*
T: Looks at mother.
M: *In the church?*
T: 'Yes' (nods).
M: *Do you mean last Sunday? Were there fish in that church in Smalltown?*
T: 'No' (mimics).
M: *No, is there something else?*
T: *BUS.*
M: *Bus.*
T: *FISH.*
M: *Did you go by bus to look at fish?*
T: *MUSEUM.*
M: *At a museum?*
T: *BIG.*
M: *Big.*
T: *FISH.*
M: *Big fish.*
(Time elapsed, 1:20).

(10)  The current topic was the location of the museum.
M: *Was it in Keytown?*
T: 'No' (mimics) *COUNTRY.*
M: *It was a country.*
T: <u>S.</u>
M: *Now, think, what country was it?*
T: <u>S.</u>
M: *Sweden.*
T: 'No' (mimics).
M: *No.*
T: <u>D.</u>
M: *Denmark, was that the excursion with the class, when you went to look at a museum with fish, was that what you were thinking about?*
(Time elapsed, 0:39).

(11)  The current topic was sharks at the museum.
T: *BIG.*
M: *Were they big?*
T: *FISH.*
M: *Fish*

T: H̲. (looks up at mother).

M: *Sharks, were there sharks?* ('haj' in Swedish).

T: 'Yes' (nods).

M: *Yes, were they alive?*

T: 'No' (mimics).

M: *No, that is good.*

T: Folds the right-hand part of the communication board.

M: *Don't you want to talk about sharks? But you were the one*
   *who started to talk about it.*

T: 'No' (mimics, looks at the camera).

M: *No, well then you can talk about something else.*
   (Time elapsed, 0:35).

For the conversations of Olof and Tina, the entire transcription for each topic was presented. For Sven, due to the length of the dialogues, only minor parts were presented. However, common to all three conversations is that the topics were closed and that the initiatives were taken by the speaking partner most of the time. The conversations were maintained by the speaking persons and the interpretative work was mainly done by them. The three non-speaking adolescents all had extended practice with Blissymbols and used them in the interaction, but Blissymbols were only used to a limited extent by all of them.

For Sven and Olof, the interactions were 'successful' in the sense that the parents and the adolescents reached a common understanding of what was meant. In the conversation between Tina and her mother, such a common understanding was not reached.

Sven's conversation was very long, not because much information was communicated during the exchange, but because it took a substantial amount of work to reach a common understanding of the different topics introduced by him. In this conversation both parties seemed determined to come to a common conclusion concerning what was meant, and they finally succeeded. This interaction was also characterised by Sven's consistent use of facial expressions to indicate 'yes' and 'no' or agreement and disagreement. Sven also used individual letters to a large extent, and the mother, as she said herself in the transcript, took short cuts by guessing. Blissymbols were rarely used in this interaction, in spite of the fact that the introduced topics were always closed with mutual understanding. Sven also obtained the highest scores on the Raven test. It is tempting to suggest that for Sven the Blissymbols were only one of several means of communication, including gestures, bodily movements and vocalisations, and he chose effectively among the communication possibilities. The mother was very active in suggesting interpretations and the two parties were engaged in an efficient collaborative process.

In the conversation between Tina and her mother, no common understanding was reached on one of the main points in Tina's message.

However, as external observers we were able to understand what was intended and can show what went wrong. A recurrent theme in the interaction was 'fish', both in the usual or literal sense, but also in a particular expression which the mother was not able to recognise. This was due, we would suggest, to a lack of relevant background knowledge (which we had), but also to Tina not being able to provide this knowledge. Tina wanted to tell her mother that she had visited a fish market. This fish market is located in a building known as the Fishchurch by the people in the town where it is situated. The mother was not familiar with this expression, the family lived far away from Tina's residential school, and the mother was therefore unable to understand the intended message.

Tina failed to get the message across by using the Blissymbols and finally gave up, indicated by her folding a part of the communication board. Ironically, the mother remarked that Tina did not seem inclined to continue, and somewhat reproachfully said that after all it was Tina who originally had suggested what to talk about. The situation might be described as Tina not being able to find a suitable metalevel of communication where she would have been able to explain and paraphrase her intended message. She obtained a low score on the Raven test, and her failure to use supplementary and inventive ways over and above the Blissymbols might perhaps be ascribed to limited cognitive resources.

Tina's situation was in contrast to that of Sven described above. Sven seemed to use Blissymbols as one of several communication possibilities and was able to establish a collaborative situation, together with his mother, which profited from his entire repertoire of communication acts. This impression is, of course, relative to Tina who did not turn to any supplementary means of expression when her communication board failed. Both had similar vocabularies of Blissymbols.

Olof was successful in his communication, but very different from Sven in the sense that much of the communication work was done by his parents who were very active in structuring the conversation and, most important, more or less knew the answers to the questions from the leaflet that described the excursion which Olof was going to take part in. The interaction resembled a lesson where the teacher knows the answers and mainly checks the student's knowledge. Some of the difference between Olof and Sven may be due to the fact that Olof communicated with both his parents while Sven communicated only with his mother. The number of participants in a conversation may influence the dynamics considerably.

## Conclusions

There is one general feature of the free interactions in the present study which stands out clearly and has been illustrated by the three conversations, namely, the amount of laborious collaborative work when considering the communication potential and capacities of the non-speaking adolescents in the structured tasks. These results pertain to all aspects of language use, not least to the discourse.

All the free dialogues were characterised by difficulties in establishing a conversational discourse where the non-speaking adolescents would take the initiative and not only react to the speaking persons' initiatives and suggestions for interpretation. Compared to the referential task, a main problem was to get access to relevant mutual knowledge (cf. Clark and Marshall, 1981) on the basis of what was communicated with Blissymbols and with spoken words. Alternatively, the topics introduced by the speaking person were trivial in the sense that the mutual knowledge was not used for any conversational 'work'. This was in contrast to what happened in the referential task where the relevant mutual knowledge was, in part, explicitly defined.

The picture that has become apparent is the result of a complex interaction between the characteristics of the communication system used (i.e. Blissymbolics), the non-speaking individuals, their learning history and experiences, and their speaking communication partners. The adolescents' experiences with face-to-face interaction had taught them to be passive, relatively speaking, in the interpretative work and, so it seemed, to provide minimal information before allowing the speaking person to start the interpretative work. It might be argued that this behaviour is in fact well adjusted to the communication situation, and fits with the general principles of spoken communication. Lindblom (1990) has emphasised the variability of spoken communication as an aspect of adequate adaptation to the demands of the situation, not least to the listener, and that consequently casual, informal, reduced pronunciation is a normal feature of talk in some situations but not in others.

The major difference between people who speak and the non-speaking adolescents in this study seems to be that the latter group varied their communication expressions only to a limited degree. They used very reduced forms of communication, remaining at one end of the continuum from reduced to overexplicit communication forms.

The communication patterns of the interactions between the adolescents and their parents confirm, on a general level, previous research (e.g. Light, 1988; Light et al., 1985a,b,c). Metacommunication was often explicit and the 'negotiation' of meaning (cf. Rommetveit, 1974) was painstakingly evident, but the explicitness is found almost exclusively among the parents, that is, among the speaking partners in the conversation. Also, the typically reported slow pace of interaction was found. The individual variation among the speaking conversation partners was nevertheless considerable. Some parents put less effort into the explicit interpretation work but tried to get the non-speaking adolescent to be more explicit in the communication.

The general conclusion, though, is that the discourse activities exhibited by the non-speaking adolescents in the spontaneous conversations did not exhibit to a full extent the potential shown in the structured settings of the experimental parts of the study. Maybe this is an adequate adaptation to the demands for a certain pace in the interaction, but it might also reflect that the adolescents lacked sufficient skills in applying their discourse knowledge.

The results raise questions concerning the everyday experiences of non-speaking people and the possibilities of instructional influence. Non-speaking people learn to rely on the speaking partners for much of the interactional work. This is to some extent rational. It makes the communication more rapid and in this sense more effective. An important question is, however, if, and when, this communication strategy may become detrimental for the non-speaking individual in the sense that initiatives are not taken and intentions not expressed because the relevant skills and knowledge are lacking.

## Acknowledgement

This study was financed by a grant from the Swedish Council for Social Research.

# Chapter 9
# A psycholinguistic approach to graphic language use

HANS VAN BALKOM AND MARGUERITE WELLE DONKER-GIMBRÈRE

The use of graphic language representation in augmented communication has only recently become the subject of more comprehensive investigation (Levelt, 1994). As a fledgling research field, it sorely lacks an accepted theoretical framework, and consequently a uniform approach to planning of assessment and intervention. This chapter explores the applicability of psycholinguistics as a theoretical framework to study graphic language representations in aided communication, and the way in which graphic signs are used in concept formation and message construction in particular. It will be argued that visual and linguistic information processing rely on similar mental, computational procedures, and that, due to this processing similarity, speech comprehension may somehow provide a ready entry for a syntactic learning process to use graphic signs in linguistically identifiable sequences. The application of psycholinguistic research in the area of aided communication, may contribute to a better understanding of the underlying mechanisms that non-speaking persons use to acquire language through graphic sign systems. It may also provide information about the structure and working principles of models that explain the normal speech communication process. Studies of natural and spontaneous compensation in aided communication may help to verify models of the processes involved in speech and language processing and performance and lead to the development and evaluation of intervention and assistive techniques.

Aided communication is in fact – first and foremost – language intervention; an area that needs a better theoretical basis in order to understand, explain, improve and evaluate the actual learning strategies of users and the intervention programmes that are supposed to teach such strategies.

## Psycholinguistics and graphic language use

Over the past four decades psycholinguistics has evolved as an influential field of study for the exploration of several domains of language:

structure, language processing (language and thought or mind), language use or function, first and second language acquisition or learning, and language pathology. Psycholinguistic research has developed through contributions from linguistics, neuropsychology and cognitive science. Psycholinguistics covers research in the areas of language production, language comprehension and language acquisition in typical and atypical circumstances within and across cultures (Fodor, Bever and Garrett, 1974). It is this broad orientation that makes the psycholinguistic perspective important for studies of augmentative and alternative communication in general, and graphic sign communication and intervention in particular. Within the scope of psycholinguistics and aided communication, there are three main research questions related to graphic language representations and interventions:

- What mental processes are involved in comprehending and learning graphic language representations?
- What mental processes are used to express meanings and intentions with graphic language representations?
- How do graphic sign users acquire language and literacy skills?

These three questions will be addressed in the two studies reported in this chapter. The first study focuses on the actual use of graphic signs in the Netherlands and North America. The second study addresses the issues of language performance and language competence of experienced graphic sign users.

## Linguistic constraints in graphic language use

The field of augmentative and alternative communication over the past decade has been influenced by a vast number of interaction studies and an emphasis on research on particular graphic sign characteristics in learning (Light, 1988, 1989; Sevcik, Romski and Wilkinson, 1991; van Balkom and Welle Donker-Gimbrère, 1994). These studies indicate striking differences in language performance, language competence and language development between graphic sign users and natural language users; for example in the organisation of turn exchanges, the number of initiations between communication partners and communication functions.

Most explanations suggested for these differences can be traced to the considerable obstacles graphic sign users meet in acquiring and learning the social and linguistic skills necessary for adequate retrieval of information from their communicative environment. These problems have mainly been attributed to limitations imposed by the individual's specific impairment (e.g. physical, cognitive or multiple), the characteristics of the communication aid and the sign system used. The studies of graphic symbol use indirectly led to an increased interest in research regarding the way in which graphic sign users acquire language and process information. The communication aid actually functions as a message-assembling and message-transmission device. The linguistic message itself consists of specific tokens (or graphic symbols; e.g. alphabetic characters, graphic signs or photographs), displayed on the input part of the communication aid (e.g. keyboard or chart with graphic signs). The study of the linguistic characteristics of these tokens has revealed important information relevant for research in processes of language comprehension and production, and language acquisition of non-speaking, aided communicators. The typology of the characteristics found provides information about the linguistic compensatory strategies and the specific constraints encountered in the use of graphic signs for message formation and communication.

This research is of primary interest to clinicians and educators because it may support the development, improvement and evaluation of intervention and language programmes. However, little is still known about how graphic signs are functionally utilised to represent meanings and intentions. The results of the two projects presented here may contribute to a better understanding of the psycholinguistic processes involved in aided communication.

## The use of graphic signs

During the eighties, graphic signs became more widely used in the Netherlands and Flanders. However, little was actually known about the people communicating with graphic signs and the systems they used, and a need for more knowledge had been expressed by funding agencies as well as user organisations. In January 1989, a study concerning the use of graphic signs in the Netherlands was initiated as part of a collaborative project by the Institute for Rehabilitation Research, Indiana State University and Purdue University (van Balkom and Welle Donker-Gimbrère, 1994; Welle-Donker Gimbrère and van Balkom, 1995; Welle Donker-Gimbrère, von Blom, van 't Hoofd and van Balkom, 1991).

The study, called Grasycom (Graphic Symbol Communication) set out to survey the actual use of graphic signs for communication, identify graphic sign characteristics, make an exploration survey of criteria used to describe graphic signs and underlying theories, and gain insight into the relevance of the various graphic sign characteristics for the users. In November 1991, the study was completed. Its results are of particular interest to professionals involved with improving assessment and intervention of augmentative and alternative communication through the use of graphic sign representations.

Table 9.1: Respondents in the Grasycom study (percentages in brackets).

| Facilities | N | Phoned | Use graphics | Participants | Returned |
|---|---|---|---|---|---|
| Habilitation and rehabilitation centres | 25 | 25 (100) | 23 (92) | 23 (100) | 21 (91) |
| Activity centres | 35 | 26 (74) | 6 (23) | 6 (100) | 5 (83) |
| Schools for physically disabled children | 30 | 15 (50) | 13 (87) | 13 (100) | 13 (100) |
| Schools for intellectually impaired children | 107 | 72 (67) | 43 (60) | 41 (95) | 26 (63) |
| Daycare centres for children | 107 | 60 (56) | 29 (48) | 28 (97) | 19 (68) |
| Institutions for intellectually impaired people | 152 | 40 (26) | 17 (43) | 17 (100) | 16 (94) |
| Group homes for physically impaired people | 40 | 39 (98) | 4 (10) | 4 (100) | 4 (100) |
| Daycare centres for intellectually impaired people | 210 | 44 (21) | 20 (45) | 19 (95) | 12 (63) |
| Nursing homes | 341 | 39 (11) | 26 (67) | 25 (96) | 19 (76) |
| Diagnostic teaching settings | 4 | 1 (25) | 1 (100) | 1 (100) | 0 (0) |
| Total | 1051 | 361 (34) | 182 (50) | 177 (97) | 135 (76) |

## Method

Information was gathered by means of telephone interviews, written questionnaires and structured personal interviews. Five different questionnaires for five kinds of respondents were constructed, targeting:

- developers of graphic sign representations (N = 50, respondents N = 15);
- speech therapists working with graphic signs (N = 182);
- speech therapists working with a primary user. Both the therapist and the aid user took part in personal interviews (N = 175, respondents N = 139);
- users of graphic signs, to take part in personal interviews (N = 135);
- communication partners of the aid users selected. The communication partners were also asked to take part in the personal interview session (N = 135).

The telephone interviews, combined with the first two types of questionnaires, provided general information concerning the types of graphic signs used. The other three questionnaires, combined with personal interviews, provided information about individual communicative practice and graphic sign intervention.

## Results

Possible graphic sign systems (or collections or sets) were identified by telephone interviews of 363 randomly chosen facilities out of 1051 possible sites in the Netherlands (see Table 9.1). These facilities comprised special schools, daycare centres, habilitation and rehabilitation centres, institutions for people with intellectual impairment, nursing homes and group homes. Approximately half (182) of the facilities reported that they used graphic signs to assist communication for their clients or students.

A questionnaire was sent to the 177 facilities who in the telephone interview had indicated that they used graphic signs. A total of 135 questionnaires (76%) were returned. The answers showed that the population using graphic signs was extremely diverse in age, cognitive, linguistic and physical abilities, and that the use of graphic signs was equally varied. For some, the graphic signs were the only means of communication (temporary or permanent). For others, the graphic systems functioned as didactic tools, stimulation for communication, assistive devices for oral expression, indicators for activities (calendar), and alternatives to reading. Typically 1–3 out of a group of 12–15 clients would depend on graphic signs for face-to-face communication.

The decisive factor stated for introducing graphic signs was usually severe motor impairment and poor prognosis for speech. The decision to introduce graphic signs as the primary means for communication appeared to be made with some hesitation as 0–3-year-olds and 3–6-year-olds were under-represented in the Netherlands, compared to reported use in North America (Welle Donker-Gimbrère et al., 1991). Graphic signs were often described as a last resort.

## Systems

A total of 34 documented graphic sign systems have been identified in the Netherlands. Yet the clinicians were on the average well acquainted with two or three systems, while using only one, or occasionally two. Mostly they used self-made graphic signs, obtained from advertisements, illustrations in magazines, packing materials and the like. Best known in the Netherlands were Blissymbolics, Taalzakboek (pictures and word lists, mainly meant for people with aphasia) and Picto, which turned out to be a generic term for several pictographic sets (see Introduction). Recently, an increase has occurred in the use of the Vijfhoek Pictogrammen Systeem (based on PIC), Bèta-prenten and PCS. Rebus was not reported to be used.

Among the developers of graphic sign systems, transparency and visual clarity were the most frequently mentioned design characteristics. The degree of transparency tended to be overrated, though. Only a minority of the developers provided instructions, guidelines or rules for expanding the original graphic sign lexicon.

The graphic sign users in this study communicated with the help of eight different sign systems: Blissymbolics (11), Vijfhoekpictogrammen (2), Picsyms (4), Maria Roepaan Beeldlezen (pictographic reading system) (5), Van Geijtenbeek Beeldplaatjes (pictographic images) (5), Beeldtaal (pictographic language) (3), Taalzakboek (Language book or folder with pictures and words) (10) and 'Grafisch Gesprek' (graphic conversation, based on finger spelling) (2) (cf. Welle Donker-Gimbrère and van Balkom, 1995).

## Communicative use

Structured interviews were conducted with each of the 42 users of the five most widely used graphic sign systems, their speech therapist and a significant communication partner, in order to obtain information concerning their physical, cognitive and linguistic abilities and skills, vocabularies, modes of expression and preferences with regard to graphic signs. The group of graphic sign users comprised people with severe motor impairments (congenital and acquired); people with normal cognitive abilities and with moderate to profound intellectual impairment, with and without accompanying physical impairments; people with hearing impairments; people with acquired language impairments like aphasia; and people with multiple impairments. Their ages ranged from nearly 4 to 87 years.

In spite of the diversity in graphic signs described above, the communication had a number of typical features. With the exception of one person, all the graphic sign users could understand the spoken language of their environment. A large majority never combined elements of the graphic signs in order to create meanings they lacked in their sign lexicon (cf. von Tetzchner and Martinsen, this volume). Even the most expert users had access to a relatively restricted vocabulary of approximately 1000 graphic signs, while some vocabularies contained only a few dozen signs.

The vocabularies were thus very restricted compared to the 20.000 or so different words that make up the spoken vocabulary of an adult, the 5000 words of the average five-year-old, or the 3000 words considered essential to talk about everyday occurrences in a foreign language (Bloom and Lahey, 1978; Schaerlaekens and Gillis, 1987). The graphic sign lexicons contained a large proportion of content words and very few graphic signs would allow utterances to be syntactically structured. More than half of the respondents produced messages that on average did not exceed two graphic signs in length (cf. Collins, this volume; von Tetzchner and Martinsen, this volume). When required to choose between graphic signs with varying characteristics, the users' choices differed markedly from those made by their clinicians and communication partners (Figure 9.1). Most noticeable were a preference for realism, detail and colour, and a lack of governing rules, across intellectual ability, age and the current graphic sign system used.

There was little overlap between the graphic sign lexicons of the users, even within the groups that used the same graphic sign system. All graphic sign users were in fact multimodal communicators.

## Discussion

Though many of these communicative characteristics in isolation might be explained by motor restrictions or time pressure on the side of the user, they do suggest a lack of overall organisation, either cognitive or linguistic. These tendencies may have been exacerbated by the training approach which predominated at the time, which emphasised use of single sign-concept associations. Since the time of the survey, the situation may have changed in the Netherlands through a heightened awareness of augmentative and alternative communication and the implementation of early intervention programmes including alternative communication forms (cf. Heim and Baker-Mills, this volume). Still, in order to achieve graphic sign intervention parallel to normal language

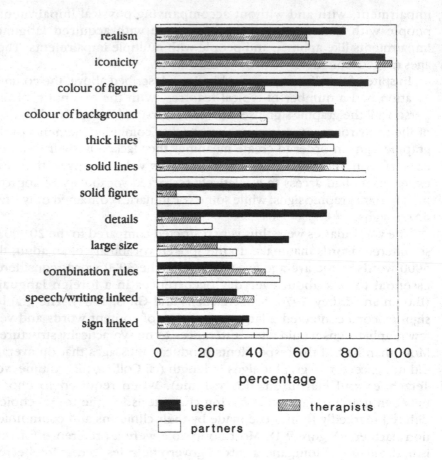

**Figure 9.1** Preferred characteristics of graphic signs according to users, speech therapists and communication partners

development, more in-depth studies are needed of the linguistic characteristics of graphic sign performance in diverse situations with various degrees of structure, across different languages and age groups. The Grasycom study actually did provide basic user-oriented information about the daily use of graphic signs, derived from a cross-cultural and cross-linguistic perspective. The next section presents a pilot for forthcoming in-depth studies of the linguistic characteristics of graphic sign use.

## Linguistic performance in graphic sign use

In order to realise any communicative intention, language users must create messages whose expression will effectively reveal their intentions. According to Levelt (1989, 1994) a message is *not* the utterance or otherwise linguistically realised output, but some mental, conceptual representation still to be formulated, still to be expressed in a representational language form. This implies that a hearing person with a speech or language disorder who understands spoken language and uses a visual language representation (manual or graphic signs) as an alternative expressive means, develops a receptive capacity for spoken language. Through this receptive capacity word meanings (mental concepts) may then be translated or coded into visual signs, and the visual language representations function as codes for spoken language. Seen from that perspective, graphic sign users have developed a linguistic compensation technique (through their graphic signs) for their incapacity to speak. Graphic sign users in fact behave as natural language users. Hypothetically, one may therefore presume that they process incoming linguistic information similarly to speaking persons but are restricted in language output due to the limited linguistic resources of their communication aids (cf. also von Tetzchner et al., this volume).

Studies of the spontaneous language output of non-speaking graphic sign users may reveal significant characteristics of the linguistic strategies they employ in message creation. However, this graphic sign output should not be elicited through spoken input (e.g. by asking question, story retelling task, etc.). Elicitation techniques based on spoken language require auditory processing and thus prepare or frame lexical access, word-finding and formation of meaning in the mind of the graphic sign user. Hence, non-verbal elicitation tasks based on graphic input should be used for spontaneous production of messages in graphic signs. This non-verbal elicitation technique offers better opportunities for discovering the specific characteristics of linguistic strategies used by non-speaking graphic sign users in the mental process of concept and message creation (cf. Cromer, 1991; van Balkom and Welle Donker-Gimbrère, 1994). In-depth studies of the linguistic characteristics of typical and atypical performance may enhance the understanding of the ways in which language is represented in the minds of non-speaking communication aid users, and addressed more specifically:

- the development of methods and techniques for assessing language comprehension in non-speaking persons;
- the development of intervention programmes for language acquisition and language learning (e.g. literacy);
- the development of a new generation of communication aids based on language engineering (e.g. prediction techniques, semantic compaction and automatised techniques for transducing restricted language input into text or synthesised speech).

## Method

The four adolescents with cerebral palsy, Danny, Berny, Angela and Charly, were experienced graphic sign users. They were video recorded at a school for children with cerebral palsy in Philadelphia while they were describing pictures in a children's book to their primary speech therapists, using their own communication boards with graphic signs (cf. Table 9.3). The book contained pictures that could be retold with the graphic signs of the four students. The students were selected because they were experienced graphic sign users.

Each student was instructed to describe the pictures as if telling a story to younger children. The speech therapist was instructed to repeat each word as it was selected by the student, paraphrase the sentence when it was completed, and then ask the student to confirm the paraphrased sentence. A single camera was used to videotape both student and speech therapist (cf. McCoy et al., 1994; Vanderheyden et al., 1994).

## Transcription

The graphic sign users actually combined vocalisations, gestures and graphic signs in multimodal messages. In order to capture as much as possible of this multimodal content the transcriptions comprised vocal productions (words and non-words), hand and arm gestures (pointing and miscellaneous gestures), facial expressions (eye contact, agreeing and disagreeing) and head gestures (nodding, shaking and looking elsewhere). However, in the examples below, only the graphic signs of the messages are presented.

## Graphic sign vocabulary

The number of graphic signs on the communication boards of the four students varied from 215 to 400. One hundred and fifty graphic signs appeared on all four communication aids. These 150 graphic signs had been used to check for the students' possibility of retelling the content of the picture book (Table 9.2).

## Results

The four students took between 11 minutes and one hour to retell their stories. The total number of graphic sign messages used to retell the stories of 11 pictures in the picture book was 104. The average was 26 messages (range 14–38). A total number of 202 graphic signs was used to produce the 104 messages, an average of about 2 graphic signs per message. The speech therapists produced the same number of paraphrases, but inserted more words. The total number of words used in the 104 paraphrased messages was 769 (range 79–255), an average of about seven words per paraphrase (see Table 9.3 for individual results). Table 9.4 shows the frequencies of the main categories of content words and function words used by the four students.

Table 9.2: Graphic signs available to all four students

**People**

| | | | |
|---|---|---|---|
| *BABY* | *BOY* | *DADDY/FATHER* | *DOCTOR* |
| *FRIEND* | *GIRL* | *I* | *JILL* |
| *MAN* | *NURSE* | *MUMMY/MOTHER* | *TEACHER* |
| *THERAPIST* | *WOMAN* | | |

**Verbs and activities**

| | | | |
|---|---|---|---|
| *BE* | *BREAK* | *COOK* | *DRAW* |
| *DRINK* | *EAT* | *FIX* | *GIVE* |
| *GO* | *HAVE* | *HELP* | *KNOW* |
| *LOSE* | *LOVE* | *MAKE* | *OPEN* |
| *PAINT* | *PLAY* | *WANT* | *WASH* |
| *WORK* | *WRITE* | *COME* | |

**Adjectives and prepositions**

| | | | |
|---|---|---|---|
| *ANGRY* | *BAD* | *CLEAN* | *HOT* |
| *DOWN* | *GOOD* | *HAPPY* | *NEW* |
| *IN* | *LITTLE* | *MORE* | *UP* |
| *OFF* | *ON* | *SICK* | *WET* |

**Objects**

| | | | |
|---|---|---|---|
| *ARM* | *BED* | *BOOK* | *BREAD* |
| *CAR* | *EAR* | *EYE* | *FACE* |
| *FOOT* | *HAND* | *ICE/ICE-CREAM* | *JUICE* |
| *LEG* | *LETTER* | *MUSIC/CD/TAPE* | *ORANGE* |
| *PAPER* | *PENCIL* | *PEANUT-BUTTER* | *PIZZA* |
| *SHOE* | *TABLE* | *TELEVISION* | *WATER* |

**Places**

| | | | |
|---|---|---|---|
| *BATHROOM* | *BEDROOM* | *DINING-ROOM* | *HOME* |
| *OT-ROOM* | *OUTSIDE* | *PT-ROOM* | *PARTY* |
| *PLAYROOM* | *ST-ROOM* | *SCHOOL* | *STORE* |

**Time**

| | | | |
|---|---|---|---|
| *AFTERNOON* | *BIRTHDAY* | *HOLIDAY* | *MORNING* |
| *NIGHT* | *MONDAY* | *TUESDAY* | *WEDNESDAY* |
| *THURSDAY* | *FRIDAY* | *SATURDAY* | *SUNDAY* |
| *TODAY* | *TOMORROW* | *YESTERDAY* | |

**Question words**

| | | | |
|---|---|---|---|
| *WHAT* | *WHEN* | *WHERE* | *WHO* |
| *WHY* | | | |

**Phrases**

| | | |
|---|---|---|
| *I DON'T KNOW* | *PLEASE* | *THANK YOU* |

Table 9.3: Student and speech therapist productions

| System | Danny Single words | Berry PCS, Single Words | Angela Oakland Rebus Single Words | Charly Oakland Rebus Single words |
|---|---|---|---|---|
| Vocabulary | 352 | 252 | 413 | 352 |
| Total signs used (tokens) | 182 | 125 | 119 | 36 |
| Different signs used (types) | 64 | 66 | 46 | 26 |
| Per cent used | 18.2 | 26.2 | 11.1 | 7.4 |
| Type-token ratio | 0.4 | 0.5 | 0.4 | 0.7 |
| Mean length of message | 6.1 | 3.3 | 5.4 | 2.6 |
| | Therapist of Danny | Therapist of Berry | Therapist of Angela | Therapist of Charly |
| Total words used (tokens) | 255 | 229 | 206 | 79 |
| Different words used (types) | 83 | 96 | 80 | 46 |
| Type-token ratio | 0.3 | 0.4 | 0.4 | 0.6 |
| Paraphrases | 30 | 38 | 22 | 14 |
| Mean length of utterance | 8.5 | 6.0 | 9.4 | 5.7 |

Transcripts of graphic sign representations produced by the four students are described in order to uncover linguistic strategies in the sequencing of graphic signs to achieve interpretable messages or sentence types. In the examples, 'S' refers to the student, 'T' to the speech therapist. Three aspects of the graphic sign output will be discussed: word order deviations, phrase structure characteristics and meta-linguistic skills. In addition, the interaction strategies of the conversation partner and their use of the extra-linguistic context are discussed. Adjustments and insertions in the speech therapists' paraphrases are underlined (for other notations, see Table 0.1).

## Word order deviations

There were two kinds of word order deviations: 'One position deviations' comprise one-word or two-word positions in one syntactic clause or between words of two syntactic clauses. 'Multiple position deviations' comprise the crossing of several word positions in various syntactic clauses. (1) and (2) are examples of one position deviations:

(1)    S:  *BOY WILL PUSH TO STORE GIRL.*
       T:  *The* boy will push the girl to the store.
(2)    S:  *CLEAN GIRL MUMMY DESK.*
       T:  *They* (girl and mummy) *clean the* desk.

Examples (3) and (4) show multiple position deviations:

(3)    S:  *GIRL BLUE BOX HELP BOY IN SHOPPING CAR.*
       T:  *The* girl helps the boy putting the blue box in the shopping-car.
(4)    S:  *TWO BED SLEEP BOY ONE GIRL WHITE BED BROWN BED.*
       T:  *The* boy and the girl are sleeping *in* two beds; one in a white and the other in a brown bed.

## Phrase structure characteristics

The majority of the graphic sign messages were characterised by a succession of nouns. The four students made a total of 462 graphic sign selections, and 336 of these (73%) consisted of nouns. The nouns occurred in both subject and object positions, as in (5) and (6):

(5)    S:  *MUMMY GIRL SHOES.*
       T:  *Mummy is helping the* girl with her shoes.
(6)    S:  *BOY GIRL BREAD CHEESE SANDWICH.*
       T:  *The* boy and the girl are making bread, a cheese sandwich.

Table 9.4: Frequency of word categories used

| Frequency of word categories used | |
|---|---|
| Action verbs | 70 |
| Auxiliary verbs | 7 |
| Adverbs | 25 |
| Nouns | 336 |
| Adjectives | 11 |
| Pronouns | 10 |
| Prepositions | 42 |
| Negations | 5 |
| Conjunctions | 11 |

In some cases a noun or a combination of nouns was used in a position marked for an action verb, as in (7), or circumscribed an action verb, as in (8) and (9):

(7)   S:  *GIRL GREEN GRASS WATER.*
       T:  <u>The</u> girl water<u>s</u> <u>the</u> grass <u>for it to be</u> green.
(8)   S:  *FOOD WATER MUMMY HOT STOVE.*
       T:  *Mummy <u>uses</u>* water <u>to cook.</u>
(9)   S:  *GIRL STORE EAT MONEY FOR.*
       T:  *<u>The</u>* girl <u>pays</u> money for <u>the food in the</u> store.

### Meta-linguistic skills

The graphic sign users demonstrated overt meta-linguistic skills in some of their messages. These meta-linguistic skills were made explicit through self corrections, repetitions of self, and semantic bypasses.

    Self corrections and repetitions of self are explicit strategies for correcting or repeating a previously indicated graphic sign (the erroneous sign is put in brackets []).

(10)  S:  *[COOKIES] PIE GIRL.*
       T:  *<u>The</u> girl <u>is making a</u> pie.*
(11)  S:  *BOY [BAG BROWN] MAKE BREAD.*
       T:  *<u>The</u> boy make<u>s</u> <u>a sandwich.</u>*
(12)  S:  *GIRL [SIT] IN A GREEN OPPOSITE-OF SIT.*
       T:  *<u>The</u> girl <u>is standing on the</u> green.*

Semantic bypasses were used to overcome semantic restrictions in the graphic sign vocabulary. These consisted mainly of paraphrases or analogies of the meaning of graphic signs not available on the communication board.

(13)   S:   *PUT CLOTHES IN MOTHER A WASH WALL.*
         T:   *The* mother puts clothes in the washing machine.
(14)   S:   *GIRL MAKE BREAD BOY MAKE WHITE FOOD.*
         T:   *The* girl makes the toast and the boy makes the eggs.
(15)   S:   *GIRL PUT CLOTHES OPPOSITE-OF GREEN.*
         T:   *The* girl is putting the clothes on the clothesline.

## Partner strategies

The examples presented above also indicate some of the strategies used by the speech therapists to enhance and interpret the students' sign sequences in their paraphrases (cf. also McCoy et al., 1994). Among the most frequently used strategies were word order adjustments and conceptual or semantic inferences.

(16)   S:   *BOY GIRL STORE GO HOME.*
         T:   *The* boy and the girl were in the store and go back home now.

In (16) the speech therapist inserted the verb to be in past tense, *were*, the conjunction *and*, the determiner *the*, the preposition *in*, and the adverbs *back* and *now*. The paraphrase was framed in Subject-Verb-Object (SVO) word order. The fact that they knew the picture books actually helped the speech therapists to interpret the graphic sign sentence and transduce it into a correct and fully specified spoken sentence. The four speech therapists mostly used the SVO order of the graphic sign sentences to interpret and to build their paraphrases. This SVO standard rule for paraphrasing seemed to be very robust. Graphic sign sentences that deviated from this word order were mostly changed into an SVO word order (see the examples above).

## The extra-linguistic context

In order to study the role of extra-linguistic contextual information in the interpretation process, five interpreters were given a random selection of 30 transcribed graphic sign messages, without the paraphrases of the speech therapists and without information about the picture described. The informants were asked to convert the graphic sign messages into grammatically correct sentences. The results of this small study indicated that 108 (72%) of the 150 interpretations were semantically identical to the paraphrases provided by the original speech therapists. This high percentage of correct interpretations might be attributed to the semantic redundancy framed in the sequences of content words, especially of nouns.

# Discussion

The discussion of the results from these studies addresses linguistic issues regarding the meaning of words as they may be used in the selection and processing of graphic signs in augmentative and alternative communication.

### Inferences based on literal meaning

The graphic sign vocabularies on the communication boards of the students were limited in size and variety. Their output was semantically restricted, indicating that limited access to lexical items might have made it difficult for them to match a conceptually framed message in the mind with a message of graphic signs. As indicated earlier, the process of selecting graphic signs approximating as much as possible to a conceptually framed meaning may sometimes lead to semantically strange selections of graphic signs (or semantic bypasses). The speech therapists were quite successful in arriving at or guessing the correct interpretation, as evidenced by explicit confirmations given by the students.

The speech therapists seemed to use a conceptually based inferencing process. However, their interpretations were, at least partially, based on extra-linguistic, contextual knowledge, about the picture book and the associated description task. It is also likely that the high proportion of content words offered redundant semantic information which facilitated correct interpretations.

These kinds of interpretation strategies have been studied in more detail within the area of linguistic semantics (e.g. Frawley, 1992). Linguistic semantics is concerned with literal, decontextualised meaning. Literal meaning is determinable outside of context; it comes with its own set of facts. Its opposite is implicational meaning, which is not so decidable; everything must be calculated by the interpreter, working from the expression in relation to perceived intentions and circumstances.

Implicational meaning is thus said to be contextualised. The issue of literal meaning helps explain the way in which graphic sign users conceptually plan their messages, on the basis of which communication partners interpret the telegraphic messages. Literal, decontextualised meaning is associated with the grammatical structure of language. Grammatical structure exists, similar to literal meaning, outside the contexts in which it is used. This association of literal meaning was used in the paraphrases of the speech therapists and the interpretations given by the five new interpreters. Apparently, the propositional content of the graphic sign sequences provided sufficient literal meaning to infer correct interpretations. Almost all paraphrases and interpretations were in SVO word order. Interpretations were probably based on the predominant grammatical knowledge that the subject frequently (but not always) correlates with the actual actor, generally precedes the verb (frequently, however not always), which in turn usually precedes the object, which frequently (but not always) denotes the actual receiver or beneficiary. The robustness of this association between literal meaning and grammatical structure is applicable to almost every natural language, as well as languages in which formal facts differ and word order matters less (Frawley, 1992).

## The meaning of nouns

According to Langacker (1987a) 'a noun ... is a symbolic structure whose semantic pole instantiates the schema [THING]; or ... a noun designates a thing' (p. 189). Jackendoff (1989) indicates that the projected (perceived) world is clearly divided into things and entities with certain kinds of spatial and temporal integrity. Nouns are encoded as the most temporally stable, verbs as the least temporally stable, and adjectives in between (Givón, 1984). Givón further observes that whereas all languages have both concrete and abstract nouns, the latter are always derived, usually from verbs.

Frawley (1992) suggests that the basic noun in any language is that which encodes physically anchored, spatially bound entities. In contrast, verbs typically have existence only in time and denote dynamic, temporal relations. These 'temporal' and 'non-temporal' domains polarise experience and map respectively onto the major class division in languages: verbs and nouns. Nouns denote more non-temporal, more concrete, stable relations, and according to Givón (1984) and Langacker (1987a,b), this explains why nouns are remembered better, acquired earlier, translated more easily from language to language, less subject to encoding variability across languages, and more stable under paraphrase. The internal stability of nouns allows them to be relatively immune to linguistic context. These conclusions also get some support from cross-cultural and cross-linguistic child language studies (Bates, Bretherton and Snyder, 1988). The acquisition and use of nouns versus verbs and syntax have also been discussed by Armstrong, Stokoe and Wilcox (1995) and Johnson-Laird (1993). They argue for the prerequisite of experiential learning and visual-spatial processing of movement patterns for the development of syntax. The meaning of verbs especially seems to depend on the acquisition of dynamic, temporal entities.

These theoretical notions about nouns and verbs indicate that the typical motor disabilities and associated visual-spatial problems of the majority of non-speaking persons might limit a successful development of the prerequisites for language and syntax learning. Nouns seem to be easier to learn, to use and to acquire than verbs, adverbs, adjectives and prepositions. The function of adjectives and sometimes of action-verbs seems to be taken up by the nouns. The speech therapists nearly always produced the nouns denoted by the students' graphic sign in the same order in their paraphrases. The examples in which the students marked nouns as action verbs and the ways in which the students used their meta-linguistic skills to correct nouns and invent semantic bypasses seem to give support to the notion that nouns are easier than verbs. However, the lack of in-depth studies of language productions of non-speaking, graphic sign users makes these statements intuitive and subjective.

## Parallel processing of language representations

Most graphic sign users have limited opportunities for getting involved in social discourse and various discourse situations. This implies that they have little access to new information, and therefore also have difficulties with the formation of new concepts and elaborated conceptual meanings. Besides these limited opportunities to interact, graphic sign users have to represent their knowledge in the form of an artificial and restricted form of language representation. Graphic signs might not be related to the (innate) knowledge of the language faculty in the same way as speech and manual signs.

This could mean that graphic sign users have to learn two different forms of language representation simultaneously; the speech-auditory language representation (receptive language) and the graphic-visual form of representation (expressive language). A possible mismatch in language representations can occur, necessitating the implementation of a mental translation process, which may function along the lines of Jackendoff's proposal for visual and linguistic processing. However, this translation process would imply a continuous extra mental load on the graphic sign user. Besides that, the graphic sign user is also constrained in ways to create novel messages due to having a restricted number of graphic signs available on his communication device and possibly due to a lack of linguistic and communicative competence and experiences. The proportion of graphic signs actually used in the pilot study varied from 7.39 to 26.19 per cent, indicating little variation in sign categories used. (Type-token ratios varied between 0.35 and 0.72). Further research is needed in order to sort out the possible effects of these constraints on the cognitive and linguistic development of graphic sign users. Cross-linguistic and cross-cultural studies of environmental input of information to graphic sign users through different media may increase the knowledge about how graphic sign users in different language communities generally retrieve information and develop conceptual knowledge from speech-auditory language representations mapped on to graphic-visual forms of representation.

# Chapter 10
# Being an interesting conversation partner

NORMAN ALM AND ALAN F. NEWELL

The development of electronic devices and computer-based systems to provide aided communication for non-speaking people has led to improvements in the quality of synthetic speech, and the ease of use of the interface. Manufacturers and researchers continue to seek out new methods for improving the effectiveness and efficiency of operation of these systems. The problem remains, however, that most aided communicators have significant difficulty in taking part satisfyingly in social interactions (Blackstone, 1991; Merchen, 1990; Murphy, Collins and Moodie, 1994). One reason for this is that, in order to allow communication to take place successfully, the aided communicator's conversation partners must alter the conversational rule that participants take equal shares of the conversation.

## The effort in partnering an augmented speaker in conversation

Where a word and letter board is in use, the board user's conversation partner typically employs extensive context knowledge in order to expand very abbreviated messages from the board user into a full utterance. The development of electronic and computer-based speech output versions of word and letter boards has given users more independence in actually creating the message, but often fairly cryptic short messages are produced, because of the slowness and difficulty in constructing them. These must then be interpreted by the other person, using context knowledge. This, of course, makes good use of the listener's human ability to perceive context, and apply it to guessing what the communication may be, a task which is still far beyond the capabilities of computers.

All conversations involve the participants using context knowledge to infer meaning in what is being said. With aided communication, however, the balance is very unevenly tipped. The aided communicator's conversation partners must take responsibility not only for their own contribution, but also, to a large extent, for the augmented communicator's successful participation. Strategies which are employed include guessing words from initial letters, guessing sentences from initial words, and formulating full sentences from telegraphic output by the aided communicator. An example which shows all three strategies is given below. It is taken from a transcript, recorded by one of the authors, of a conversation held between a person, Adam, using a word-board, and a speaking conversation partner, Charles (see Table 0.1 for notations).

(1)    Adam is describing a swimming competition he has just returned
       from in Malta, using a letter and word board.
       A:   I at M-A.
       C:   *At the competition in Malta?*
       A:   'Yes' (indicated with vocalisation and facial expression).
            Brown W-I-N.
       C:   *You won a medal? A bronze medal?*
       A:   Yes' (indicated with vocalisation and facial expression).
            In 1-0-0.
       C:   *In the 100 metres.*
       A:   B-A.
       C:   *Backstroke?*
       A:   'Yes' (indicated with vocalisation and facial expression).

A notable feature of this example is the non-speaking person leading the direction of the conversation. This is, in fact, not typical of aided communication. In addition to reliance on a speaking conversation partner for expanding most contributions, a non-speaking person's communicative output typically consists of responses to questions (Light, 1988; Merchen, 1990; von Tetzchner and Martinsen, this volume).

It has been argued that it is up to the speaking conversation partners to make the necessary adjustments to allow for satisfying interaction. This point appeals on the basis of human rights, and certainly, all might hope that more accommodation could be made for non-speaking people by speaking people. Those who are very close to non-speaking people can provide this level of commitment to making the communication process work, but the experience of people who cannot speak is often that their social world is largely restricted to family and paid carers (Murphy, Collins and Moodie, 1994).

It has been pointed out that the very difficulty which requires collaboration in constructing communication can be seen as a positive, engaging experience by communication partners. Collins (1994) argues that 'the challenge ... is potentially motivating for both participants' (p. 27). Similarly, Kraat (1985) has pointed out that successful augmented communication may need to be judged in relation to its effectiveness, and not in comparison with unimpaired conversation. However, this does raise the question of how many potential conversation partners can be relied upon to have the level of commitment and competence which this approach requires.

In any case, relying entirely on an increased effort by all potential speaking partners is unlikely to be a successful strategy. As will be described below, interaction between people is something which already requires considerable effort on all sides. This is generally true for all interactions between natural speakers. Interaction is not something which 'just happens'. It is prepared for, engineered, and guided by the participants throughout.

## Interaction as work

Most people acquire the skills necessary for successful interaction from birth to early adolescence, and then use them automatically, without giving them conscious attention. The mechanisms and the very real work involved in interaction become apparent however when a problem emerges in an interaction, and the participants must decide how best to cope with it. For instance, as a general rule, silences in a conversation carry a negative implication (Newman, 1982; Tannen and Saville-Troike, 1985). When a silence is too long, therefore, participants notice the problem, and, in deciding what to do about it, become aware of the normally non-conscious rule that conversations ideally move smoothly from topic to topic in an organised way. They might therefore begin to think about the topics which have just been discussed, and to search for another contribution to make which is relevant. Or they might settle for a topic which is not relevant, but which is otherwise suitable, and preface its introduction with an apologetic statement that they know they are breaking the usual rule, such as *Oh, on a completely different subject* ....

Since interpersonal interaction takes significant effort individuals choose to interact or not with another person partly on the basis of how much effort it will be, sometimes saying *I saw _____ but I just didn't have the energy to deal with her today, so I made sure she didn't see me.* Interaction with others also produces a degree of stress. Even the arrival of another person into one's awareness can cause a measurable response, an increased stress level due to having to prepare for the effort of interacting.

Interacting with others can often seem relatively easy, but there is never a complete lack of effort. The rewards outweigh the effort expended, but people will sometimes need to calculate whether the effort needed to interact out-weighs the benefits resulting from it. Part of the work involved results from taking responsibility for keeping the communication partners interested in, and, if appropriate, enjoying, the conversation. Humour can play a large part here, particularly in informal conversations, which usually need to be entertaining. Much of our story-telling consists of events which the speaker hopes the listeners will find amusing. As well as humour, shock or surprise may be the expected reaction to a story being relayed, or perhaps mutual condemnation of another's actions. These are all attention-getting and interest-holding devices. They are employed because the speaker takes responsibility for holding the listener's interest.

Where does this leave the aided communicator? It has been noted that people interacting with communication system users must do more work to make the interaction possible, and they can generally expect less of the usual 'rewards' from the conversation, given the non-speaking person's obvious difficulties. Clearly there are occasions, such as intimate discussions about matters of great importance between people who know each other well, where the strength of the encounter means that all the above considerations are not necessary. People are prepared to make an effort for high points or crises, but non-speaking people can easily be left out of the everyday social communicative world which most people are immersed in most of the time (McGregor, 1991).

Goffman (1959, 1963) demonstrated that these everyday, continual encounters are extremely important. A person's very concept of self is bound up with their social persona which is projected out to the world through each day, through interacting with a wide variety of people. It is not enough for people to have interactions with family and close friends. The roles which they play out on the wider public stage every day are vital in establishing people as valid participants in the social environment.

## Social identity is mainly created through casual conversation

Individuals spend a great deal of conversational time presenting and then maintaining a social 'front', that is, a consistent presentation of self in the way the person would like to be perceived by others:

> 'When an individual appears before others, he knowingly and unwittingly projects a definition of the situation, of which a conception of himself is an important part' (Goffman, 1959, p. 213).

Goffman calls the skills and techniques used to accomplish this the 'arts of impression management'. These skills are more often called for with strangers. When with family and close friends, it is possible to relax and be less concerned with this. However, the fact is that for most people a great deal of their daily interaction takes place outside this close circle. Using theatrical terms to describe interaction:

'The more information the audience has about the performer, the less likely it is that anything they learn during the interaction will radically influence them. On the other hand, where no prior information is possessed, it may be expected that the information gleaned during the interaction will be relatively crucial' (Goffman, 1959, pp. 195-196).

Each person carries, from interaction to interaction, a definition of self which is affected by all their social contacts. When someone does not fulfil expectations in a social encounter this is a cause of discomfort in others:

'.. the social interaction ... may come to an embarrassed and confused halt; the situation may cease to be defined ... and participants may find themselves without a charted course of action' (Goffman, 1959, pp. 213-214).

If this failure is a chronic one, it can have serious consequences for that person's ability to be socially effective. When someone is unable to project accurately a social identity, this will tend to lead to them being reduced in the minds of others from the position of being a whole person, to a discounted position. A consequence, which will be recognised by people with physical impairments, is that others will 'tend to impute a wide range of imperfections on the basis of the original one, and at the same time to impute some desirable but undesired attributes, often of a supernatural cast, such as "sixth sense", or "understanding"' (Goffman, 1963, pp. 15-16). Thus non-speaking people will often be assumed to be deaf, and cognitively impaired as well, and disabled people are often idealised. An example of this last tendency is given by a blind writer:

'You develop a "philosophy". People seem to insist that you have one and they think you're kidding when you say you haven't. So you do your best to please and to strangers you encounter on trains, in restaurants, or on the subway who want to know what keeps you going, you give your little piece' (Chevigny, 1962, pp. 141–142).

Another result of stigma is that any minor failings or incidental problems tend to be interpreted as a direct result of the stigmatised differentness.

'.. if a person of low intellectual ability gets into some sort of trouble the difficulty is more or less automatically attributed to "mental defect" whereas if a person of "normal intelligence" gets into a similar difficulty it is not regarded as symptomatic of anything in particular' (Dexter, 1958, p. 923).

A common experience of non-speaking people is communication going wrong because of the unease of speaking partners. For instance, as noted above, it is an expectation among English speakers that silences in a conversation be quite short. A severely physically impaired non-speaking person using a communication system is in the position of not being able to take part appropriately in the rapid give-and-take of conversational interaction. With strangers, it may be impossible to avoid giving an impression of lack of intelligence, lack of interest, or negative feelings about the interaction, none of which may be the case. Similar problems occur when a participant is unable to control facial expressions appropriately.

A further problem for someone with a severe physical impairment who cannot speak is, not only that they have difficulty in producing conversation, but also that they are continuously giving out inappropriate messages. For people who know the impaired person well, allowances are made, and the rules of interaction operate differently when that person is involved, but when interacting with a potentially large number of people every week who do not know them intimately, such a special understanding would be an unrealistic expectation.

If, through a disability, a person is unable to project an acceptable or accurate picture of themselves, they are liable to be stigmatised. Goffman (1963) argues that the status of 'normal' is lost when an individual cannot appropriately perform these roles. In a description of her experiences after a glossectomy, Pettygrove (1985) found Goffman's analysis an accurate picture of the dramatic alteration in her ability to function socially. She summarises this analysis thus:

> 'Stigmas are particularly painful for persons with disabilities, because they may lack the ability to provide appropriate cues, and their disability elicits inappropriate stereotyped responses from others. In anticipating such stereotypes, one may attempt to conceal a disability, withdraw from the social setting, or provide additional cues ('disidentifiers') to correct or deny misinterpretations associated with the stigma. Repeated experiences with being socially stigmatised become a personal struggle to preserve and present an unstigmatised definition of self' (p. 107).

To summarise: All social encounters require a significant degree of effort by all participants. They do not 'just happen'. Non-speaking users of communication systems have a particular problem in taking part in social interaction because of their physical difficulties in producing utterances easily. This can lead to social isolation, or at least a very restricted range of conversation partners. Another profound effect of a communication problem is the inability to create and maintain a social identity through language.

The aspect of language use which is being discussed here is pragmatics (Levinson, 1983). The work of Goffman and others highlights that pragmatics is not only an important factor in aided communication: it may often be the crucial factor.

# Pragmatics in aided communication

The development of aided communication systems began with the simpler aspects of language. This was a sensible way to proceed, given that the work has been largely exploratory. Thus, lexical considerations have been apparent in attempts to develop appropriate dictionaries (e.g. Beukelman, Yorkston, Poblete and Naranjo, 1984). The syntactic aspect of language has also been addressed, with systems such as Blissymbols (McNaughton and Kates, 1978), and syntactic word predictors (Morris, Newell, Booth and Arnott, 1991). The semantic level appeared in systems such as Minspeak (Baker, 1982), and in hierarchical topic storage methods (Blackstone, 1986; Beukelman and Mirenda, 1992).

In the past, researchers tried to build up an understanding about how language is structured and used by analysing it from the 'bottom up', from lexical analysis to syntactic, semantic, and finally pragmatic analysis. This was partly because actual spoken language was considered too complex and unruly to be subject to careful analysis. Work on conversation analysis over the past decades, however, has shown that a careful study is possible of how language is actually used in real contexts (Atkinson and Heritage, 1984; Garfinkel, 1967; Stubbs, 1983). Also, philosophers of language in this century have pointed out that language is very much a social construction. Human beings learn to communicate by being immersed in communication situations with others (Vygotsky, 1962). As Wittgenstein (1953) puts it, there is no such thing as a private language.

The importance of a stronger emphasis on pragmatics in aided communication has been argued for some time by, among others, Kraat (1985), Newell (1984) and Calculator (1988). In a survey of the state of the art in interaction using aided communication, Light (1988) suggested that aided speakers might want to achieve the communication goals of: communicating needs and wants, information transfer, social closeness and social etiquette.

McKinlay (1991) makes the point that a non-speaking communication system user often needs to create a correct first impression quickly with listeners, and then might be able to drop back to communicating more slowly, once they have established important social facts about themselves. McKinlay calls this the necessity of 'perceived social competence'. He argues that:

'A "technical" approach to this problem would begin with text generation and work toward improvements in perceived social competence. A "social" approach, on the other hand, would begin with a model of perceived social competence and then work back to a text generation model' (p. 204).

One of the most important barriers to establishing social competence for a non-speaking person is the rate of communication. It is very difficult to establish and maintain a social presence at a rate of 2–8 words per minute (Beukelman and Mirenda, 1992). In other words, poor communication rate results in poor communicative pragmatics. It would seem at first that this is an insuperable problem, since fluently spoken language is infinitely variable. It is difficult to see how this fluency and infinite variability could be produced given the limitations a disabled user will have in employing any sort of control device. In fact, even non-disabled persons would not be able to use any currently available input device to even approach the speed of communication possible when using their natural unimpeded vocal apparatus.

## Research prototypes based on pragmatic considerations

A number of prototype communication systems have been developed at Dundee University to test out different ways of improving the pragmatic aspects of conversation using a communication system (Newell and Alm, 1994; Newell, Alm and Arnott, 1993). Each has been designed to examine different aspects of the problem or different methods for overcoming the difficulties which aided communicators' experience. What all the prototypes have in common is an approach which tries to model aspects of social and conversational interaction in software, in order to provide the user with predictive help throughout the conversation.

Two assumptions lie behind all of these prototypes. Firstly, it is often the case that it is more important to say something which is more or less appropriate than to be absolutely precise about what you say, and miss the right moment. Secondly, while it is true that language can be infinitely varied, in fact people tend to use a finite range of conversational gambits for much of their conversation (Gumperz, 1982).

Each of the research prototypes requires that the user create a large store of personal conversational contributions. This is done in their own time, perhaps with help in entering the text into the system. During future conversations, the prestored items are made available at appropriate moments by the system. The user can thus mix in this 'reusable' material with utterances being created word-by-word or letter-by-letter. The advantage of the prestored material is, of course, the relative speed with which it can be produced.

One prototype provided users with quick ways of accomplishing basic and often-needed social routines, such as greeting and parting utterances and a continual stream of feedback remarks to another speaker. Having a facility such as this, it was proposed, might begin to provide users with the ability to take part more fully in social etiquette routines, and thus establish a better social identity, as described above. The prototype was developed to explore a number of questions. These included the feasibility of having a communication system whose ultimate unit was not words, or phrases, but speech acts (Austin, 1962; Searle, 1969). Another question was whether users would find it acceptable for the system to select an utterance from their store for them on the basis of a requested speech act, and if this meant a significant increase in communication rate (Alm, Arnott and Newell, 1989).

Trials of this prototype were carried out over a six-month period with four non-speaking volunteers. Three of the evaluators had cerebral palsy, and had been non-speaking since birth, and one had been deprived of speech through muscular dystrophy. After an initial training period, the evaluators used the prototype and also their current communication method in four communication situations: meeting in a corridor, receiving some information, having a general conversation, and taking part in a group conversation. The other speakers in these situations were volunteers drawn from people the evaluators knew well and also people who were strangers to them. The conversations were all tape recorded and transcripts were made of them.

The results showed the prototype gave users an increase in conversational rate, conversational participation, and range of speech acts compared to their existing methods of communication. Questionnaires established that both the prototype users and their conversation partners felt the prototype improved the quality of the conversations except in one regard: when the user was called upon to contribute something to the conversation other than following the given routines (Alm, Arnott and Newell, 1992; Alm, Brophy, Arnott and Newell, 1988).

Another system has been developed which predicts sentences from a large prestored collection, using knowledge about the user, the user's frequent conversation partners, and the topics they like to talk about (Broumley, Cairns and Arnott, 1990). The users, in their own time, create a store of sentences, and label each one with a number of facts about its potential usage. In conversation situations, the sentences are then predicted based on the context of the conversation, including the topic, and the conversation partner(s) involved. Semantic networks are used to hold the information needed to make the predictions. The system thus attempts to simulate the (largely non-conscious) way in which speakers arrive at an appropriate thing to say next in a conversation.

The prototype was developed over a one-year period, with the participation throughout of two non-speaking people. These two people then assisted with an evaluation of the finished prototype, using it with three types of conversation partner: their spouse, another relative who they saw occasionally, and an acquaintance who they saw only occasionally. Sessions with the prototype were compared with sessions using the existing communication methods. All sessions were tape recorded and transcripts made.

Compared with their current communication methods, the users with the prototype were producing longer utterances, taking more of a proportion of the interaction, taking more control of the conversation, and spending less time repairing conversational breakdowns. This prototype, however, produced no significant increase in communication rate, or in the range of different speech acts employed (Broumley, 1994).

Further research work is continuing to find other ways in which a user might be presented with predicted texts, based on the context of the conversation. A number of approaches are being investigated which rely on linking stored texts in relevant and flexible ways. One prototype uses a method called 'fuzzy information retrieval' to make it possible for the system to produce a set of texts closely related to the one being spoken, where the relationship does not have to be clearly defined. This would have the advantage of allowing the user to move flexibly from topic to topic. For instance, following a joke about cars, the user might then want to tell another joke on cars or on another subject, have some more discussion about cars, or talk about trains or other forms of transport. The 'fuzzy' method of retrieval has the useful feature that the system will always produce a set of candidate utterances, no matter how small or disparate the store of utterances is, and the set produced will be the best fit possible to the existing utterance (Alm, Nicol and Arnott, 1993).

Another project is investigating ways of helping non-speaking communication system users to accomplish everyday tasks which involve speaking by offering predicted conversational routines and subroutines to the user at appropriate points (Alm, Dye and Harper, 1995). This project could be said to be investigating language as a tool for accomplishing tasks other than just interacting. Such tasks might include travelling around, shopping, or getting a restaurant meal. An advisory group of potential users is attached to this project. The point they have made about this approach to an aided communication system is that what it may offer is not just a chance for them to perform some tasks better, but a chance for them to do the task themselves for the first time.

The prototypes described above, and other new systems under development in Dundee and elsewhere, represent attempts to have more 'intelligence' built into aided communication systems. More and more initiative can be taken by the system on behalf of the user, but it is important that the balance be optimal between what the computer controls and what the user controls. Each must contribute what they are best at, but the user must remain in ultimate control (Arnott, 1990).

## Conclusions

It is important to find imaginative ways to help non-speaking users of communication systems to take more responsibility for accomplishing a range of pragmatic functions. Unless this is done, they are likely to find full social participation very difficult. Their social world will be restricted to people who are willing and able to collaborate with them extensively in communicating. Their ability to create and maintain an accurate social identity through communication acts in public will remain constricted. What many of these pragmatic functions have in common is the speaker taking responsibility for keeping up their end of a mutually constructed interaction. Being an interesting conversation partner should not be seen as a desirable but largely unobtainable goal for non-speaking people. It is an essential part of maintaining a full social presence.

As children learn to communicate, a great deal of practice, repetition, and getting it wrong goes into acquiring communicational and interactive abilities. Thus the mere provision of pragmatics based communication systems will not of itself allow many non-speaking people to take part immediately in the social network. It may be that where such systems find an equally important application is in their use in training non-speaking children and adults in the processes of interaction.

# Chapter 11
# A semiotic analysis of the possibilities and limits of Blissymbols

SERENELLA BESIO AND MARIA GRAZIA CHINATO

Vast international use of the Blissymbolics system within the field of habilitation and its growing popularity are proof of its practical validity. Initially, it was mainly used as an instrument of communication for children with cerebral palsy (Kates and McNaughton, 1975; Udwin and Yule, 1991a,b) but Blissymbols have also been employed to support education and habilitation of people with intellectual impairment (Abrahamsen, Romski and Sevcik, 1989; Gava and Montalto, 1991; Sansone and Tagliapietra, 1983) and people affected by other language pathologies, such as aphasia (Johansen-Horbach et al., 1985; Ross, 1974).

In this chapter, the code of the Blissymbolics system is analysed, as it was presented by Charles Bliss (1965), by considering its semiotic nature. A code is 'a system of signals (signs, symbols) which, conventionally, is devoted to represent and transmit information between the sender and the receiver. Semiotically, a code is a system of correlations or correlation rules, between a codifying system and a codified system' (Eco, 1975, p. 47). The analysis of the code, from a semiotic point of view, concerns the specification of the system of descriptive parameters, of the sign characteristics and of the relationship between the *signifier* and the *signified*. It does not imply an analysis nor a judgement of the pragmatic value and use of the code itself; hence, possible limited versions and uses will not be considered. In the second part, the communication context of each of the characteristics found will be examined in order to see whether they can explain the success of the system in this sense. Shifting from analysing the code itself to its use, a particular concern is whether points of theoretical weakness may actually become points of pragmatic strength.

## An international a posteriori language

Throughout the history of mankind, numerous attempts have been made within every culture to achieve the utopia of global communication, namely the finding or construction of a perfect language (cf. Eco, 1993; Pellerey, 1992a). Some of these are constructed as 'a priori' plans for a language and seek to reflect the very nature of things. For this reason, they are also defined as 'philosophical a priori languages', as the ontological order of reality they seek to mirror derives from a global epistemological perspective (such a language can assume the values of both a method and an organising principle). Other languages (particularly universal ones) are constructed as 'a posteriori languages'; meaning that they take a natural language as their model and become parasites of it, especially of its grammatical and syntactic aspects.

Blissymbolics was created as an 'international a posteriori language', but has developed in an unexpected fashion and taken on life in a field that is quite distant from subsidiary languages. It has been used to facilitate dialogue, not so much among distant peoples as among people with special communication needs. From a semiotic point of view, we have singled out three characteristics that help to determine and define Blissymbolics: it is an a posteriori system, an international language and icon-based. For the purpose of this study of Blissymbolics as a code from a semiotic point of view, these characteristics are used as parameters of analysis.

## Blissymbolics as a parasitic system

From the morphological, grammatical and syntactic point of view, Charles Bliss (1965) conceived Blissymbolics as a parasite of the English language. He is likely to have considered this language an ideal model due to its simple inflections and derivations of structure, and then simplified the model even further. The grammar of Blissymbolics could thus be defined 'laconic' as it seeks to apply a principle of economy at all costs (for similar considerations for Esperanto, see Zinna, 1993). Hence, in *morphological* terms, no difference in gender is considered and, as a consequence, no concord of any kind is necessary. In addition, although differences in number are considered (via the use of a plural marker), they do not demand further inflection. In particular, as with English, correct interpretation of the verb (in this case its graphic sign) demands that it be always coupled with its subject. Moreover, the verb has only one possible conjugation and the categories it can signify (mood, tense, etc.) are extremely simplified. The case of the infinitive mood, which does not differ from the present indicative, is a typical example.

As to *syntax*, the strict basic order of Blissymbolics (subject, verb, object) proposed by Bliss is further evidence of the link with English, but also harks back to the mythical idea of a language that can reflect a universal, natural logic, where word order must follow the structural logic of thought and respond to the demands of common sense (Couturat and Leau, 1903; Dalgarno, 1661; Eco, 1993). Nevertheless, this supposed subdivision of the world into universally valid categories clearly refers only to the local perspective, that of the Western world (and not to the perspective of a 'natural syntactic structure', as claimed by Jones and Cregan, 1986). From this point of view, it is clear that Blissymbolics is not based on the English language alone, but more broadly might be considered as a product of Western culture.

This fact is also mirrored in its *content model* and the 1400 lexical items presented by Bliss. For example, strictly referring to this basic lexicon and omitting for the moment combined graphic signs, among the graphic signs (the 'lexemes' of the lexicon), there is one for 'beer' but not for 'sake'; there are signs to define professions which are far from universal, like *SOCIAL-WORKER*, and to symbolise concepts like 'dieting', 'wage-earning' and 'time table', which are hardly widespread in parts of Africa and Australia. Likewise, the graphic structure, particularly the iconic representations chosen by Bliss, often recalls images of objects of Western culture and traditions: *BED, FEELING,* and *WARDROBE* are examples of this.

Parasitism on Western culture is especially evident in the construction rules of the so-called 'complex graphic sign' (superimposed or in sequence). These are expressed through periphrases (e.g. 'house of God' for *CHURCH*) based on a kind of logic that is influenced by the linear causality and values which Western culture traditionally adopts to fragment reality. In the case of the graphic signs in sequence, in the positional order prescribed by Bliss, signs that define the nature of what is being represented (a person, an animal, a thing, a feeling, or a more specific typology of any of these) are generally placed first, followed by their function or main characteristic. In this way, each complex graphic sign seems to reproduce, in a contracted and more immediate form, the direct syntactic order of the general code: a sort of hologram of the whole system. This continuous cross-reference to the culture within which a system has been created has the unavoidable, but perhaps imperceptible, power of reinforcing the culture itself. Blissymbolics is similarly defined and self-contained, as are the Western natural languages, and plays a role in maintaining the logic and mentality from which it derives.

## Blissymbolics as a closed system

The code of Blissymbolics seeks to gain the status of an international communication system. It therefore contains advantages linked to structural simplicity, as well as limitations inherent in the universality principle. Like all international languages, Blissymbolics owes its long-term survival to unyielding defence of the system's structure, which must remain as it is, at the risk of losing its basic universality and strictly denotative power. The organisations that today supervise the use of Blissymbolics are aware of the importance of maintaining a standard structure. They control not only the graphic quality of existing signs but also the logical and graphical coherence of new signs introduced to enrich the vocabulary. This imperviousness curtails the risks of parallel development: 'the inexorable law of historical evolution would reduce the language into a series of dialects in the space of a few years' (Pellerey, 1992a, p. 121).

This lack of transformability also distances Blissymbolics from natural languages (Albani and Buonarotti, 1994), which, conversely, are constantly subject to uncontrollable evolution, modifications, and to the process of continental drift that gives rise to languages, dialects and idiolects. While linguists once pursued the idea of a perfect, immutable language, today they attribute the power and value of natural languages to this very transformability. However, the richness of natural languages is also brought about by the inventive possibilities of the various linguistic codes: peoples, or individuals (particularly poets) can make creative use of this, thus entering into an original relationship with their own language that not only describes but invents the world. By contrast, it is forbidden to mess about with the basic elements of Blissymbolics, that is, construct new graphic signs using the basic graphic features, as this might generate anarchy in sign production.

One could point out that Blissymbolics nevertheless allows a kind of light-hearted inventiveness through the use of combined graphic signs. But even this characteristic reveals a controlled use of the system, because this pseudo-creativity has to respect rigorous parameters. The resulting combinations may serve to represent concepts related to real-world objects for which there are no corresponding Blissymbols but cannot use graphic Blissymbols to create concepts outside this sphere. On the other hand, this lack of inventiveness seems to be implicit in the linearity of the code rules. Each inventive relation is based upon mental operations which are far from linear, such as hyperencoding, abduction, transcoding, etc. (Bonfantini, 1987).

## Aspects of semiotic analysis in Blissymbolics

Languages based on icons or pictures have always attracted Western researchers in quest of the perfect language, if such a thing were to exist (Eco, 1993). The main characteristics of Chinese writing that originally attracted Bliss were the high clarity and comprehensibility of ideograms for large sections of neighbouring populations, independent of languages spoken and geographical location. With further simplification, this led to the idea of an international icon-based system and it was on this that Bliss placed his bets for the creation of a universal peace-making language.

## Iconicity and arbitrariness

The pictographic signs within Blissymbolics correspond exactly to the authoritative definition of 'icon' proposed by Peirce (1931–1958). According to this author, an icon is 'a particular sign which bears a likeness to external reality and which presents the same property as the denoted object' (p. 220). This definition led to discussions, and Eco (1975) suggested several modifications: 'To represent an object iconically means to transcribe the cultural properties attributed to it through graphical (or different) artifices' (p. 272). In this sense, at least in a given culture, Blissymbolics icons can be defined as transparent; they are widely understandable without any need of further mediation. Nevertheless, as an object encompasses numerous properties, it is hard to believe in a universal point of view from which an image can be adjudged as similar to something, so the choice of the system inventor is bound to a specific cultural background. The cultural parasitism of Blissymbolics icons has been underlined above.

The problem of iconicity is linked to the principle of *arbitrariness*, that is, the need for the relationship between the signifier and the signified to be unjustified. Formalised by de Saussure (1977/1916), with time this principle has become a parameter for the evaluation of languages: when a communication system is arbitrary, there are no limits to what can be communicated (Hockett, 1960). By the end of the seventeenth century, the principle had already been formulated in order to re-examine the myth of a language capable of expressing the nature of things. From that time on, it has represented the basic principle for assigning language status to a wide range of sign systems (Radutzky, 1981). Within Blissymbolics, this issue largely concerns pictographic signs, which are systematically drawn as similar as possible to the reality of objects,

Iconicity usually diminishes, resulting in increased arbitrariness of the idiographic signs, where the contribution of real invention is stronger, and the relationship between the signifier and the signified must necessarily be mediated by convention. So, Blissymbolics ideograms propose a new form of parasitism, as they are affected by what has been defined as the 'drama of ideography' (Pellerey, 1992b). They may identify and describe their contents, that is, ideas themselves, but only in the sense of naming them with natural language words.

The leap towards complete code arbitrariness is taken by the third type of Blissymbols (more recently McNaughton (1985) has divided them into four classes), the 'arbitrary' signs, which, within semiotic terminology would be better defined as 'conventional' signs. However, these signs have been assimilated from outside (dollar, medical, arrows, etc.) and indicate autonomous creation, as well as concepts of arbitrariness and convention that are external to Blissymbolics.

## Lack of metaphor

The system's concreteness (defined above as denotative rigidity) prevents the formation of *metaphors*. That is, the relationship between the graphic sign and its meaning is not modifiable or ductile (see below about polysemy). Many researchers have assigned a propulsive function to the metaphorical form within natural languages, identifying it as one of the foremost sources of inventiveness. The possible forms of metaphor have been classified according to their level of complexity and relation with a linguistic habit (Eco, 1971; Le Guern, 1975). The lowest level is lexicalised metaphor, which is similar to the figurative sense, for example, *you dog!* The highest level is when the metaphor generates meaning. This occurs usually in poetry, such as, *a skein of streets.*

There is considerable variation in the individual use of these forms. And this is one of the channels through which a personal style of communication becomes original and recognisable. As to Blissymbolics, it cannot make allowance for individual rhetoric. As mentioned earlier, to survive as a system it must avoid deviance from the norm.

The Blissymbol *METAPHOR* is used to mark the beginning of a word or sentence to inform the reader that what follows should not be taken literally. To be more precise, it does not introduce the possibility of constructing metaphors, but indicates a slight connotative amplification of the sign's meaning towards figurative sense. For example, the sentence *YOU ARE AN ANIMAL* preceded by *METAPHOR* should be read in a figurative sense. If the system considers even the figurative sense dangerous, it cannot make allowance for another aspect of natural languages: the semiotic series (Eco, 1975). No element of a natural language dwells on its immediate interpreter, but enters a multilevel structure in which the connections never progress in a linear fashion, while the denotations transform into connotations through the individual's invention. This is another prohibition of Blissymbolics that frees the user and reader from doubts of interpretation and forces them to remain on a strictly literal level.

## Polysemy

Polysemy is another aspect of Blissymbolics that apparently contradicts its denotative rigidity and identifies it as a source of simplicity. Even if it does not allow metaphoric or inventive use, Blissymbolics is constructed so that no graphic sign corresponds to only one meaning, but to three, four or more that are related according to a criterion of synonymy or semantic contiguity. The same graphic sign may be interpreted as *ENCOUNTER, ASSEMBLY, MEETING, GATHERING-OF-PEOPLE, CONFER-ENCE*, etc. Another graphic sign may in various settings be translated as *HEAR, LISTEN, APPREHEND, PERCEIVE*, etc. No mechanism within the system permits correct interpretation of graphic signs or suggests the most appropriate synonym in a given context. In order to guide the reader and anchor the polysemy of Blissymbols more solidly, it is essential to resort to spoken language or alphabetic writing support, on which the code must largely depend.

This generalisation of meanings has a considerable impact on the expression of those who use the system to communicate. Similarly to many other artificial languages (a priori or a posteriori), Blissymbolics is unable to express all the connotative and, even more importantly, denotative subtleties of a natural language. It was to this very characteristic Giacomo Leopardi (1823/1956–1966) once ascribed the nature of any strictly universal language, which, in his opinion, was servile, poor, timid, monotonous, uniform, dry and hideous. Assuming a less drastic position, in an age when discussion about languages of this kind is no longer a live issue, one can still point to how the condensation of synonyms reduces meaning and seriously weakens the system.

## Limits of Blissymbolics

This semiotic analysis highlights serious limitations of the structure of Blissymbolics. The one that most seriously affects the whole code is its extreme simplicity at every level, that is, in lexicon, morphology and syntax.

First, the aforementioned vocabulary reduction is a source of severe impoverishment, and, while polysemy appears to be a solution to overcome this problem, it also introduces serious inaccuracies in the relationship between sign and meaning. The enlargement of the semantic field that polysemy appears to offer remains only hypothetical if another code does not intervene to provide a clearer definition of the meaning. Simplification carried out at the levels of code construction seems to produce functional effectiveness and validity. Nevertheless, where users take advantage of the possibility to eliminate particles such as articles and prepositions, there is a risk of introducing excessive ambiguity in the communicated message.

Another, rather contrary, characteristic of Blissymbolics is that the system leans towards an intuitive relationship between sign and meaning. This is the system's iconicity. On the one hand, it maintains close links with the culture it emerges from (Eco, 1975), and, on the other, leads to non-arbitrariness of the code, a fact that in itself jeopardises its very nature as a language. An aspect of the pictographic representation is the fact that an image cannot assert the non-existence of the thing it represents; as Worth (1975) put it: 'Pictures can't say ain't'. This increases the linearity of Blissymbolics because it draws on the straightforwardness of icon meaning and leads to the assumption that sentences are more likely to be constructed in the positive rather than negative form.

One could retort that Blissymbolics provides the possibility of affirming non-existence through the use of signs like *OPPOSITE* and *NOT*. However, as the system relies on another code for interpretation – that is, the Blissymbolics needs to refer to the negative construction of the natural language – it lacks autonomy and becomes parasitic on the semantic universe of the reference language.

For the reasons outlined earlier, such a code cannot permit an inventive approach. It does not embrace the form of ambiguity in discourse on which unexpected sense generation is based, nor does it allow for metaphorical creation.

## From language of peace to code of survival

Since Blissymbolics was introduced into the field of habilitation and rehabilitation, a great deal of research has been devoted to its operational validity, which lies at the heart of its world-wide growth in popularity (Biancardi, 1985). On the level of theoretical definition, the most outstanding effect produced by Blissymbolics has been its shift from a universal language to a communication code (Archer, 1977; Vallini, 1981). This shift in the context of use, from an international language for all to a support code for those incapable of conventional verbal expression, casts off any pretension of universality and removes the need to decide about the status of Blissymbolics as a language.

In the transition from a conceptually and structurally defined system to a communication instrument, the parameters for system evaluation also have to be modified. In this evaluation context, other questions may be considered for analysis. When approaching Blissymbolics as a practical tool, it is important to stress its operational effectiveness. This means that some linguistic judgement criteria are confined to the background, and others are sought that directly concern the tool's properties, such as efficiency, efficacy and functionality (Cannao, 1991). Henceforth, the elements of Blissymbolics that have been extrapolated from the above analysis (and that represent limits from the semiotic point of view) will be compared with the communicative purposes of its use as an alternative code. One may find that the very points of theoretical weakness become, in this new context, points of pragmatic strength.

Two clinical conditions will be used as examples: the use of Blissymbolics as alternative communication for intellectually impaired children and the potential benefits Blissymbolics may offer adults with aphasia (Avent, Edwards, Franco and Lucero, 1995). These examples have been chosen because they are sufficiently different to be treated as a paradigm. The first case involves the issue of language learning and cognitive skills, while the second concerns the loss of previously-acquired functions. The first case concerns habilitation and development, the second case rehabilitation and recovery.

# When cons become pros

### Structural simplicity

The main characteristic of Blissymbolics revealed by semiotic analysis is its utter simplicity. However, while seen as a limitation from a semiotic perspective, in the habilitation field it becomes an advantage. Besides being simple in nature, Blissymbolics can be useful at various levels of structural complexity and thus at various levels of cognitive complexity. As it is flexible, it can be reduced in lexicon and internal organisation, allowing the interventionist to match it to a person's cognitive skills and communicative needs. For people with intellectual impairment, syntactic and grammatical simplification may be maximised, reducing the set of graphic signs to an absolute minimum. These may nevertheless be sufficient to break a person's communicative silence.

Moreover, the communication board may be organised according to strategies which differ substantially from the norm. Commonly used approaches are a semantic contiguity criterion and a perceptive evidence criterion (Cannao, 1991; Gava and Montalto 1991). It is also possible to avoid assigning a precise grammatical value to the graphic signs, relying on the communication context to mediate interpretation. For example, the situation will determine whether a person wants to say *LEGS, FEET* or *GO*. The possibility of constructing sentences without using articles and prepositions offers advantages for people with intellectual impairment because it simplifies the communicative task.

The role this characteristic may play in rehabilitation of adults with aphasia is not so straightforward. Although the use of a communication board with Blissymbols could prove useful as visual support for production of spoken sentences, it may also to some extent encourage a sort of underestimation of the particles of discourse and foster production of grammatically incorrect sentences. This may be a problem in the case of non-fluent aphasia with agrammatism.

The rigid direct syntactic order on which the system is based plays a major role in characterising the simplicity of Blissymbolics (Hind, 1989). The form this assumes in intervention, that is, the colour scheme recommended for use with Blissymbolics, may be an important aid to sentence production (Besio and Chinato, 1991). However, for people with severe intellectual impairment, the use of a communication board divided into such areas will only be a long-term goal. In the case of people with aphasia, the fact that the order of the expression is guided in a predetermined direction has rehabilitative value (Ross, 1974). In rehabilitation of people with aphasia, some methods simply use specific aids, such as cards and tokens, to facilitate visualisation of the typical grammatical scansion of the sentence. This is to avoid the elimination of some sections of speech and encourage correct collocation (e.g. Gudi and Gore, 1993; Pradatdiehl and Bergego, 1994).

Finally, structural simplicity also implies simplicity in the system's internal graphic strategies. Many complex graphic signs are based on the constant re-use (redundancy) of the 100 elements of which the system is composed, for example, *CHURCH, SCHOOL, CONCERT-HALL,* etc. The advantage offered by redundancy consists in a memory aid which helps to 'fix' the relationship between the sign and its meaning. While this characteristic of economy helps anyone who wants to learn the system, it has even greater value for both people with intellectual impairment (where memory difficulties are common) and adults with aphasia, who are offered a visual source for mnemonic 'anchorage' of word strings (Hartje and Sturm, 1987; Wilson, 1987). Still, the main interest in the particular structural form of complex graphic signs lies in the linear logic that constructs and distinguishes them. This logic represents an elementary form of reasoning which may assume a particular meaning and play a role in promoting the cognitive development of people with intellectual impairment (Cannao and Moretti, 1982; Stella and Biancardi, 1987).

## Iconicity

It is well-known (for the semiotic field, see Barthes, 1986) that images may be easier and more immediate to understand than linguistic messages. One may assume that the iconic image, of a higher logical level, can be a valid mediator for learning towards symbolisation (but see Allen, 1975, for a review of contrasting views). Discussing sign language for deaf people, Brown (1978) maintained that it is was easier to learn than spoken language because of its iconic features. Pictographic signs give the relationship between sign and meaning an immediacy that allows simple recognition and rapid memorisation of the graphic sign. This has been demonstrated for iconic signs in American Sign Language (Bellugi, Klima and Siple, 1975). In addition, it adds a symbolic level, however elementary, to the person's cognitive world. In habilitation, this is the most important benefit in reaching for a denotative (thus symbolic) level which can support the subject's development (Piaget, 1951; Spradlin, 1963; Sansone and Tagliapietra, 1983).

But it also offers advantages in the communication of adults with aphasia. Pertinent images and highly significant contexts or suggestions may help them with their spoken or written production, with control of these (Basso, 1981, 1987; Ross, 1974). In the same way, Blissymbolics, like other methodologies used in speech therapy with aphasic people, can be an essential evocative context of words, precisely because of the low-level symbolisation of its iconicity. Moreover, practically all pictographic Blissymbols depend upon the concreteness of the object they represent. As already argued, this makes the system an inadequate vehicle of innovative creativity and abstraction. On the other hand, it poses less difficulty in communication for subjects with intellectual impairment. Furthermore, it supports learning of pictographic signs, in particular when they refer to objects ordinarily in the immediate surroundings.

Sometimes, it may even be necessary to emphasise this characteristic of concreteness in order to facilitate memorisation of the graphic signs. For some people, the representational immediacy of the sign – or signs – in relation to the object may still be too abstract. Consequently, decoding may be difficult. In this case, the interventionist emphasises the iconic characteristics of the sign using specific devices such as colouring, addition of graphic details, etc.

Iconicity also possesses expressive and representative strength, a 'power of attraction' towards other meanings. For example, a person may incorrectly but successfully use the graphic sign *GLASS* to signify a desire to drink instead of the existing signs *DRINK or THIRSTY*. In this, as in other cases of Blissymbols use, a sort of limited agreement is created within a small or tiny group. The fact that this agreement is not universally recognised is immaterial because the communication works.

Idiographic signs, on the other hand, demand a different sort of cognitive effort of the user because their relation with the object involved is more arbitrary. This difficulty, together with the abstract quality of the concept these signs generally refer to, can sometimes prevent people with severe intellectual impairment from learning and using them. In the case of adults with aphasia, a simple but important relationship of graphic evocation of verbal strings can be established by idiographic signs, in a similar way but to a lesser extent than with graphic signs of greater iconic content.

## Polysemy

As discussed earlier, Blissymbols are polysemic, as are the basic elements of many other graphic codes (Biancardi, 1985). This imposes serious limitations on their expressive potential. In the field of disability, this is particularly true of their use by people with aphasia. The extreme uniformity of signifiers, the compacting of synonyms into a single semantic field, and the reduced number of concepts that may be referred to when using this code are all disadvantages in communicative expression. In addition, people with aphasia might not manage to control this synonymy competently, so as to benefit from having the communication board at hand. Each graphic sign is more likely to be memorised and used in the communication, only for its one-to-one relation with a single significance, and not with a collection of significances. The problem is not so serious with regard to people with intellectual impairment, where the issue of polysemy is too refined to be of particular relevance (Gava, 1991). In this case the lexicon of the input – as well as the output – is severely reduced. In clinical practice interventionists tend to follow a principle of parsimony in verbal communication.

When the code is employed at an elementary level, the first graphic signs used inevitably correspond to semantic fields with uncertain boundaries, such as WATER, LIQUID, DRINK, JUICE, etc. This may be an advantage in communication, since Blissymbolics may fulfil the same functions in development as the speech code for a child who is learning to talk (Musselwhite and St. Louis, 1988; Vanderheiden and Grilley, 1977). Lastly, when Blissymbolics is used as a means for educational activities, polysemy may allow increased language understanding for children with intellectual impairment who can learn in this way, for example, that some words belong to the same semantic field (Abbeduto, Furman and Davies, 1989).

## Parasitism

Earlier in this chapter, the conviction was expressed that the dependence of the Blissymbolics code on other codes confirms the view that, as a language, it has a parasitic nature. As a matter of fact, the aspect of parasitism has increased when the code has been subordinated to the requirements of habilitation and rehabilitation. Within this context, graphic signs lose their vitality and acquire a particular form, always being coupled with a corresponding written gloss (cf. also Besio and Ferlino, 1992, 1993). The system's lack of autonomy and the ambiguity of sense it might entail are solved unilaterally but decisively by association with another code. In intervention, this aspect of Blissymbolics is often a real advantage.

It may play an incidental role in literacy acquisition of people with intellectual impairment (sight-word learning), and a more important role in the recovery of reading and writing functions in people with aphasia, possibly due to the repetitions produced by the use of the communication board (Cubelli, 1986; Cubelli, Foresti and Consolino, 1988; Deloche, Dordain and Kremin, 1993).

# Conclusions

The present chapter has demonstrated how disadvantages of Blissymbolics as a universal language may become advantages if the perspective from which the system is observed changes, and if a pragmatic point of view is taken. Blissymbolics has become a system for augmentative and alternative communication, and has acquired greater value, more strength and even more credibility. When a code is used as an operational (and in this case, communicative) tool, it becomes, in practice, the mediator for a new state of mind, which may lead to unexpected consequences.

The first and most prominent of these is that the Blissymbolics code loses its nature as a universal language because of the limitations that have demonstrated how, on the pragmatic level, it essentially lives within dialogue. The reason for this lies not only in its becoming the mediator for communication of at least two individuals, but above all because it brings into play a new, concrete and very powerful possibility for disabled people: the capacity to 'take the turn' in a conversation (cf. Goffman, 1969, 1981). Being able to access a symbolic mediation also means being able to intervene and to join in the dialogue, to begin a conversation, to answer, to interrupt, etc. These are basic acts in human dialogues but without symbolic mediation they cannot be performed because they are entrusted to communication means of a lower order, which are easily overlooked by the interlocutor (such as facial expression, movement, body posture, vocalisations, etc.). These acts also contribute to identifying a person as an individual.

If these characteristics constitute the great strengths of Blissymbolics as a communication tool, they should also represent crucial parts of intervention programmes, not only for communication purposes, but also to mediate the construction of the person's world. This will be a very concrete world, easy to understand and represent, a world based on a small number of straightforward rules that in some cases may be broken. The graphic signs will be limited in number, express a restricted number of concepts and be closely linked to the individual's experience. But even given these limitations, Blissymbolics may nevertheless represent an important tool for breaking a communication impaired person's silence enabling a more active role to be played in human relationships. With a lot of work and a pinch of luck it may also be a good springboard towards more elusive but more promising goals.

# Chapter 12
# Augmentative and alternative telecommunication for people with intellectual impairment – a preview

JANE M. BRODIN AND STEPHEN VON TETZCHNER

Telecommunication is playing an increasingly important role in shaping the patterns of human co-operation and communication in modern society. Telecommunication is a prerequisite for, or may facilitate, many forms of social participation. Telecommunication is changing or replacing some of the earlier ways of establishing and maintaining social relationships, and may even create completely new forms of social interaction. These changes will have consequences for people with intellectual impairment, but until now, little attention has been given to their telecommunication needs. People with intellectual impairment tend to have low social status, and in many countries their needs are given low priority by health and social service providers. As a consequence, they may have limited access to technical devices which might compensate for their disabilities.

Part of the reason for the limited focus on telecommunication may be the fact that many people with intellectual impairment have lived their whole life in large institutions or within their family with few contacts outside the institutions and if they had any telecommunication needs, staff or family would have taken care of these for them (e.g. Holm, 1993). However, this pattern is currently changing in many countries. The large institutions are being abolished and people with intellectual impairment do not to the same extent have all activities organised in one place. They tend more often to live in smaller houses, hence needing telecommunication to keep contact with work, friends and relatives, and for organising visits and other social events.

People with intellectual impairment may have a range of difficulties using a telephone: they must be able to operate the telephone, have somebody to call, be able to carry out a conversation over the telephone, be motivated to communicate and realise the benefits of using the telephone (Brodin, 1994; Frederiksen et al., 1989; Roe et al., 1995). Access to telecommunication for people with intellectual impairment is an essential part of their desegregation and equal participation in society. Knowledge about various forms of telecommunication and the demands they make on the users, as well as knowledge about communication skills and problems among people with intellectual impairment, are therefore essential for making adaptations that may make telecommunications accessible for a larger part of this group. For example, telephones with large buttons, short numbers and a large keyboard with pictures of the people who may be called may make the telephone easier to operate. Cellular telephones may increase security and make independent travel possible for some people.

The present chapter is concerned with the medium itself, that is, how transmission of visual signals may augment telecommunication for intellectually impaired users. In addition, it is discussed how new forms of telecommunication technologies may be used to enhance services for this group of people. Since few studies have addressed these questions and most relevant knowledge is lacking, we have called this chapter a preview.

## Characteristics of telephone conversations

There are many forms of telecommunication but the most common example is ordinary telephone contact. Telephones make people available at a distance, but the quality of the conversation is not the same as in face-to-face interaction. Telecommunication is characterised by fewer mutual *situational cues*, as compared with face-to-face conversations and other situations where the parties can see each other. This leads to a lower degree of what Short, Williams and Christie (1976) call 'social presence'. These distinctions are not due to differences in physical stimulation but to the kind of relations the various forms of telecommunication may create between the communicating parties (Moscovici, 1967).

Because of limited access to situational cues, telephone conversations make special demands on the user's communicative competence. For example, the partners cannot see each other, and the one who calls does not know for sure who will answer the telephone, and the one who answers the call cannot be sure who is calling. Telephone conversations therefore usually start with an introduction:

    J:   *Hello, this is John.*
    M:  *Hello, John, this is Mary.*

The visual parts of the non-verbal communication in face-to-face conversations, such as direction of gaze, eye contact, gestures, body posture and facial expressions, serve as cues for regulating the discourse, taking turns in speaking, etc. Such cues are important for organising the conversation because it is difficult to listen and speak simultaneously. Nevertheless, the regulation of the discourse does not break down even when the parties rely only on hearing, as in the use of ordinary audio telephones. In ear-to-ear conversations, sentences are usually shorter, there are fewer interruptions and there is less overlap, that is, both parties speaking at the same time. There are not as many pauses, since the pauses are filled by the other party who take them as opportunities for speaking (Butterworth, Hine and Brady, 1977; Rutter, 1987).

In addition to having to rely on acoustic conversational cues only, in telephone conversations it is not possible to use situational cues for understanding the other or making oneself understood. The communication partners cannot point at people, objects and events but instead have to describe them entirely in words.

Thus, telephone conversations make higher demands on the user's communicative competence than conversations face to face. Together with the lack of visual cues for interaction and access to situational information, this may make telephone conversations inaccessible or difficult to participate in for people with intellectual impairment.

## Intellectual impairment and telecommunication

A large and heterogeneous group of people are labelled intellectually impaired. Many different conditions and combinations of conditions may contribute to their learning difficulties. All forms of physical, sensory and cognitive impairments are more frequent in this group than in the general population. Linguistic competence and other skills that are important in telecommunication vary considerably (Bloom and Lahey 1978; Granlund, 1993; Kirman, 1985; Rosenberg and Abbeduto, 1993). It is not the case, however that all intellectually impaired people have difficulties using the telephone. Many understand how it functions and make good use of it. Others have such limited spoken language that even with considerable training, they will not be able to make use of it. Some may be able to speak but have difficulties understanding that someone they know is speaking and that this person is in another location and can hear what they are saying. For them, the difference between the radio, audio tapes and telephones may not be clear. Some people with intellectual impairment can use the telephone but have difficulties remembering the telephone number and pushing the right buttons.

Situations may suddenly be changed for the person picking up a ringing telephone or making a telephone call. This makes demands both on speed and the ability to adapt to new situations. People with intellectual impairment often react more slowly than others and may need more time to adapt to the situation established by a call.

People with intellectual impairment are often dependent on context when communicating. They tend to communicate about matters relating to the immediate situation. Even people with moderate intellectual impairment may have difficulties in keeping conversational control, taking turns and following the tacit rules of conversational interaction (Bedrosian, 1988; Rosenberg and Abbeduto, 1993). These are skills that are particularly important in telephone conversations.

Conversations are often grounded in events which are currently taking place. If one of the conversation partners is intellectually impaired, a lack of situational cues may make it difficult for the partners to find a common topic to talk about. Conversations usually start by one person suggesting a topic that the other accepts. Alternatively, if the partners disagree or have different expectations of the conversation, there may be negotiations, whereby the parties to some extent take each other's perspective. Without situational cues, such negotiations may be too abstract and difficult to grasp for people with intellectual impairment. They may also have difficulties understanding the words of the communication partner and making themselves understood without the situational support they usually receive in conversations face to face. In addition, people with intellectual impairment and autism tend to interpret words literally (Happé, 1994). This may be reinforced by difficulties adapting to the situation of the person at the other end.

Lastly, people with intellectual impairment often have little experience with independent use of the telephone. In this area, as in many others, they are dependent on being taught skills other people acquire without being taught explicitly. In the literature, transport is often discussed (Edgerton and Gaston, 1991; Syse, 1992) while the fact that the telephone is typically used for organising visits and transport, and may be useful for people with intellectual impairment in other ways, is often overlooked. They may not have received appropriate training in telephone behaviour, and hence do not know how it works, how to make a call, and the social rules that apply to establishing and maintaining telephone conversations.

# New developments in telecommunication

Through the transition from letters and telegrams to telephone conversations, telecommunication users have been enabled to use more of their communicative competence, thereby improving and expanding distance communication. When the audio telephone was invented in 1876 by Alexander Graham Bell while he was attempting to design a hearing aid for his wife, telecommunication was advanced significantly compared to the use of letter code of the telegraph. It became easier to use and gave new groups of people access to independent telecommunication because it was no longer necessary to be literate in order to take part. This was a necessary requirement for the telephone becoming a general household device in industrialised countries. In recent years, vision-based forms of telecommunication have become important supplements to the audio telephone. These allow alternative visual communication forms and may serve to augment spoken conversations. They include *fax, picture telephones, videotelephones* and *computer networks.*

Fax may be considered a form of distance copying, as reflected in the original name of the service, *facsimile transmission.* Today, it is the most commonly used means for transmission of text and graphics, although it is not as interactive as picture and videotelephone technology. Like electronic mail and other computer-based telecommunication forms, it is asymmetric (simplex), that is, communication goes in one direction at a time only, making it more like mail than telephone conversations.

Picture telephones are add-ons to telephones and hence the communication is functionally symmetric (duplex). They include a small camera that takes a still picture and transcmits it in a few seconds, during which the telephone is mute and the partners are unable to speak.

Videotelephones transmit live pictures and sound simultaneously. This renders both speech and more visual cues – though still not all the cues that are present in face-to-face conversations – making telecommunication more 'natural'. It removes some of the previous limitations of telecommunication, creating situations more similar to face-to-face conversations which make fewer demands on linguistic and communicative competence. Like audio telephones, videotelephone communication is symmetric, allowing both parties to communicate at the same time.

Computer networks include electronic mail and computer conferences. The term 'electronic highway' is today used about transmission of information via a high-capacity, digitised telecommunication network (Cullen et al., 1995).

The development of new telecommunication terminals is presently focused on *multi-media terminals* which can transmit data, pictures, video and sound at the same time. When this is applied in communication, the receiver may get other cues, and more cues, than those normally present in face-to-face conversations. This development could improve the quality of telecommunication in general, and it may be vital for people who can make little use of communication with speech alone.

Both multi-media terminals and videotelephones depend on an upgrade of the current analogue telephone network. A new international telecommunication standard, *Integrated Services Digital Network* (ISDN) with a basic access of two 64 kbit/s (kilobits per second) channels and one 16 kbit/s channel for signalling, is available in many European countries and elsewhere, and this is the basis for transmission of live pictures via the telecommunications network today. A *broadband* version of ISDN (B-ISDN) is being developed, with transmission rates from 64 to 150–620 kbit/s. In the future, this will make high quality sound and video transmission possible. However, while ISDN may be implemented in the present physical network, broadband communication requires optic fibres in all parts of the network, making general implementation unlikely in the near future. In addition to increasing the capacity of the network, advanced telecommunication services are made possible by techniques for compressing the information that is transmitted (Cullen et al., 1995; Emiliani and Stephanidis, 1995; Mathisen, 1991; Møllerbråten, 1991).

The utility of the new telecommunication modes for people with various forms of disabilities has been investigated in a number of research projects. For example, deaf people who are able to write may use text telephones. Picture telephones may provide still pictures of the communication partner, objects, graphic signs and locations, and cues about the situation of the speaker. Videotelephones give broader situational information, provide live pictures, and allow lip reading and use of sign language, making telecommunication available to people who depend wholly or partly on these modes of communication. Transmission of Braille or touch makes telecommunication accessible to people with combined vision and hearing impairment. For people with motor impairments, computer communication makes it possible to prepare and send messages written in orthographic script or Blissymbols and other graphic systems without spending a long time at the telephone (for reviews, see Roe, 1995; von Tetzchner, 1991b). However, a search based on key words related to telecommunication and disability in the major data bases of educational, psychological, sociological and medical literature in the autumn of 1995 produced very few references on telecommunication for people with intellectual impairments.

## Augmented telecommunication conversations

Alternative and augmented telecommunication implies the use of other telecommunication modes to replace or support audio communication. For people without comprehension of spoken language, the audio channel may be essentially redundant but most hearing individuals included in studies of vision-based communication are able to speak. Studies of alternative and augmentative telecommunication conversations comprise the use of fax, still picture telephones and videotelephones.

### Fax

Brodin (1993) investigated the use of fax for facilitating and supporting distance communication. It was hypothesised that the speed of telecommunication compared to traditional mail would make faxing easier to understand and more interesting to use than writing letters. Four men and one woman with moderate intellectual impairment participated in the study for a period of 1½ years. According to the staff, they could understand simple spoken language. One used single-word utterances, but not in a functional manner, while the others were unable to speak. They expressed themselves through manual signs, PIC signs (cf. Introduction) and gestures. Two of them had a few times listened to a relative speaking to them over the telephone while the others had never used a telephone at all. Due to the lack of functional speech and telephone experience, the fax was not used to complement spoken conversations but to send letters. The equipment consisted of eleven fax machines, placed at four day centres and in the participants' group homes. In one case, a parent was the communication partner. For the others, staff or peers at the day centres participated. The staff and relatives were interviewed before the project was initiated and regularly during the duration of the project. A questionnaire was filled out at each end after every call, and supplemented with bi-weekly notes provided by the staff.

A total of 653 faxes were sent during the 1½ years, averaging a little more than one per day and slightly less than two faxes per person per week. The topics in the faxes included previous and future activities and food (for ethical reasons no detailed content analysis was made).

The major advantage of the fax was the fast reply, sometimes via fax but occasionally over the telephone, thereby approaching the dialogue function of ordinary telephone exchanges. The swiftness of the reply seemed to make it easier for the intellectually impaired users to understand the function of fax than the slower services of the mail, and it was more motivating. Interviews with the staff indicated that using the fax stimulated and developed the participants' communication skills: they asked for more PIC signs, their interest in writing letters to friends increased, and they began to send faxes on their own initiative. However, the participants were entirely dependent on the staff's attitudes to the use of fax, and their willingness and time to support it. Transmission was fast, but it sometimes took a long time to prepare the message. Changes and shortages of staff proved critical for the number of faxes sent and statements such as *This week, we have not used the fax very much because of....* were not unusual. There may sometimes be natural reasons for not being able to send a fax, but it nevertheless seemed as if the fax was underused and that the prospects of the participants for putting their newly won skills into use were limited.

## Picture telephones

Many people with intellectual impairments understand verbal information better if it is accompanied by pictures. Brodin and Björck-Åkesson

Table 12.1: Characteristics of the individuals using the picture telephones.

| Person | Age in Years | Sex | Intellectual Impairment | Communication modes |
|---|---|---|---|---|
| Anders | 22 | Male | Mild/moderate | Understands speech but has severely limited speech. Uses manual signs and Blissymbols. |
| Britta | 34 | Female | Moderate | Speech of limited complexity. Some manual signs. No communication board but uses contact book with pictures of activities and events that she participates in for communication. |
| Carina | 38 | Female | Moderate | Speech. Does not use manual or graphic signs. |
| Daniel | 30 | Male | Moderate | Speech supplemented with manual signs, pictures and PIC. |
| Eva | 30 | Female | Moderate | Speech supplemented with manual signs, pictures and PIC. |
| Fredrik | 12 | Male | Moderate | Poor speech, supplemented with manual signs and gestures. |
| Greta | 10 | Female | Moderate | Limited speech and some manual signing. |
| Hanna | 6 | Female | Moderate | Speech, but has used manual signs before. |

(1991, 1995) used a still-picture telephone (Panasonic WG-R2) to augment telecommunication by intellectually impaired subjects. The system was attached to an ordinary audio telephone and consisted of a camera and a small graphic display. Both parties in the conversation needed to have this installed. It was then possible to show a still picture of the person who was talking or to transfer drawings, photographs and graphic signs. The transfer of one picture took less than ten seconds, during which the audio channel was mute. The telephone had a memory which stored the last six pictures transferred.

The study involved three children and five adults and lasted for a period of five months. All except one could speak fairly well but several supplemented the speech with manual signs, pictures or graphic signs (Table 12.1). All of the subjects could reply on the telephone, six of them could recognise voices, and two could make a call independently.

Twenty telephones were placed in the subjects' homes, day centres they attended, and in the homes of friends, relatives and relief care families. Each person had at least one partner to call (Table 12.2). The focus of the study was the effect of picture support in telephone conversations, that is, whether the still picture improved comprehension and production of language and might be considered a communication aid for people with intellectual impairment. Each telephone conversation was registered by the person who helped the subject making the call. Notes were made at the end of each week, the staff and the parents were interviewed regularly during the project period, and video recordings were made at the day centres. A total of 601 telephone calls were registered and analysed.

All of the participants were observed to transmit at least two pictures per conversation and some many more. This is given as a minimum number because the helper – whether parent or staff member – did not want to supervise the whole conversation. The pictures transmitted included the user and other people present, as well as objects, photographs and PIC signs held in front of the camera (Table 12.2).

Four of the adults and two of the children increased their frequency of using the telephone. They learned to operate the picture telephone fairly easily and used the equipment more adequately over time. They have since used the telephone in a functional way and seem to have made gains in independence and self-confidence. Calling to ensure that someone is home is a very common everyday function of the telephone. For example, for ten-year-old Fredrik, calls from his mother – including her picture – telling him that she was home from work made it possible for him to walk home independently from the day centre, something he did not dare to do before the picture telephone was implemented.

Table 12.2: Picture telephone use by the individuals participating in the study.

| Person | Number of partners | Number of conversations (minutes) | Mean length of conversation transmissions | Minimum number of picture transmissions | Content of picture |
|---|---|---|---|---|---|
| Anders | 1 | 59 | 5 | 5 | Himself, members of staff, manual signs, photographs, PIC, objects, letters and text. |
| Britta | 1 | 15 | 8 | 4 | Herself, members of staff and objects. |
| Carina | 2 | 58 | 12 | 2 | Herself, members of staff, friends and objects. |
| Daniel | 2 | 145 | 10 | 5 | Himself, members of staff, photographs, PIC, objects and waving 'good bye'. |
| Eva | 3 | 184 | 10 | 5 | Herself, friends, PIC, gestures and objects. |
| Fredrik | 3 | 77 | 8 | 2 | Himself, friends, relatives and parents. |
| Greta | 1 | 51 | 11 | 2 | Herself, communication partners. |
| Hanna | 1 | 12 | 13 | 3 | Herself, grandmother, friend. |

Two of the subjects did not complete the trial. One was a six-year-old girl whose mother found it too tiring to arrange systematic telephone training in the evenings after long working days. A 34-year-old woman withdrew from the trial after only one month. She showed anxiety and was tense when using the picture telephone. The staff attributed this to her intellectual impairment and somewhat impaired vision. However, the insecurity may also have been caused by too little support during training. Training and initial support were needed in order for the users to gain full benefit from the additional visual cues. This may, however, have restricted the use of picture telephone more than necessary. As with the fax study cited above, the staff tended to regard telecommunication more as a training activity than as an integrated part of the intellectually impaired users' communication options. In spite of the fact that the telephones were easy for the staff to operate, if the occupational therapist responsible for the training in the day centre for some reason was absent, the augmented telecommunication was not usually maintained by other members of staff.

In a similar study, Brodin and Björck-Åkesson (1992) used still-picture telephones (Panasonic WG-R2) in a six month trial with two men and two women with profound intellectual impairments, aged 25–39 years. None of them could speak or use manual and graphic signs. They communicated with vocalisations and gestures. The telephone exchanges were 'dependent', that is, they were made together with staff and parents. The aim of the project was to investigate whether this means of communication would be of any use at all for people with such profound impairments. Ten telephones were placed in the participants' group homes and in their parents' homes. The same procedures were used as in the study cited above, and in addition, the intellectually impaired users were video recorded during exchanges.

The picture telephone exchanges lasted 3–8 minutes and consisted in sending pictures of greetings, objects and food. It is not clear how much the intellectually impaired users actually understood of the exchanges but they were generally motivated to participate. Of the 123 registered telephone calls, sixteen were initiated independently by the impaired users and thirteen more after an initial encouragement. Recognition of faces seemed to increase as well as understanding of a few PIC signs. One mother said that she had discovered communication skills in her daughter which she had not expected. The social standing of the participants increased among the other residents but the attitudes of the staff were less positive. The participants needed considerable assistance, so the staff's understanding and attitude to using the picture telephones were decisive for their functionality. One staff member said that she believed that it was a *luxury for intellectually impaired individuals to have a picture telephone*. Another thought that *there were others who would benefit more from the telephones*. Nevertheless, two of the participants were allowed to keep the picture telephones and are still using them.

Still-picture devices for standard audio telephones are fairly simple to use and do not require that the user has an ISDN connection like videotelephones do. It is, of course, necessary that the communication partner has a similar device. The two studies reported here indicate that picture telephones may augment telecommunication conversations and help people with intellectual impairment overcome some of their difficulties in using ordinary telephones. The small number of subjects studied, however, warrants caution in generalising the results. On the other hand, the positive interest shown by most participants in spite of the limited number of persons each of them was able to call suggest that a still-picture device may enhance and facilitate telecommunication for this group of people and motivate them to use distance communication.

## Videotelephones

While picture telephones only allow transmission of individual still pictures at a low rate and with limited detail, videotelephones transmit live and more detailed pictures. Studies involving deaf people suggest that videotelephones may be used for manual signing (Blohm and Mühlback, 1990; Delvert, 1989; Dopping, 1991; Lindström and Pereira, 1995; von Tetzchner, 1991c; Whybray, 1991). There is not yet a detailed study of videotelephones used to augment everyday telecommunication similar to the picture telephone studies cited above, with the exception of Brodin and Alemder (1995) which concerns telecommunication in daily living. Videotelephone studies have concentrated on issues related to distance education and service provision.

A simulated videotelephone trial was conducted at a special school for intellectually impaired children and adolescents in a rural area in Portugal (Pereira, Matos, Purificação and Lebre, 1992). The aim of the study was to examine whether the students were able to use videotelephones in an educational setting. A major reason for the study was the fact that students with intellectual impairment were often absent from school and it was assumed that the reason for this was the long travelling distances. It was hoped that videotelephones might be used to increase their participation in school work via distance education.

Two television monitors and video cameras were placed in separate classrooms and linked by coaxial cable which provided transmission of sound and live pictures of television quality. Fifteen students, aged 8–23 years, participated. Eight functioned in the mild range of intellectual impairment, six in the moderate range, and one in the severe range. All used spoken language. During the trial, they were taught breathing exercises, spatial organisation and basic arithmetic – addition and subtraction.

Observations of the teacher-student interactions and interviews with staff and students showed that the students rapidly adapted to the medium; only one of them found the use of videotelephones difficult. The others readily understood the teacher's instructions and questions without difficulty and there were no significant differences between the reported quality of teaching directly and via the simulated videotelephone. The results indicate that videotelephones may be used to supplement education by teaching students who are often absent in their homes, constituting a substitution for travelling for those who live far away from school.

While one reason for the children's absence was the long travelling distances, another reason may have been the parents' attitude to what the school could offer their children. If parents do not feel that education is important for their children, they will let them stay at home now and then. Distance education offers the possibility of allowing the parents to participate in the teaching process and hence increase their understanding of their children's educational needs. Long distances to school are a problem in many countries and there may be a risk that parents who do not recognise the value of education will let their intellectually impaired children stay at home more, isolating them from the social training they would get in interaction with teachers and pupils.

Another Portuguese experiment was aimed at identifying transmission needs and user requirements, and investigating whether existing equipment was useable for people with intellectual impairment (Pereira et al., 1993; Pereira, Vieira, Rocha and Cidade, 1994). Twenty-eight individuals, aged 16–30 years, participated. Five had severe, twelve moderate and eleven mild intellectual impairment. Each of two workplaces had a videotelephone (with a personal computer attached) and an ISDN connection. The aim was to examine the subjects' ability to discriminate, classify, match, describe and name different objects presented on the videotelephone, and relate it to the performance of similar tasks in the normal classroom. The results showed that all participants were able to use the videotelephone, but only the mildly impaired ones could use it without difficulties. The others needed assistance and verbal instructions during the tasks. The subjects with severe impairments showed more difficulties performing the tasks than the others. However, no significant differences were observed in the performance in the videotelephone setting compared with direct face-to-face situations.

An Irish study used cable television network for delivering distance support services to 44 adults, four with severe, sixteen with moderate, and twenty-four with mild intellectual impairment, living at two different sites (McEwan, 1995). In this study, the cable television functioned essentially as a videotelephone and had a better sound and picture quality, but the potential network was much smaller (cf. Perälä and Lounela, 1991). The participants had previously attended either pre-vocational or vocational training centres and this training was followed up in community housing where they were living. The services included conversations and recreational services, that is, games and instructional programmes that would have been impossible without transmission of live pictures.

Preliminary results showed that the social networks appeared to be enhanced. The users were able to utilise the visual information provided by the screen, although some of them needed considerable assistance when using the equipment. Communication was more effective than with the audio telephones alone. It functioned best when the users interacted with familiar people. Younger people felt more comfortable using the equipment than older people.

Two men with moderate intellectual impairment, aged 32 and 35 years, participated in a Swedish ISDN multi-media minitrial designed to evaluate the technical use of videotelephones (Tandberg Vision) and computers, as well as the duration and methods of training needed by such users. The computers were attached to the videotelephones and used for transmitting PIC signs simultaneously with the live pictures on a separate monitor. One of the men had unintelligible speech, while the other had no functional language. They communicated with gestures, vocalisations and manual and graphic signs. During a period of six weeks, 40 videotelephone calls were registered, 28 between the two participants and twelve between a participant and a staff member. The results indicated that the users were stimulated by using the videotelephone, but unstable ISDN connections at this time made the quality of sound and image non-optimal for communication for this kind of user. However, the technical problems related to unstable ISDN lines have now been sorted out and the main remaining problem is related to the fact that the staff found the time needed for training too long (Brodin, Fahlén and Nilsson, 1993).

In an ongoing Swedish study of videotelephones, participants were 24 adults, aged 23–60 years, with moderate intellectual impairment, from six different day centres (Brodin and Alemder, 1995). Most of the users had some spoken language but supplemented this with graphic and manual signs. Three of the day centres were located in the north and three in the south of Sweden. Each participant could call the eight people living nearby. The participants, living in different group homes and working at different day centres, did not know each other beforehand. Attempts to get users acquainted via videotelephones were an explicit aim of the project.

The project continued for a period of three years. Documentation consisted of questionnaires and interviews with staff and relatives, as well as with participants when possible. Preliminary results showed that the participants in general increased their social network and managed to make new friends via videotelephones. In the beginning, they made pre-arranged calls at fixed times. After some time, they started taking the initiative to call friends at the other day centres. During the project they got to know each other better and developed individual preferences with regard to whom they liked to call. Telephones are typically used to organise face-to-face meetings and social contacts (von Tetzchner and Nordby, 1991). Some participants extended the videotelephone acquaintance to parties arranged by the staff and local public dances arranged for people with intellectual impairment, and some participants asked the staff to help them arrange meetings on a a more personal level.

In the interviews, the staff said they felt the participants had become more interested in peers and staff at the centre. Visitors had became an interesting issue for the participants; it might be a friend they were waiting for or an unexpected visit from somebody they had met on the videotelephone. This apparent greater interest in other people may reflect an earlier social deprivation and be related to the fact that they had obtained greater choice of companionship, in particular with regard to people outside their own day centre.

The need for assistance in making calls and maintaining the dialogue decreased and many of the participants became able to operate the equipment by themselves. In general, their communication skills seemed to have improved. Sometimes they communicated about subjects the staff did not recognise and they needed new words and graphic signs to express themselves. Thus, it seems a warranted conclusion that in some respects the participants increased their quality of life through gaining access to videotelephones.

## Service provision

Limited resources and setting priorities are central issues in habilitation work in most countries. They may be particularly important in rural areas where often more time is spent on the road than in providing the services, but with the present density of traffic, even in cities travelling may consume many of the working hours. The same access to situational information and other visual cues that could augment or make telecommunication accessible for disabled people also provides new possibilities for supervising professional work at a distance, and hence for reducing travelling time and costs, and making the intervention more efficient.

In a study of supervision of habilitative intervention, two videotelephones (Tandberg 4001) were placed in a national habilitation centre in Oslo and a nursery school in Valdres, 250 kilometres from the city (von Tetzchner, Hesselberg and Langeland, 1991). Intervention supervision was carried out for five children from one to five years of age (mainly motor impaired but three were also intellectually impaired). When the project started, the children had recently been assessed, either at the Centre or during a team visit. Two of them were in the early phase of intervention, while three were in a follow-up phase. The project lasted three months, and there were 2–7 supervisions for each child.

Among the intervention activities that were supervised, physiotherapy had a central position. In a typical supervision session, the local physiotherapist went through the exercises with the child, while the physiotherapist in Oslo watched and commented during or following the treatment. After this, new exercises or interventions were discussed, which the physiotherapist in Oslo demonstrated with a doll. The local physiotherapist then went through the new exercises with the child while being helped by the specialist in Oslo. Language training was another important area. Similar supervision was given in sign teaching, sound articulation and language stimulation in general. To some extent toys and other material were shown on the videotelephone. Since the child was usually present, the supervision also implied a limited but continuous assessment of the child's skills.

At the habilitation centre in Oslo, the more frequent supervision placed greater demands on the staff in terms of concrete and focused supervision that would not have been possible with the traditional written reports following assessments once or twice a year. Intervention could be followed up in more detail, and the increased knowledge about local conditions made it possible for the professionals at the Centre to make allowances for conditions that they otherwise would not have known about. For example, one of the children developed more quickly than expected. This was seen during the videotelephone sessions, and the interventions were altered in such a way that the positive change was taken into account. Normally, the same general intervention would not have been carried out until the next assessment at the Centre. This would not have been adapted to the child's present needs. It would probably have become boring and the child might have developed negative feelings towards the training.

The more immediate follow-up led to misunderstandings being cleared up, and the local professionals felt more confident that what they did was right. They felt it was possible to ask questions that would have been difficult to put in a letter or an ordinary telephone conversation. It was also easier to express disagreement and discuss the intervention measures with the people at the Centre. This last point was particularly important, because local professionals often sabotage interventions that they do not understand the point of, do not agree with, or do not know how to carry out.

The quality of the supervision via videotelephone was not considered equal to supervision in the same room, but it was regarded as being significantly better than via an ordinary telephone, and a greater sense of nearness was reported by the participants. The difference between an ordinary telephone and the videotelephone became manifest when there were ordinary telephone contacts between supervision sessions. The impression of the work and the skills of the child that the supervisor formed from these telephone conversations sometimes turned out to be quite wrong when the child was seen over the videotelephone. With the videotelephone, the impression was more correct, hence the supervision was more in accordance with the actual needs. One of the physiotherapists in Oslo said that she *could not have given better supervision without holding the hands of the local physiotherapist*. The videotelephone was a pre-ISDN prototype with a rather poor picture quality, but even this quality was considered good enough by the participants. This probably reflects the fact that they really needed the visual information, without which supervision would have been impossible. The fact that the various professionals knew each other beforehand probably also contributed to the success of the videotelephone supervision.

The same pre-ISDN prototype (Tandberg 4001) was used for supervision from an autism unit in Bodø to a nursery school in Mosjøen, both located in the North of Norway (Holand, von Tetzchner and Steindal, 1991; Steindal, 1993). At Mosjøen, there were two intellectually impaired and autistic children, aged three and five years, who had not learned to speak. For both of them manual sign teaching was initiated but the local professionals had little experience with teaching manual signs to autistic children and needed both sign instruction and supervision of teaching. However, shortage of human resources, long travelling distances and many cancelled flights due to bad weather in the winter limited direct follow-up. A special education teacher used the videotelephone connection for teaching manual signs to professionals and parents and supervising the sign instruction for the two autistic children in Mosjøen. The two children went to different nursery schools, and the work was supervised individually, making a total of 22 supervisions over a period of nine months.

In spite of the fact that the picture quality of this first prototype was much poorer than present-day videotelephones, it was possible to supervise manual sign intervention. In subsequent interviews, the teachers said that they often found themselves confronted with issues which they did not know how to solve, and that it was not easy to find these discussed in the literature. It might have been possible to discuss on some of these problems on an ordinary telephone, but they found that many of the issues were difficult to explain without being able to demonstrate with the child present. Thus, the availability of visual information made a crucial difference. At present, videotelephones are used to supplement direct observations and face-to-face meetings in the follow-up of projects under the Norwegian national programme for building up competence related to habilitation services for autistic people (Harald Martinsen, personal communication, August 1995).

# Conclusions

The small number of studies presented here suggest that new telecommunication technologies – transmitting visual as well as acoustic information – may make distance communication accessible or easier to access for people with intellectual impairment. One firm conclusion of this preview is that visual cues seem to be important for many intellectually impaired people. For some, the quality of telecommunication was improved, as well as their motivation and satisfaction when using it. For others, visual cues were a necessary requirement for using telecommunication at all.

Even the limited function of add-on still-picture devices made a significant difference. Transmission of moving pictures has made telecommunication even more adaptable to the communicative competence of people with intellectual impairment, so both picture and video telephones may be considered technical aids for this group. Several studies have showed that videotelephones and picture telephones reinforced, facilitated and supported telecommunication. Many of the participants improved their communication and commenced taking the initiative in respect of distance communication. However, requirements for optimal use of the new telecommunication technologies that have become apparent are proper adaptation of the equipment and sufficient training and assistance from parents and staff. Importantly, there seems to be a need for change of attitude: staff and parents must regard telecommunication as part of intellectually impaired people's everyday communicative options. This will contribute to empowering people with intellectual impairment and improve their quality of life.

Also the studies of distance education and supervision showed positive results, indicating that new telecommunication technologies may be utilised for distributing expert knowledge and building up local competence on disability and habilitation in rural areas, improving follow-up, and reducing time and resources professionals and parents spend on travelling.

All studies involving picture telephones and videotelephones had a limited number of participants, primarily because of the price of the equipment. The high cost compared to an ordinary telephone implies that it may take several years before this kind of equipment is in regular use, and probably even longer before it has become common in the homes of people with intellectual impairment. One may only hope that this prediction is proven wrong.

## Acknowledgement

Brodin was supported by the Swedish Transport & Communications Research Board during the work with this chapter.

# Chapter 13
# Enhancing communication skills of children with Down syndrome: Early use of manual signs

KAISA LAUNONEN

Early intervention of intellectually impaired infants and young children is a quickly expanding field and new methods are being developed around the world. Early intervention can be defined as 'systematic strategies aimed at promoting the optimal development of infants and toddlers with special needs and at enhancing the functioning of their families and caregivers' (Mitchell and Brown, 1991, p. xii). These preventive strategies can be considered as primary or secondary. *Primary prevention* is concerned with averting the conditions which cause disabilities. This chapter addresses *secondary prevention* which has to do with the early identification of conditions which are likely to place a child's development at serious risk, and the implementation of measures to ameliorate or reduce the severity of any disability which might result from such factors (Mitchell and Brown, 1991).

The assumption behind starting an early intervention programme is usually that the sooner one begins specialised activities with the infant, the more likely one is to prevent or reduce future problems of development (Cunningham, 1988). Intensified activities, together with the plasticity of the developing organism, are thought to produce positive outcomes (Casto, 1987). There are great hopes for the effects of early intervention and it is a general finding that early intervention programmes do have substantial immediate benefits for disabled populations (Casto, 1987). There are, however, many questions which have to be answered, in particular whether there are any beneficial long-term effects of early intervention programmes for impaired infants. For the time being, there is a lack of well-designed, controlled evaluation studies which can demonstrate that the intervention programmes, those already in use and those being developed, really do have long-term benefits and are cost effective.

People who have Down syndrome have been found to display distinctive problems in language development and use which cannot be explained by the intellectual impairment alone (Cardoso-Martins, Mervis and Mervis, 1985; Mundy, Kasari, Sigman and Ruskin, 1995; Smith and von Tetzchner, 1986). They are further behind in their language development than are mental-age-matched, normally developing children or other groups of intellectually impaired children. Besides the general language deficiency, the development of speech seems to be especially delayed in children with Down syndrome (Bray and Woolnough, 1988; Dykens, Hodapp and Evans, 1994). The reason for these difficulties is not yet properly known, and considerable individual variation is evident in the development of children with Down syndrome (Dykens et al., 1994).

Previous studies emphasise that acquisition of preverbal communication skills provides an important foundation for the emergence of language in both normally developing children and children with Down syndrome (Bates, Camaioni and Volterra, 1975; Goldin-Meadow and Morford, 1990; Mundy et al., 1995). Many researchers share the observation that the communication of children with Down syndrome is already deviant in the early preverbal phase (e.g. Mundy et al., 1995; Smith and von Tetzchner, 1986). Children with Down syndrome tend to be more passive and show less initiative in their interactions than normally developing infants (Cardoso-Martins and Mervis, 1985; Fischer, 1987; Levy-Shiff, 1986). Parents seem to be more directive in their interactions with their child with Down syndrome than with other children (Cardoso-Martins and Mervis, 1985; Maurer and Sherrod, 1987), and, in some cases, surprisingly blind to the communicative behaviour of the infant with Down syndrome (Smith and Hagen, 1984). The opinion about children's passivity seems to be more generally accepted than the lack of communicative skills of parents, where there seem to be larger individual differences. The concept of maternal directiveness, as such, has been called into question (e.g. Pine, 1992), and the findings of several studies suggest that parents of children with Down syndrome are able to adjust their communicative style according to the child's skills (Fischer, 1987; von Tetzchner and Smith, 1986).

Several researchers have reported deviant auditory processing in persons with Down syndrome (Marcell and Weeks, 1988; Pueschel, Gallagher, Zarter and Pezzullo, 1987; Varnhagen, Das and Varnhagen, 1987). In the study by Marcell and Weeks (1988), subjects listened to or looked at increasingly longer sequences of digits and attempted to recall them either orally or manually. The results suggested that normally developing persons and other groups of intellectually impaired people typically show better memory for sequences of auditory than visual information while individuals with Down syndrome display either the reverse pattern or equivalent auditory and visual recall. Pueschel and associates (1987) used the *Kaufman Assessment Battery for Children* to investigate sequential and simultaneous processing in children with

Down syndrome, their siblings, and a group of children matched for mental age scores. The children with Down syndrome performed significantly less well on subtests which included auditory-vocal and auditory-motor tasks than on subtests with visual-vocal and visual-motor tasks.

However, the communicative abilities of individuals with Down syndrome are not characterised solely by difficulties and weaknesses. Their pragmatic skills are often good and they tend to use compensating strategies in order to be understood: mimicry, gestures, actions, and – if possible – signing (Bray and Woolnough, 1988). Several studies suggest that it is easier for people with Down syndrome to learn manual signs than spoken words, at least in the early stages of language development (e.g. Abrahamsen, Lamb, Brown-Williams and McCarthy, 1991; Johansson, 1987; Layton and Savino, 1990; Le Prevost, 1983).

If the primary reason for the difficulties in speech and language learning has its origin in early preverbal communication and failure in early interaction, early intervention should concentrate on guiding parents in supporting the development of interaction in the best possible ways. And if one reason is poor auditory processing, an aim of intervention should be to develop more profitable methods, building on the possible strengths of the child, namely visual-motor means of communication. These were the main starting points for the early intervention project with manual signing presented here.

In 1988–93, speech therapists of Helsinki City Social Services Department carried out *The Early Signing Project: Enhancing the development of the early communication and language skills of children with Down syndrome*. The aim of the project was to find out how intervention with children aged between six months and three years, based on the use of manual signing, gestural communication and action, along with speech, would affect the development of language and communicative skills of children with Down syndrome. The main focus of the study was the effect of the intervention two years after the programme was terminated. Through the project, new early communication intervention methods were also developed for general clinical use.

# Method

## Subjects

The project consisted of two parts. In the first part, the development of communication of 29 children was followed. The second part was a controlled study in which a subgroup consisting of 12 of the 29 children was compared with a control group.

*Intervention group.* There were 36 families in the first ten family groups of the intervention programme. Of these families, 29 were included in the intervention group. Seven families were left out, either because they did not follow the programme regularly or the children had severe epilepsy which seriously affected their development. There were 17 girls and 12 boys in the intervention group. All came from urban families of which 27 were Finnish-speaking, and two were bilingual (Finnish/Swedish and Finnish/English; in the latter case, the language used with the child at home was Finnish. Finland is an officially bilingual country, and the Swedish-speaking minority in the Helsinki area is 7.1 per cent).

*Research group.* The twelve oldest children of the intervention group, six boys and six girls, made up the research group. All of them had trisomy 21 and no other disability which could have had an effect on the intervention. Five of the children had a congenital heart defect which was surgically corrected at an early age. Seven of the children were first-borns. By the age of five, two were single children while the others had one or two siblings. All came from Finnish-speaking families and attended day-care outside their home; seven children from the age of one, four children from the age of three, and one from 4½ years. For most of the children, individual speech therapy started soon after the programme was terminated at the age of three. For one child, speech therapy continued to the age of four and for another child to age five years. For the rest, it went on at least until school age, which for disabled children in Finland is six years (for other children seven years).

*Control group.* For ethical reasons, after it was initiated, the intervention programme has been offered to all families living in the Helsinki area with a new-born child with Down syndrome. This caused some problems for forming a contemporary control group which did not participate in the programme. The control group therefore comprised the 12 oldest of the preceding age group of children with Down syndrome in the Helsinki area, of whom all the families agreed to participate in the project. In the control group, eleven children had trisomy 21 and one had translocation trisomy. None of them had other impairments. Four children had a congenital heart defect; one of them could not have an operation. There were nine girls and three boys in the group. Three of the children were first-borns. By the age of five years, the children had 1–4 siblings. All came from urban families; eleven were Finnish-speaking and one was bilingual (Finnish/Swedish). By the age of five, the ten remaining children attended day-care outside their homes, having started between the ages of one and four years.

Services other than the early signing programme (see below) were the same for the two groups. Early intervention for the children in the control group consisted of services given to all families attending the clinic for disabled children, including the intervention group. For most families, these services included two yearly visits to the clinic where a team of professionals examined the child, consulted with the parents, and gave them advice, both orally and in writing, on how to enhance the development of the child in different skill areas. Nine children in both the research group and the control group were given physiotherapy before learning to walk without support. For the control group, individual speech therapy was initiated between 2½ and 5 years, with an average of 3½ years. For these children, speech therapy continued at least until they reached school age.

## Procedures

All families with an infant with Down syndrome, living in the Helsinki area, were, if willing to participate, included in the early signing programme. The programme started when the child was about six months old and ended at the age of three. The speech therapists' part in the intervention was mostly indirect. They gave advice to the parents who trained their own children. Direct contact between the child and the speech therapist was included in the programme in order to follow the development of the child and to ensure that the intervention was carried out according to the individual needs of each child and its family.

Family groups of 2–4 families met with two speech therapists; during the first six months, groups met every second month, and, after that, once a month (see Table 13.1). In the course of the 2½ years of intervention, there were 25 sessions with each family group and at each session the families were assigned tasks and given advice for training at home. Besides the family groups, the child and the parents had individual appointments with the speech therapist every second week. If possible, the day-care personnel were included in the programme. Training, however, was the responsibility of the parents.

Table 13.1: Follow-up of the programme according to the age of the child

| Age in months | Stage of the programme | |
| --- | --- | --- |
| 6–12 | Daily: | Training at home |
| | Bi-monthly: | Family session |
| 12–36 | Daily: | Training at home |
| | Bi-weekly: | Speech therapist meets the child |
| | Monthly: | Family session |
| | | Evaluations made by parents and the speech therapist |
| | Semi-annually: | Portage assessment |
| | | Three questionnaires |
| | | Video recording |
| 36–60 | Annually: | Portage assessment |
| | | Three questionnaires |
| | | Video recording |

Parents were advised to have daily brief 'training sessions', in order to make the use of the signs explicit. Signing in daily situations at home was, however, emphasised. In the beginning, training consisted of a variety of shared activities, aimed at encouraging the child and the parents to take part in mutual activities. Many of these were traditional games (such as 'See-saw Margery Daw', 'Round and round the garden', and 'This little piggy'). In the beginning, activities in which the focus is on the use of hands were emphasised, and in the course of the first six months, the focus shifted gradually to conventional manual signs. From the age of twelve months, the monthly programme included 6–10 new manual signs, suggestions for training at home, and a song which was sung with signs. The last ten monthly programmes consisted of games and play designed to encourage the children to actively use their different means of communication. During this period, teaching of new manual signs was related to individual needs with the help of video tapes and instructions given to parents by the speech therapists.

The family group sessions, each lasting 45–60 minutes, usually started with singing the 'signing song' of the previous month, followed by the new manual signs and strategies. Parents were given drawings and verbal instructions for each new sign and pictures from children's books on the same theme, and advised to collect the graphic material in a book which the child could use as a picture book when together with other people. In addition, they were given oral and written suggestions for the training of each new sign. The new song, with its signs, was taught to families. After going through the new programme, there was usually a brief period of 'free conversation', and the session was finished by singing the song of the month.

Initially, parents were advised to train with one of the parents opposite the child, giving the model, and the other sitting behind the child, hand guiding it to make the manual sign when necessary. At the same time, parents were advised to be sensitive to the child's reactions and to keep help at a minimum. After the child had learned some manual signs, imitation was emphasised as a way of learning new signs. Parents were told to speak normally when using signs and to sign the 'key words' of the spoken utterance, according to the language skills of the child.

Even if the routines of the signing programme were structured, the purpose was not to make the parents slavishly follow the routines. They were told that learning manual signs was not a goal but a tool. One of the main themes in the programme was to reinforce the child's active behaviour and initiative from very early on. The parents were given varied information, both orally and in writing, about conditions that may enhance language development and on how to encourage the child to use its early means of communication. The systemic, interactive nature of all communication and learning was emphasised, as well as the fact that infants are competent individuals, responsible for their own part in communicative interactions. It was also pointed out that children need a range of interesting challenges which can encourage them to explore the world. The child's characteristics and communicative strengths were discussed by the parents and the speech therapists. The family was always encouraged to use its own individual style in communication.

In addition to being an empirical basis of the project, the assessment methods and video recordings (see below) had aims closely linked to the intervention itself. Through taking part in assessments, evaluating their child's development, and watching the video tapes when at home or with the speech therapist in the clinic, parents learned to observe both their own and the child's behaviour. They learned to search for the strengths of the child and identify useful intervention strategies (cf. Ballard, 1991).

## Measures

The evaluation of children in the intervention group was made every sixth month from 1 to 3 years of age. Follow-up assessments were made when the children were 4 and 5 years old (and will be made at the age of 8 years). General development was evaluated with *The Portage Assessment Scale* (Tiilikka and Hautamäki, 1986) which gives a profile of the child's skills in five areas: *social, language, self-help, cognitive,* and *motor.* The Portage scale is not standardised. It can, however, be used to evaluate the developmental level, and its reliability and validity have proved to be good in studies of intellectually impaired populations in Finland (Arvio, Hautamäki and Tiilikka, 1993). Scoring was adapted to the needs of the project in order to show effects of signing skills separately. Because some children mastered a skill only by using signs, children who used signing were given two values: with and without signing, mainly for the areas of social development, language and cognitive development. For self-help and motor development, signing skills as such did not make any difference. The Portage assessments of the intervention group were mostly made at the clinic by the speech therapist and one or both of the parents.

*Three questionnaires* were created for assessing the development and efficiency of the child's expressive communication. One of the questionnaires was filled in by the parents and the speech therapist separately once a month; the other two were used in half-yearly evaluations. The parents usually filled in the questionnaires at home and if there were any unclear points, they were discussed during the next session or soon afterwards. In addition, parents made notes of the daily training at home. At the half-yearly assessments, the children were video recorded playing with the speech therapist and sometimes also with one of the parents. At the present time, some of the children in the intervention group have not yet reached the age of 4 years. Hence, this age level includes only 21 children.

Except for video recording, the control group was assessed in a similar way once a year. Because the project started when the oldest children in this group were almost three years old, many of the early observations are not complete. Five children were assessed with the Portage scale at the age of one and seven children at the age of two. All twelve children were assessed at the ages of three and four years, and ten children at the age of five. One family moved away and one family did not want to take part in the project when the child was five years old. Thus, the most complete comparisons are available for the time when the programme was terminated for the research group, at the ages of three, four and five years. Although at this stage, some children did and some did not use manual signing, the principles of intervention were the same for both groups.

The assessments of the control group were made mostly in the home by the speech therapist and one or both of the parents. The questionnaires were usually filled in together on the same occasion. Parents of the control group were not as accustomed to making evaluations of their child as were parents of the intervention group.

Several milestones in the early development of communicative skills of the intervention group were registered: early gestures (waving 'byebye' and clapping hands), pointing with index finger, first manual sign, first spoken word, and the number of manual signs and spoken words yearly from 12 to 48 months. These measures were based on information given by the parents. A checklist of specific items such as waving 'bye-bye' or clapping was not provided. Instead, parents were asked to write down all the early gestures that the child was using. For this reason, this information is missing for some children. For pointing with the index finger, it was required that the child pointed to an object out of its reach, not just touched an object or a picture with the finger. Determining when a child for the first time used a manual sign purposefully proved to be difficult. The first imitation of a manual sign, recognised by the parents and the speech therapist, was accepted. Determining the 'first spoken word' proved even more difficult (cf. Bates et al., 1975). Some parents reported the first word of the child approximately at the age of one, but could – maybe a year later – state that the child had not yet said its first word. If parents corrected their evaluation, the later age was used – if not, the first one. Thus, the estimates of first words are only suggestive.

The expressive vocabularies of manual signs and spoken words were based on records made by parents. Because active use was difficult to define, parents were asked to write down all the manual signs and spoken words that the child could produce when asked to. In the later evaluations, when some children used dozens or hundreds of signs and words, parents were asked to estimate the vocabulary size. Pure imitations were not counted because some children in the intervention group could imitate signs almost indefinitely without understanding their meaning. The way that an individual family collected this information was not checked; parents of the intervention group knew that they would be asked for the information at the half-yearly assessments. Some parents asked for help from the speech therapist for these evaluations but both in the intervention group and the control group the final numbers were always the parents' estimates. In the evaluations at three and four years of age, the vocabularies of some children were so large that their parents just wrote 'hundreds'. In these cases it was decided to give them a size of 300, which for some children might be somewhat low.

For comparing the research group and the control group, analyses of variance was made of the yearly Portage scores from one to five years of age and repeated measures of analyses of variance from three to five years of age. The number of manual signs and spoken words are compared at three and four years. By the age of five, expressive language had for many children reached such a level that it was impossible to estimate the number of individual signs and words. When estimating the number of symbols (manual signs and spoken words), parents also gave examples of *first combinations of symbols* that the children had used.

# Results

Milestones in early communicative skills of the intervention group and the research sub-group are shown in Table 13.2. There was considerable individual variation with regard to when the children were reported to clap hands, wave 'bye-bye', and point. All the children participating in the programme started to use manual signs and the mean age for the first sign was 17 months. At the age of 1½ years, most of the children (23) used some signs, and by the age of two years, all the children used some manual signs for communication (Table 13.3). There were large individual differences with regard to both the number of signs and how actively and varied were the signs used. The increase in the number of manual signs was notable until the age of three. By that age, some children began to speak quite clearly, and by the age of four, the average number of spoken words had surpassed the number of manual signs. Seven of the 21 children in the intervention group used more spoken words than manual signs in their communication at the age of four.

Table 13.3 indicates that, at ages of three and four, children of the research group were using more communicative symbols, both manual signs and spoken words, than the children in the control group. When manual signs and spoken words were counted together, the size of the average vocabulary of the research group at age three was as large as that of the control group at age four. All children in the research group used manual signs in their communication. In the control group, three children communicated by signing (at age four) and these three were among the most advanced linguistically of the control group.

Table 13.2 Age in months at appearance of early communicative skills of children who participated in the early signing programme; intervention group (IG, N=29) and research group (RG; N=12).

| | | Mean | Std | Range | Median | Missing |
|---|---|---|---|---|---|---|
| Clapping | IG | 11.4 | 2.6 | 6–16 | 11 | 12 |
| | RG | 11.0 | 0.6 | 10–12 | 11 | 7 |
| Waving | IG | 14.7 | 3.4 | 9–23 | 14 | 7 |
| | RG | 13.6 | 3.4 | 9–21 | 13 | 4 |
| Pointing | IG | 16.0 | 2.3 | 10–22 | 16 | 0 |
| | RG | 16.7 | 1.9 | 14–22 | 16.5 | 0 |
| First sign | IG | 17.0 | 2.2 | 14–22 | 17 | 0 |
| | RG | 17.8 | 1.8 | 14–21 | 17.5 | 0 |
| First word | IG | 18.8 | 4.6 | 12–30 | 18 | 0 |
| | RG | 19.3 | 4.8 | 14–30 | 18 | 0 |

At the age of three, all except one of the research group joined two or three symbols (signs, signs and words, or words) together, two of them only occasionally. In the control group, three of the children joined two spoken words together, and two children joined two manual signs occasionally. At the age of four, four children in the research group used spoken sentences, four joined manual signs or signs and spoken words together, and four used such combinations occasionally. In the control group, seven children joined two or three spoken words together. At the age of five, six of the twelve children in the research group used spoken sentences, one used manual signs and spoken words in all three ways of combination, one joined signs and spoken words together, and four used combinations of two signs or signs and gestures. In the control group, five children used spoken sentences, one combined signs, signs and words, and words. Four out of ten remaining children in the control group did not join symbols together at the age of five (Table 13.4).

On the first Portage assessment at 12 months, the two groups did not differ significantly. The children in the control group (N=5) seemed to be slightly ahead of the research group (N=11) in all areas except self-help (Table 13.5). At the age of two, the research group (N=12) was ahead of the control group (N=7) in all areas except self-help. The difference was greatest for language development with signs, the area where the intervention programme could be expected to have the most immediate effect.

From three to five years of age, the profiles of the Portage assessments of the research group and the control group clearly differed from each other, the children in the research group being ahead in all areas of development (Table 13.5). The difference was evident even when signing skills were not taken into consideration. The difference between the two groups was most marked at age three, when the intervention

Table 13.3 The number of manual signs, spoken words, and signs and words counted together (total) of children of the intervention group (IG; N=29, at 48 months N=21), research group (RG; N=12), and control group (CG; N=12). (Med = median; 'None' = number of children without any manual signs or spoken words).

| Age | Group | Manual signs | | | | | Spoken words | | | | | Total | | | |
|---|---|---|---|---|---|---|---|---|---|---|---|---|---|---|---|
| | | Mean | Std | Range | Med | None | Mean | Std | Range | Median | None | Mean | Std | Range | Med |
| 12 | IG | 0 | 0.0 | 0 | 0 | 29 | 0.2 | 0.5 | 0-2 | 0 | 25 | 0.2 | 0.5 | 0-2 | 0 |
| | RG | 0 | 0.0 | 0 | 0 | 12 | 0.2 | 0.6 | 0-2 | 0 | 11 | 0.2 | 0.6 | 0-2 | 0 |
| 18 | IG | 7 | 9.8 | 0-40 | 3 | 6 | 1.3 | 1.7 | 0-6 | 1 | 13 | 8.3 | 9.9 | 0-41 | 4 |
| | RG | 5.3 | 8.1 | 0-30 | 2.5 | 4 | 1.1 | 1.6 | 0-4 | 0 | 6 | 6.3 | 8.4 | 0-31 | 3.5 |
| 24 | IG | 31.4 | 25.6 | 3-110 | 20 | 0 | 5.7 | 6.7 | 0-32 | 3.5 | 2 | 37.1 | 26.6 | 4-111 | 29 |
| | RG | 34.2 | 21.1 | 10-74 | 27 | 0 | 3.9 | 3.3 | 0-10 | 3.5 | 2 | 38.1 | 21.7 | 11-81 | 31.5 |
| 30 | IG | 73.3 | 55.1 | 5-200 | 65 | 0 | 11.9 | 18.3 | 0-100 | 8 | 1 | 85.1 | 61.6 | 8-220 | 74 |
| | RG | 74.2 | 42.6 | 15-150 | 80 | 0 | 7.6 | 5.9 | 0-20 | 7 | 1 | 81.8 | 43.2 | 19-158 | 87 |
| 36 | IG | 101.7 | 79.0 | 10-300 | 100 | 0 | 17.3 | 20.1 | 1-100 | 10 | 0 | 119.1 | 84.2 | 17-318 | 102 |
| | RG | 93.3 | 65.0 | 15-250 | 100 | 0 | 17.3 | 17.0 | 1-50 | 11.5 | 0 | 110.7 | 73.2 | 20-300 | 106.5 |
| | CG | 3.3 | 4.6 | 0-17 | 2.5 | 5 | 10.3 | 11.2 | 0-40 | 6.5 | 3 | 13.6 | 11.2 | 0-40 | 12 |
| 48 | IG | 151.0 | 104.1 | 20-350 | 200 | 0 | 105.0 | 122.0 | 3-300 | 200 | 0 | 255.9 | 141.1 | 25-500 | 305 |
| | RG | 108.3 | 69.1 | 20-250 | 90 | 0 | 128.2 | 131.8 | 3-300 | 50 | 0 | 236.5 | 141.6 | 30-500 | 220 |
| | CG | 35.7 | 82.8 | 0-300 | 1 | 6 | 75.8 | 98.2 | 0-300 | 45 | 1 | 111.4 | 121.8 | 0-355 | 65 |

Table 13.4 Number of children in the research group (RG) and the control group (CG) who made different combinations of symbols at the ages of 36, 48, and 60 months. W = combinations of spoken words; W+S = combinations of spoken words and manual signs; S = combinations of manual signs.

|  | 36 months | | 48 months | | 60 months | |
| --- | --- | --- | --- | --- | --- | --- |
|  | RG | CG | RG | CG | RG | CG |
| W |  | 3 | 4 | 6 | 6 | 5 |
| W, W+S |  |  | 1 | 1 |  |  |
| W, W+S, S | 2 |  | 1 |  | 1 | 1 |
| W, S | 2 |  |  |  |  |  |
| W+S, S | 1 |  | 3 |  |  |  |
| S | 6 | 2 | 4 |  | 4 |  |
| No combinations | 1 | 7 |  | 5 |  | 4 |

Table 13.5 Comparison of children in the research group (RG) and the control group (CG) on the means of the Portage scores at 12, 24, 36, 48 and 60 months (* p< .05; ** p< .01; *** p< .001).

|  | RG | CG | df | F |
| --- | --- | --- | --- | --- |
| 12 months |  |  |  |  |
| social | 11.36 | 12.57 | 1,14 | .43 |
| language | 5.01 | 7.54 | 1,14 | 2.68 |
| self-help | 9.97 | 8.76 | 1,14 | .51 |
| cognitive | 5.07 | 6.34 | 1,13 | .76 |
| motor | 6.81 | 7.96 | 1,14 | .78 |
| 24 months |  |  |  |  |
| social | 26.50 | 23.50 | 1,17 | 1.28 |
| social + signs | 27.78 | 23.50 | 1,17 | 2.34 |
| language | 14.91 | 12.03 | 1,17 | 3.58 |
| language + signs | 17.90 | 12.03 | 1,17 | 11.42** |
| self-help | 21.45 | 22.10 | 1,17 | .09 |
| cognitive | 18.75 | 16.01 | 1,17 | 2.53 |
| cognitive + signs | 19.88 | 16.01 | 1,17 | 4.15 |
| motor | 20.60 | 19.14 | 1,17 | .28 |
| 36 months |  |  |  |  |
| social | 42.63 | 37.29 | 1,22 | 2.85 |
| social + signs | 45.50 | 37.29 | 1,22 | 6.54* |
| language | 24.34 | 18.77 | 1,22 | 4.69* |
| language + signs | 29.78 | 18.77 | 1,22 | 22.34*** |
| self-help | 38.93 | 35.26 | 1,22 | 1.44 |
| cognitive | 30.89 | 23.61 | 1,22 | 23.76*** |
| cognitive + signs | 32.28 | 23.61 | 1,22 | 30.52*** |
| motor | 37.94 | 33.14 | 1,22 | 4.32* |

Table 13.5 Contd.

|  | RG | CG | df | F |
|---|---|---|---|---|
| **48 months** |  |  |  |  |
| social | 52.10 | 47.81 | 1,22 | .89 |
| social + signs | 54.60 | 48.23 | 1,22 | 2.11 |
| language | 34.41 | 23.11 | 1,22 | 7.44* |
| language + signs | 38.34 | 23.86 | 1,22 | 15.32*** |
| self-help | 47.79 | 43.29 | 1,22 | 1.39 |
| cognitive | 37.39 | 28.42 | 1,22 | 12.46** |
| cognitive + signs | 38.60 | 28.69 | 1,22 | 16.11*** |
| motor | 45.31 | 40.43 | 1,22 | 2.62 |
| **60 months** |  |  |  |  |
| social | 57.75 | 53.39 | 1,20 | .88 |
| social + signs | 59.78 | 53.63 | 1,20 | 1.93 |
| language | 41.15 | 30.53 | 1,20 | 3.40 |
| language + signs | 44.70 | 30.65 | 1,20 | 7.73* |
| self-help | 52.81 | 49.04 | 1,20 | .98 |
| cognitive | 42.58 | 34.03 | 1,20 | 5.66* |
| cognitive + signs | 43.89 | 34.08 | 1,20 | 8.13** |
| motor | 49.44 | 46.88 | 1,20 | .60 |

programme was completed. The research group ($N=12$) was significantly ahead of the control group ($N=12$) for all Portage areas except social development without signs and self-help. The difference was greatest in the areas of language with signs and cognitive development with and without signs. The differences between the groups had started to decrease at ages four and five (Table 13.5). However, significant differences were still found in the areas of language and cognitive skills. The repeated measures of analysis of variance revealed a significant difference between the groups in the development of language and cognitive skills, both with and without the help of signs, during the two-year follow-up after the intervention programme had been completed for the research group (Table 13.6).

Table 13.6 Differences between the research group (RG) and the control group (CG) on Portage at 36, 48 and 60 months (repeated measures ANOVA). (* $p<.05$; ** $p<.01$).

|  | df | F |
|---|---|---|
| Social | 1,20 | 1.49 |
| Social with signs | 1,20 | 3.27 |
| Language | 1,20 | 4.96* |
| Language with signs | 1,20 | 12.96** |
| Self-help | 1,20 | 1.38 |
| Cognitive | 1,20 | 9.87** |
| Cognitive with signs | 1,20 | 13.69** |
| Motor | 1,20 | 1.94 |

# Discussion

The results show that the early signing programme had significant immediate benefits for the children who took part and that the positive effects remained during the two-year follow-up after its completion. Compared to the control group, at three, four and five years, the children in the research group used a far wider range of communicative means and were clearly ahead both in language and general development, especially in cognitive skills.

The main difference in early intervention between the children in the two groups was the purposefully enlarged and intensified usage of nonvocal means of communication in the research group. This was developed as far as it was individually necessary and for all the children it implied some degree of signed communication. All had a period where they obtained higher scores on the Portage scale with manual signs than without. There were, however, marked individual differences in the language development of the children in the research group also. For some children, the period where signing was dominant lasted less than a year; for others, signing was their most functional means of communication at least until the age of five.

Availability of differentiated symbols for active use makes it possible for a child to interact with others in a way which may develop its communication even further. For example, at the age of three, having 93 manual signs made a big difference compared to having to rely on 17 spoken words only for communication, and even this was seven words more than the control group. The research group had an average of 111 symbols (signed and spoken) while the control group had 14. Manual signs made many communicative functions possible which would be out of the children's reach with non-verbal means of communication only, such as making requests, questions and comments, getting information, telling one's experiences, or even joking. Many of the parents in the early signing programme commented spontaneously during the active signing phase of their child that they had difficulties imagining how these communicative needs would have been fulfilled had not manual signing been available to the child.

The present findings suggest that augmented language development may enhance cognitive skills and that the developments of these two areas are closely linked. As argued above, availability of differentiated symbols provided the children with opportunities for dealing with objects, people and events on a more mature level. This cognitive growth in turn created new conditions for versatile functions of communication and language. The results support the findings of Johansson (1990), according to which preschool children with Down syndrome who had participated in an early language intervention programme had far better linguistic and cognitive competence than a non-participating control group of children with Down syndrome.

The signing is also likely to have affected the spoken input to the children in a way that made it easier for them to obtain information and understand the utterances. Part of this was probably a natural consequence of signed communication being added to the speech, but also the interaction with the speech therapist was important for the parents' learning to adapt their communication to their child's skills. When using keyword signing, parents are likely to speak more slowly, use shorter utterances and probably put stress on words they both speak and sign (Windsor and Fristoe, 1989). A significant characteristic of simultaneous signing and speaking is also that parents have to make sure that they had visual contact with the child while talking to it. The parents also had better opportunities for observing the child's behaviour and responses and reacting in an adequate manner. For instance, they waited and gave the child time, repeated the utterance, gave extra information and continued the conversation according to the child's response. The simultaneous use of visual and auditory forms of communication may also have made it easier for the child to obtain information and thus to expand its cognitive competence.

Even if the possible strength of visual processing of persons with Down syndrome is not taken into consideration, the visual-motor character of signs may be of significance, especially the possibility of adapting the speed of production when signs are taught to a child. Contrary to saying words, manually signing can be slowed down, sometimes even stopped, without loss of intelligibility. Signs can also be taught through hand guidance. Moreover, if visual skills are better than auditory skills for individuals with Down syndrome, it is likely that visual signs will catch their attention more easily than spoken words.

The results indicate that manual signing in early communication intervention, apart from advancing language and general development, also enhanced the speech development of the research group. This is evident in the Portage language scores without signing where the research group was ahead of the control group on all assessments from three through five years. Also the reported number of spoken words was higher for the research group at the ages of three and four.

Most of the children who participated in the programme started joining two or three manual signs together. The most common first combinations were, however, the joining of a manual sign and a spoken word together. According to Caselli and Volterra (1990), the capacity to use symbolic and combinatorial ability simultaneously in order to communicate indicates that the child is passing from using a general communicative capability to managing a real linguistic system. Most of these children with Down syndrome used manual signs at this transitional stage but it seems as if the signing ability never reached a 'mature' level of verbal communication even though it fulfilled versatile functions of communication. However, it is clear that the manual signs of these children, even if used only as single-sign utterances, functioned like verbal symbols in communication in the same way as single-word utterances of normally developing children. Furthermore, children who seemed to possess greater problems with speech than with language development, started to use manual signs in sentence-like structures, as a real linguistic system.

The findings of this study suggest that the early signing period was a bridge from the early preverbal phase of communication to the use of spoken language and that the transitional phase from preverbal to verbal communication may be enhanced by a goal-oriented use of the means of communication which may be available for the child prior to the verbal symbols. However, for children with Down syndrome conventional gestural communication is not enough for the transition. They need more intensive, more long-lasting, and, it seems, different stimulation than other children. The stage has to be intensified and modified qualitatively as in the early signing programme. One dimension of this modified and added quality was the use of manual signs which were easier for the child to attain than spoken words. Another important aspect was the interpretations parents made of their children's actions. These interpretations may have advanced the children's awareness of their actions, and, accordingly, the acquisition of shared meaning between them and their parents (cf. Smith, von Tetzchner and Michaelsen, 1988).

One of the main effects of the programme was thus to shape the child's communicative environment to its needs and abilities. Signed communication was an essential part of this beneficial environment. However, it is possible that introducing a new way of communication to the family might disturb the natural communication between the child and its parents. It is therefore important that parents learn to appreciate more generally the meaning of communication and its development. It was hypothesised that if parents were given adequate information on these matters, they would become aware of the importance of the child's own active role in forming a conception of the world. It is likely that this awareness was strengthened through the regular conversations with a speech therapist. It may also be assumed that the regular evaluations the parents made played a major role in the development of their communicative knowledge. Parents learned to attribute competence to the child in communication even before signing appeared, when the child was using early preverbal means of communication. In this balanced situation of interaction, the child got adequate support in its initiatives and was encouraged to be challenged in both communication and exploration. An active role from very early on may be of ultimate importance for the development of the child's image of itself as a communicating individual.

Some of the differences between the groups may possibly be explained by the general effects of early intervention. One important aspect of all early intervention programmes is the support given to parents (Cunningham, 1988; Hornby, 1991). Many parents with impaired infants feel uncertain about their parental role. They may not know what to expect of the child, generally or at a given age. When given adequate information and support they may feel more secure and relaxed and begin to gain confidence in their parental role. A more relaxed parental role may have positive effects on the interaction between the child and rest of the family and, in turn, enhance the child's opportunities for developing early communicative skills. One may question whether the general support of the parents in the control group was sufficient. It is possible that the support had more positive effects when it was provided within the more concrete frame of teaching early signing. Parents may feel more confident when they are 'doing something' for and with their child. Moreover, the value of the family groups and the support parents in the same group gave each other cannot be overestimated.

Those who criticise the use of special programmes for early intervention of intellectually impaired children often argue that what is significant is not so much the quality of the interactions as the amount of time spent with the child (e.g. Gibson and Harris, 1988). Intellectually impaired children need opportunities to learn the same skill repeatedly and in many different situations. If parents spend more time with their child, repetition becomes possible. However, children with Down syndrome are left alone to explore their surroundings more often than normally developing children (Smith and Hagen, 1984). The parents in the early signing programme were advised to have daily 'training sessions' with their child and this may have given the children more opportunities for attaining communication and other skills. However, it is not known whether the research group parents spent more time with their children than the parents in the control group. Further, knowing that the quality of the early interactions was changed by adding signed communication, the effect of a possible difference in the time spent with the child cannot be distinguished from the effects of other factors.

Because the groups were relatively small it is possible that some of the differences were due to individual variation, such as family traits or the degree of the intellectual impairment of the children. Even if the effect of the chance variation cannot be totally excluded, this would not explain the differences in Portage profiles observed between the groups. In the areas of self-help and motor development, the groups did not differ significantly (except in motor development at age three). Equal development in two areas where the intervention was not supposed to have effect suggests that the basic level of the two groups was not very different. Because the difference was largest in the areas of language and cognitive development, and clear with regard to the social area of the Portage profiles, it seems a warranted conclusion that the signing programme did have an effect in these areas.

Unfortunately, the groups cannot be compared at the earliest ages and for this reason it is not known whether the initial levels of the groups were the same. Comparisons of the intervention group and the research group show that the research group was slightly behind the total intervention group on most measures. It is thus not a 'too good' sample of the total group. In the light of the limited information available, the control group seemed to be slightly ahead of the research group at the age of one year when the first measures were made. Of the five children of the control group who were evaluated at this age, three were among the most advanced in the measures made at the age of five, suggesting that the superiority of the control group may have been due to change variation. At two years of age, seven control children were evaluated. Among them were those two children who later scored lowest on all measures. Thus the average of the control group at two years may have been somewhat too low. However, at later evaluations, the research group was consistently ahead of the control group and the difference remains even if the two low-functioning children of the control group are excluded. When the within-group variation of the two groups is compared, it shows that the research group was ahead *as a group*. Two or three of the most advanced children in the research group were ahead of the most advanced child in the control group for all Portage areas except motor development at the age of five. Even at five years, in the language area, half of the children in the research group were ahead of the most advanced child in the control group. Lastly, it should be noted that even if observations had been available for all age levels, lack of differences between the group would not have ensured equal developmental potential since the predictive value of most tests of intellectual functioning in infancy is limited (cf. Colombo, 1993).

The differences between the two groups were the most notable at the age of three years, when the intervention programme was completed. In the course of the two-year follow-up, the differences had started to decrease, but at the age of five years, there were still significant differences between the groups in the areas of language with the help of signs and cognitive development. During the follow-up period, most children received speech therapy once or twice a week, according to individual needs. For the children in the control group, this meant intensified intervention. For the children in the research group it may have meant, to some extent, less intensive intervention. However, it is probable that the early intervention had long-term effects on the interaction style of the whole family. The beneficial communicative environment did, most likely, remain once it was created.

For most of the children in the intervention group, signing was part of the continuous intervention, at least to some extent. This was also the case for some of the children in the control group. Consequently, the number of manual signs in the control group increased between the ages of three and four years. This increase came mainly from two children for whom signing was emphasised in the individual intervention and whose families had also started to use signed communication. This seems to corroborate the achievements of the research group but also shows that signing may be beneficial even when initiated at an older age. However, according to the results of this study, the vocabulary and the general language development are better when signed communication is incorporated into the child's communication from very early on.

## Conclusions

The presuppositions of this study were that children with Down syndrome have specific problems in language acquisition, and particularly in developing speech, and that the reasons for these problems lie in difficulties of early interaction and deficient auditory processing. The results of the study show that early intervention with manual signs and special attention to the active communicative role of the child had immediate and long-lasting effects. Children with Down syndrome who participated in the programme used a wider range of communicative means and were more advanced in their linguistic and overall development than the children in the control group. The results support researchers who consider early language intervention to be necessary and important for later achievements and adjustment of children with Down syndrome. They suggest that intervention methods based on manual signing as well as pointing and other pre-speech means of communication may be used similarly to prevent language problems with other groups of children who are at risk for delayed or deviant communication and language development. In this process of development, the people closest to the child play a central role. Manual signing provided the children with a means for active communication and the parents helped the child to create situations in which it could communicate actively and interactively from very early on.

# Chapter 14
# Early development of symbolic communication and linguistic complexity through augmentative and alternative communication

MARGRIET J.M. HEIM AND ANNE E. BAKER-MILLS

Researchers in the field of augmentative and alternative communication have repeatedly stressed the fact that augmented communication is a multimodal process in which the actual modes used vary widely across individual users and communicative situations. Combinations of modes, used either simultaneously or sequentially to convey a single message, have been reported not only in augmented communication in adults but also in children (Harris, 1982; Heim, 1990; Light, Collier and Parnes, 1985c). Light and her colleagues (1985c) found strong interrelationships between the modes used and the communicative functions and discourse roles in the interaction of eight young children (aged 4–6 years) and their mothers. Heim (1990) also found clear interrelationships between modes and discourse roles in the interactions of three older children (aged 8–11 years) with three different interaction partners, although the direction of these interrelationships differed in some aspects.

From a developmental point of view it is not at all clear how children learn to handle multimodality. It seems obvious that particular communication modes are used more than others in individual children related to their physical, cognitive and linguistic capacities. Because these capacities will change as the children grow older, it is not only important to investigate the possible dominance of one mode at a particular point in time, but also, longitudinally, the changes in dominance in the course of development.

The studies mentioned above all report the use of multiple modes across subjects, both across and within turns. However, how various aided and unaided modes are used in combination to convey meaning has not yet been investigated. If messages are considered in terms of propositions, the relative contribution of each mode can vary. Each of the combined modes may present the entire propositional content of the message, but it is also possible that each mode presents a different part of this propositional content. Children's control of the multimodal nature of augmented communication needs to be investigated as part of their acquisition of expressive linguistic skills.

The emergence of symbolic communication has been the subject of considerable investigation in children with the potential for speech or signing. Following Bates' analysis of early communicative development (Bates, 1979), communication using representational symbols normally emerges at some point between 9 and 13 months of age. In their first year of life, children develop from the stage of pre-intentional communication of internal states, via intentional communication using conventional signals, to the stage of intentional communication using representational symbols. In the very early pre-intentional stage children do not have the intention to communicate. They feel hunger, joy, discomfort etc., and their behaviour reflects this, without their intending to communicate their internal state. During the first year they gradually become aware of the presence of others and develop the intention to interact. Initially, this is manifested by children participating in social interaction, taking turns, reacting to the behaviour of the other person with smiles, vocalisations, etc. Later they discover that they can influence the behaviour of others to achieve their own goals. Communicative functions begin to develop, such as requests for objects and actions, or accepting or rejecting. At this early intentional stage children only use signals like reaching or directing eye gaze to achieve their communicative goals. These deictic signals are adequate for communication about objects, persons and actions which are in the immediate environment, that is, in the here-and-now. When children develop the desire to communicate about things outside the immediate situation, they need symbols: words, signs which represent referents. They enter the stage of intentional communication through representational symbols.

Little is known about the transition from pre-symbolic to symbolic communication in young physically disabled children who do not have the potential to develop functional speech. In order to become competent communicators, these children need to acquire expressive symbolic and linguistic skills, in communication modes within their own individual potential repertoire.

As linguistic skills increase, complexity of utterances also increases. Studies on the development of multimodal complexity in augmentative and alternative communication are still lacking. The emergence of intramodal complexity, that is within one particular mode such as manual or graphic signs, has been addressed in several studies (Grove, Dockrell and Woll, this volume; Udwin and Yule, 1990; Wilkinson, Romski and Sevcik, 1994) The studies of Wilkinson and associates and Grove and associates both address the development of complexity in manually signed utterances of hearing children with cognitive disabilities.

Wilkinson and associates (1994) found evidence in their study that the subjects (aged 6;2–20;2) used their vocabulary of lexigrams to build complex structures. Because the combinations of lexigrams were spontaneous and productive, they conclude that general principles of language development were operative. It was not the case that the combinations the subjects produced were present in the immediate input; the combinations were therefore judged to be creative. Grove and associates (this volume) also found evidence of creativity in the way children with intellectual impairments (aged 10;5–16;10) conveyed meaning in their multi-sign utterances, although the subjects in this study did not seem to develop a manual sign grammar. Udwin and Yule (1990) studied the communicative development of two groups of children with cerebral palsy (aged 3;6–9;8) over a period of one and a half years. Nineteen children were taught Blissymbols and 14 children were taught manual signs from the Makaton vocabulary (Walker, 1976). Although the users of Blissymbols produced more multi-term utterances than the manually signing group, both groups produced mainly one-term utterances. The use of multi-term utterances increased slightly over time.

The three studies described above address the development of complexity within one particular mode. It is possible that the results in fact underestimate the ability of the children with regard to complexity, because they were reported to use multiple modes in their communication. Research on the acquisition of augmentative and alternative communication has not yet explored the relationship between the use of different modes, despite the interest in the role of multimodality in normal language acquisition in recent years (e.g. Volterra and Iverson, 1995).

Besides these few studies, research on augmentative and alternative communication has thus far tended to address global theoretical issues or problems in children becoming competent communicators (Gerber and Kraat, 1992; Iacono, 1992; Nelson, 1992). Little work has been done on the details of the acquisition process. A better understanding of this process should have important implications for early intervention programmes aimed at facilitating the development of communicative and linguistic skills in this specific group of language users. It may also influence the process of vocabulary selection and choice of system.

The present chapter addresses the development of language skills in a young girl with severe motor speech impairment within the framework of dyadic social interaction. The main focus is on the question of whether there are aspects of linguistic development which are not directly trained, but which the girl develops spontaneously. If such aspects can be demonstrated to exist, this will be evidence of the productivity of the linguistic system this girl is developing. Her acquisition of language, as in all children, is driven by the desire to communicate but, on the other hand, it is restricted by her physical abilities. More knowledge of the processes at work in children acquiring productive language through non-speech communication modes will not only have important implications for early intervention, but may also influence general theories of language acquisition.

The case study presented in this chapter focuses on the development of symbolic communication and linguistic complexity, both in relation to the multimodal nature of augmentative and alternative communication. The data are taken from a larger research project, studying longitudinally the interactions of three children with cerebral palsy (Heim and Mills, 1992). One of the primary goals in the project is to establish the effect of intervention. An intervention programme has been developed to promote functional communication between nonspeaking children and their primary interaction partners. The programme does not involve direct training of linguistic and communicative skills in the children. It concentrates on the instruction and training of significant persons in the child's home and school environment. The main goal is that the significant persons learn to stimulate the communicative development of the children, in particular by adapting their own behaviour to the communicative needs of the child and by modelling the use of augmented modes and systems.

The study of 'Yvette' presented here concentrates on the changes in various modes of communication used over time; the changes in the frequency of representational symbols in relation to mode use over time; the relative contribution of modes to the propositional content of messages (the meaning of the message as opposed to the form); and the emergence and development of linguistic complexity, that is, multi-element messages in which each element constitutes a different part of a proposition.

## Method

### Yvette

The longitudinal study of Yvette comprises the period from age 2;7 to 5;0. Yvette has cerebral palsy (severe spastic tetraplegia with athetosis) and severe speech and physical impairment. She has no manipulation skills. With adapted testing Yvette obtained an age-equivalent score of 0;11 at the start of the project on *The Bayley Scales of Infant Development* (Van den Meulen and Smrkovsky, 1983) and 3;0 on *The Leiter International Performance Scale* (Arthur, 1952) at the end of the project, indicating a mild delay in cognitive development. Vision and hearing appeared normal. Yvette could only produce unintelligible vocalisations. She obtained an age-equivalent score on *Reynell Developmental Language Scales* (Bomers and Mugge, 1982) of 1;9 at the start and 3;8 at the end of the study. The latter score was also obtained with *The Peabody Picture Vocabulary Test* (Manschot and Bonnema, 1974). She attended a therapeutic toddler group connected to a habilitation centre where she received therapy services.

At the start of the intervention period, that is, after the second recording (see below), Yvette received a 'see-through window' of plexiglass which could be attached to the lap tray of her wheelchair, and a communication book as an extension of her available vocabulary and for situations where the window could not be used. Photographs, pictures, Blissymbols and small objects could be attached to the window and could easily be replaced with new material. She used eye gaze to select items on the window.

In the beginning period, four Blissymbols which were judged useful in many different contexts *(OTHER, MORE, HELP* and *STOP)*, were fixed on the window. In addition to these, 4–8 different graphic signs or small objects could be attached. By gaze pointing to *OTHER*, Yvette could indicate to her communication partner that she needed other vocabulary items on her window. These were kept in a small box and categorised into themes and topics. Yvette could also indicate that she needed her communication book by selecting *BLISS-BOOK* which was fixed on her lap tray. In the first two years of intervention, Yvette's total vocabulary of Blissymbols was gradually extended to a total of about 200. By using colour coding, the number of Blissymbols which were accessible on the window gradually increased to about 20 by four years of age. This number was still very limited and Yvette remained highly dependent on her partner who had to select an adequate set of Blissymbols given the context and the topic at hand.

Yvette did not receive special explicit training in the use of her communication aids nor in the meaning of Blissymbols. Her communication partners were instructed to use these aids whenever they were interacting with her in addition to speech and other communication modes like gestures, manual signs or eye gaze. Because her partners accompanied spoken words with the selection of the matching Blissymbols in meaningful communicative contexts, Yvette could infer the meaning of the Blissymbols. Communication partners also received instruction in the use of non-intrusive techniques to encourage her to use her aids whenever appropriate, given the communicative context.

**Video recording and analysis**

Yvette was video-recorded every two months in interaction with her mother at home, and with a teacher in the therapeutic toddler group, over a period of 2½ years. The recorded interactions took place during free play situations with no restrictions with regard to play-material or activities. For the analysis reported here, six recordings of Yvette and her mother were used, selected at intervals of six months. At the last analysed recording Yvette was 5;0. Intervention with her mother in the form of training started after the second recording used in this analysis, that is, at three years of age.

Segments consisting of five minutes from each video recording have been fully transcribed for both child and adult. The following behaviours were recorded: speech and vocalisations; eye gaze; gestures and actions; selection of graphic signs on communication aids; body posture; and facial expression. The transcripts have been segmented into communicative turns, which were defined by the presence of intentional behaviours directed towards the partner. A second round of segmentation was carried out at the level of proposition. In studies of normal spoken language development, underlying propositions are defined as 'all main verbs or predicates with overt (or covert) subjects' (Bellugi and Fischer, 1972, p. 184). In such studies alongside grammaticality and semantic cohesion, intonation and pause length also function as segmentation criteria. These criteria are difficult to apply in aided language interaction. Segmentation was therefore primarily based on semantic cohesion, judged on the basis of a paraphrase of the alternative communication output into spoken language. The paraphrases were made with the use of contextual information.

Each turn could consist of one or more propositions. In Table 14.1, dialogues (1), (2) and (3) contain turns by the child which consist of two propositions. Dialogue (4) consists of three propositions. There was, however, a situation in which a proposition was created across turns, as in dialogue (5). Such a situation is also referred to by Marriner, Yorkston and Farrier (1984). In this situation, the turn of the adult serves as feedback to the child that the first element of the proposition has been understood. This is particularly common where the child uses modes which are perceptually difficult for the interaction partner, such as selection by eye gaze.

For the present analysis, communicative turns and propositions were analysed on four different levels:

• the mode or modes used to convey propositions;
• the presence of representational symbols in the mode(s) used to convey a proposition;
• the relative contribution of modes to the propositional content;
• the expression of more than one element with different referential meaning within the proposition (complexity).

Following an earlier established coding scheme (Heim, 1989), *communication modes* were classified as either vocalisation/speech, selection

Table 14.1 Examples of segmentation of turns into propositions (A = adult, C = child)

| Turns | Paraphrase of propositions |
|---|---|
| (1) A: *You mean that one?* (points at book). | 'You mean that book?' |
|    C: 'No'(eye movements). | 'No, I don't mean that one'. |
|       Looks at (another) book. | 'I want that book'. |
| (2) C: Vocalises and looks at own arm. | 'Look at my arm'. |
|       Puts out tongue. | |
|       Looks at own arm. | 'My arm is dirty'. |
| (3) A: *Doll?* | 'Do you want the doll?' |
|    C: Looks at *DIFFERENT* and then at adult. | 'I mean something else'. |
|       Looks at doll trousers and then at adult. | 'Trousers should be taken off'. |
| (4) C: Vocalises and looks at photograph of Granny. | 'This is Granny'. |
|       Vocalises and looks at photograph of Mummy. | 'This is Mummy'. |
|       Vocalises and looks at photograph of Granny. | 'This is Granny'. |
| (5) C: Looks at doll and then at adult. | |
|    A: Looks at doll and then child (feedback to child). | |
|    C: Looks at bath and then adult. | 'The doll must go into the bath'. |

of graphic signs (photographs or Blissymbols), gestures/manual signs, eye gaze, or facial expression (see Table 14.2). Each proposition was coded for all the modes which are used. The category 'eye gaze' included the deictic use of eye gaze (looking at objects, persons, locations in the environment), but also the symbolic use of eye gaze (e.g. eyes directed upward to say 'yes'). In the latter case the eye gaze represents a specific referent (representational symbols: see below). If eye pointing was used to select graphic signs, only the graphic sign mode was coded. For each recording the frequencies of use of each mode and of each possible combination were counted.

Table 14.2 Coding examples

| Utterance | Modes | Propositional content | Symbolic level | Complexity |
|---|---|---|---|---|
| 1. Vocalisation | Voc | Sup | Nonrep | Noncomplex |
|    Looks at book | Gaze | Full | Nonrep | |
| 2. Looks at doll | | | | |
|    'gone' 'yes' | Gaze | Full | Nonrep+rep+rep | Complex |
|    Looks at *DOLL* | Graph | Sup | Rep | |
| 3. Looks at doll | Gaze | Comp | Nonrep | Complex |
|    Looks at *FOOD* | Graph | Comp | Rep | |
| 4. Looks at *CAR* | Graph | Full | Rep | Noncomplex |
|    Looks at car | Gaze | Full | Nonrep | |

On the *symbolic level*, the use of representational symbols was analysed in relation to the use of the various modes. Each proposition was coded according to the presence or absence of one or more representational symbols. Following Iverson, Capirci and Caselli (1994), representational symbols were defined as symbols representing specific referents. In the specific material at hand, symbols could be symbolic eye gazes or graphic signs. The basic semantic content of these symbols did not change appreciably with the context. Representational symbols could be either conventional symbols or idiosyncratic symbols used consistently and for which the meaning could be interpreted. In contrast, the meaning of non-representational signals was totally dependent on the situational context. They included deictic gestures (pointing, showing and reaching) or eye gazes (gaze pointing) and paralinguistic signals (e.g. vocalisations, facial expressions or gestures which convey feelings or inner states, vocalisations to draw attention to or stress other message elements, head nods to encourage communication, etc.). At the propositional level, modes which were only used to serve a paralinguistic function were coded as supportive.

On the *propositional level*, the use of each mode was coded according to the content expressed in relationship to the proposition as a whole. There were three categories:

| | |
|---|---|
| *Full* | A proposition is fully expressed by the mode. |
| *Supportive* | The mode expresses a part of a proposition and the content expressed in that mode overlaps totally with the content expressed by one or more other modes. |
| *Complementary* | The mode expresses a part of a proposition and adds content to make the proposition complete. The content expressed may or may not partly overlap with the content expressed by another mode. |

Finally, each proposition was coded for *linguistic complexity* according to the presence or absence of two or more elements with different referential meaning. A combination of two or more representational symbols would be coded as complex (see example 2 in Table 14.2). A combination of a representational symbol and a deictic symbol would also be coded as complex if both symbols had a different referential meaning (example 3), but as non-complex if their referential meaning was the same (example 4). A combination of a representational symbol and a paralinguistic signal was also coded as non-complex (example 1).

# Results

## Changes in modes used

Results of the analysis of modes used over time are presented in Figure 14.1. The percentages in this figure do not add up to one hundred because in one proposition several modes can be combined. Yvette's primary mode in the first two recordings was vocalisation, although she did not produce any recognisable words. Her use of vocalisation had clearly decreased at the third recording at 3;6. Her use of gesture and facial expression decreased as well, though less dramatically. Shortly after the second recording, Yvette's communication partners received instruction in recognising and responding to Yvette's gaze behaviour, as well as in using eye gaze in their own input. As a result Yvette began to use eye gaze as her main mode of communication. In the same period graphic signs were introduced to Yvette and the use of this mode clearly increased over time.

Multimodal propositions were found in all recordings, ranging from 5.3 to 44.4 percent of all propositions (cf. Figure 14.3). Combinations involving vocalisations (not speech) were the most frequent: 88 per cent of Yvette's multimodal propositions. As could be expected, the most frequent combination for Yvette was eye gaze with vocalisation (48%). From the age of 4;1, Yvette began to combine graphic signs and the use of eye gaze to form one proposition. Three-mode combinations were rare: across all the recordings Yvette produced only one such proposition.

The use of multimodality in total varied across the period studied. In Figure 14.3, the height of the bars indicates a temporary decrease, followed by an increase. The decrease in multimodality coincided with the striking increase in the use of eye gaze and the decrease in vocalisations (see Figure 14.1). The fact that Yvette's mother at this point was more focused on Yvette's non-vocal communication certainly supported Yvette's use of eye gaze. It can also explain the temporary decrease in multimodality: Yvette's vocalisations in the first recordings primarily had the function of gaining her mother's attention. Because her mother was more attentive to her use of eye gaze, Yvette no longer needed to vocalise in this way. Her use of eye gaze had become more successful. Alternatively, the temporary decrease in multimodality may be related to other aspects of development, such as the appearance of representational symbols (graphic signs and symbolic eye gaze) and the emergence and growth of complexity (see below).

## Development of symbolic communication

The second research question deals with the emergence and development of symbolic communication as demonstrated by the appearance of representational symbols: graphic signs and eye gazes which represent concepts. The results of this analysis are presented in Figure 14.2 and show a clear development. Yvette developed the capacity to produce representational symbols in her main modes between the second and

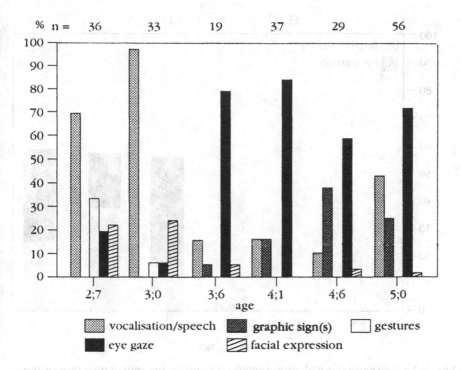

**Figure 14.1** Modes used by Yvette: per cent of total propositions

the third recording, not surprisingly since these types of symbols were absent in her input before intervention had started. Until 3;0, the input to her consisted primarily of spoken language, a mode which she was unable to use herself for representational symbols. After the second recording, the first graphic signs were introduced, which she soon learned to use productively. Between 3;6 and 4;1 symbolic eye gazes for 'yes' and 'no' were introduced into Yvette's input and she started to use these symbolic eye gazes herself consistently within a few weeks. She also developed several symbolic and deictic eye gazes spontaneously, e.g. 'gone', 'me and you', and 'do it myself'.

## Contribution of modes to propositions

In most multimodal propositions, one of the modes was used to convey the full proposition (see Figure 14.3). In these cases the second mode was used to support the content of the proposition. Modes which were coded as supportive served mainly a paralinguistic function, that is, to draw attention to a referent or to stress other message elements. The complementary use of two different modes seemed to be a later development for Yvette, with the first appearance at the age of 4;1.

The transition from vocalisation to eye gaze as Yvette's primary

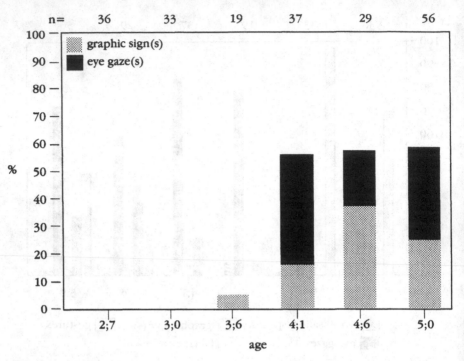

**Figure 14.2** Propositions with representations symbols: per cent of total propositions

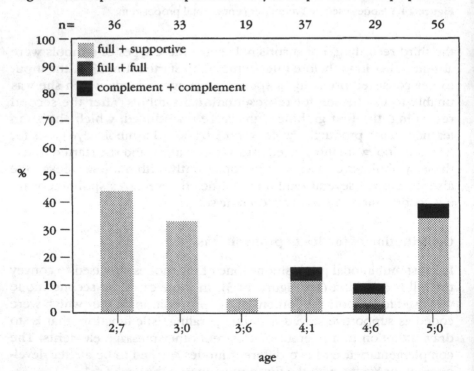

**Figure 14.3** Type of propositional construction of multimodal propositions: per cent of total propositions

communication mode has already been discussed. In the first two recordings she used vocalisation primarily to convey a complete proposition: to express feelings or to request attention. The relatively high proportion of vocalisations at 5;0 (see Figure 14.1) almost solely represented the use of vocalisation in combination with other modes (83%). In these cases, vocalisations were always used to support the proposition expressed by the other mode. Across all recordings eye gazes were mainly used to express the entire proposition and never in a supportive function. An example of such a supportive function in a two-element proposition might be where one element is expressed using both deictic gaze to an object and selection of a graphic sign, and the other element is expressed only via a graphic sign. In the course of development Yvette started to use eye gaze to complement the content expressed via graphic signs and this complementary use of eye gaze (see Table 14.2, example 3) increased slightly over time. Graphic signs were mostly used to convey a complete proposition and in the remaining cases to complement the content expressed via eye gazes. They were never used in a supportive function (Table 14.2, example 2). The use of two different modes, each expressing the same complete proposition (Table 14.2, example 4), appeared only once in Yvette's recordings.

By definition, the complementary use of modes, where each mode contributed essential content to the proposition as a whole, constituted linguistic complexity. This is the topic of the next section.

## The emergence of complexity

The last research question addresses the issue of the emergence of complex propositions, that is, the emergence of structural complexity. Before presenting the results of this analysis, we will digress and present some figures on the emergence of discourse complexity, that is, the inclusion of several propositions within one turn.

The majority of Yvette's turns consisted of one single proposition (see Figure 14.4). The production of turns with more than one proposition was only established in the last two recordings. In the last two recordings, Yvette also began to produce vertical structures, that is, one proposition across turns (cf. Smith, this volume; von Tetzchner and Martinsen, this volume). She seemed to have developed this strategy in order to avoid communication break down. Since her use of eye gaze had become extremely fast, her partner often found it difficult to follow. Yvette thus developed the strategy of expressing one element and waiting for her partner to indicate that the eye gaze had been correctly followed or interpreted. (For notations, see Table 0.1).

(6)    Yvette and her mother were playing with dolls.
       Y:    *TROUSERS* (waits for feedback).

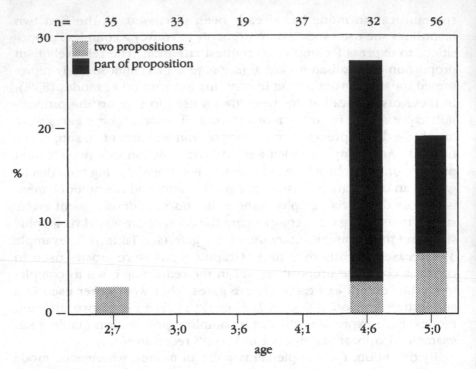

**Figure 14.4** Number of propositions per turn: per cent of total turns

M: *Trousers.*
Y: *PULLOVER* (waits for feedback).
M: *Pullover.*
Y: Looks at the doll on her lap tray.
M: *Doll.*

This proposition was interpreted as: 'The doll needs to be dressed in trousers and a pullover' (see also dialogue (5) in Table 14.1). In the last two recordings Yvette expressed a total of seven multiturn propositions: six propositions were expressed in two turns (twelve turns in total); one proposition in three turns.

The emergence of complex propositions and the changes in the use of complexity are represented in Figure 14.5. Complex propositions were present from 3;6, at the same time as the use of representational symbols. Complex propositions were unimodal at first, but Yvette soon produced multimodal complex propositions as well. Multimodal complexity necessarily implies the complementary use of modes. At 3;6 Yvette combined two deictic symbols in one proposition. At 4;1 there were also combinations of one deictic element and a representational symbol. In the last recording at 5;0, she produced the first complex propositions with two representational symbols.

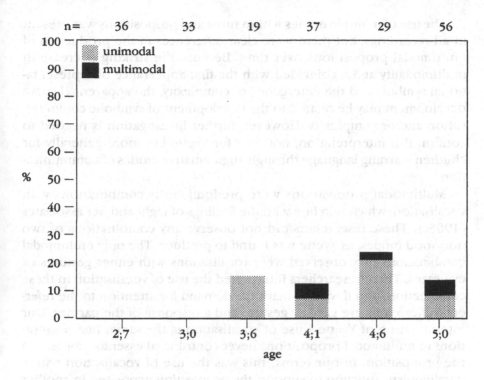

**Figure 14.5** Complex propositions: per cent of total propositions

# Conclusions

The aim of the present study was to contribute to the understanding of the role of multimodality in early communicative development through augmentative and alternative communication. Three specific issues were raised which had not been sufficiently explored in previous studies of augmentative and alternative language acquisition. The study was limited to one subject, and certainly longitudinal information of more children is needed to confirm the developmental patterns found in this girl. Yet, in our view, the results obtained provide several indications that help clarify the issues outlined.

The results showed clear changes in mode use in the course of development. The changes in preferred modes were not only related to growing cognitive and linguistic skills, but seemed also to be related to the input from the environment. When Yvette was exposed to modes which she could produce herself (eye gaze and graphic signs), she rapidly began to use these modes to convey messages. From the present study it may be concluded that the preferred mode was the mode which gave the greatest possibilities for deictic and symbolic use, given her physical capacities. Specific to the graphic sign mode was that these possibilities were restricted by the vocabulary set available to the girl.

The use of multiple modes within turns and propositions was present in all recordings, but there were clear differences in the production of multimodal propositions over time. Because the striking decrease in multimodality at 3;6 coincided with the first appearance of representational symbols and the emergence of complexity, the apparent U-curve development may be related to the development of symbolic communication and/or complexity. However, further investigation is needed to confirm this interpretation, not only for Yvette but more generally for children learning language through augmentative modes of communication.

Multimodal propositions were predominantly combinations with vocalisation, which is in line with the findings of Light and her associates (1985c). These researchers did not observe any combinations of two non-vocal modes, as Yvette was found to produce. The only multimodal combinations they observed were vocalisations with either gestures or eye gazes. These researchers interpreted the use of vocalisation in these combinations as a device to mark the demand for attention to the referent indicated by eye gaze or gesture and a response of the partner. Our interpretation of Yvette's use of vocalisation is the same: her vocalisations in multimodal propositions never contributed essential content to the proposition. In our terms, this was the use of vocalisation with a paralinguistic function to support the proposition expressed in another mode.

Further analysis of the propositional contribution of each mode within multimodal propositions revealed that the use of two modes, both of which express the complete proposition, is rare. Yvette's first multimodal propositions, in which each mode expresses an essential part of the proposition, were observed around four years of age. The relative avoidance of redundancy may stem from an economical principle of efficiency: communication requires great effort for non-speaking physically disabled children. This finding is also in line with the results of Iverson and associates (1994) who report a minimal lexical overlap between gesture and speech in speaking children.

The emergence of symbolic communication in Yvette, that is, the use of representational symbols, was closely connected with the exposure to modes with symbolic potential which she could reproduce. The frequency of propositions with representational symbols remained stable in the last three recordings between 4 and 5 years. This may have been related to restrictions in the vocabulary set available, but also to the play context of the recorded interaction.

Complexity, or multi-element propositions, appeared at the same time as the first representational symbols, first unimodally and then multimodally. Despite the absence of an apparent linear trend in the frequency of complexity, evidence was found for developmental changes in the type of complexity. In her first complex propositions Yvette combined two deictic symbols, then she combined a deictic symbol with a representational symbol, and finally she produced combinations with two different representational symbols within one proposition.

All multimodal complex propositions produced by Yvette were combinations of eye gazes with graphic signs. Most combinations consisted of a deictic eye gaze to an object, person or location in the immediate environment and a deictic eye gaze to a graphic sign, but the latter was analysed as graphic sign. Since gaze was involved in both modes, the truly multimodal nature of these combinations is somewhat questionable. Nevertheless, it is important to distinguish eye gaze used to refer to referents in the immediate situation from eye gaze as a selection method for graphic signs. The proposition was therefore coded as multimodal, in order to reflect this difference.

As mentioned earlier, the combination of gaze and graphic symbols within one communicative turn seemed to be absent in the study of Light and her associates (1985c). At least some of the eight children in this study used eye gaze as a selection method, but they also used encoding techniques (e.g. eye gaze to a block of Blissymbols, followed by eye gaze to a colour to identify the particular Blissymbol desired). Such an encoding technique was also introduced to Yvette, but within the period covered by the present study she still mainly used direct eye pointing to select graphic signs. The processing demands of encoding techniques appear to be much higher than direct selection techniques, and this might be an explanation for the absence of combinations of eye gaze and Blissymbols in Light's study.

When the development of Yvette's multimodal complexity is related to input factors, there is evidence for creativity. Although Yvette's mother modelled the use of eye gaze and graphic signs frequently, there was no indication that she modelled complex propositions in these modes, nor that she modelled the complementary use of eye gaze and graphic signs to form multimodal complex propositions. It may thus be concluded that Yvette developed these skills on her own. This is an indication of the creativity and productivity of her linguistic system. The results indicate that exposure to modes available to Yvette herself might be necessary in order for her to develop a linguistic system. But the capacity to combine different lexical elements may develop even when these combinations are absent in the child's input. According to Volterra and Iverson (1995) hearing and speaking children in the two-word stage do not combine two different representational gestures. They argue that the absence of multi-gesture combinations in the production of these children should be explained by the modality of the linguistic input to which they are exposed, that is, spoken language. Volterra and Iverson also report that deaf children of hearing and speaking parents, who had no access to a conventional linguistic input, spontaneously produced numerous combinations of two representational gestures. It seems that children who are not able to perceive the input or to productively use the modality of the input, will produce combinations in another modality.

In the seventies, researchers tended to equate non-speech communication with aid use (Light et al., 1985c). In the eighties, it became apparent that the communication of non-speaking children is essentially a multimodal process and that their communicative development should be studied within that framework. The first studies of linguistic development through aided and non-aided non-speech modes appeared in the nineties. These studies again addressed language acquisition of non-speaking children mainly from a unimodal perspective. At the same time, researchers in the field of language acquisition became interested in multimodality factors in normally developing children. In this chapter we have tried to illustrate the importance of taking into account all modalities non-speaking children use to convey meaning. The results of the studies to date, which repeatedly report very low frequencies of multi-element combinations, may in fact show an underestimation of the linguistic capacities of the children involved. Especially in the early stages of development, multimodality may play an important role in the emergence and development of more complex communication. More research is required to further explore multimodality factors in the emergence of symbolic communication and linguistic complexity. Research is also required to explore the effects of language input in aided and unaided modes, and in the interplay between input and output modalities which are so obviously different for many non-speaking children.

# Chapter 15
# Allowing for developmental potential: A case study of intervention change

SUSANNE MØLLER AND STEPHEN VON TETZCHNER

A major – but rarely addressed – concern of alternative communication intervention is the fact that it is difficult to assess whether an intervention has been successful in bringing about the potential of the individual, and when new intervention strategies should be pursued. Achievements vary considerably and there are no 'normal' functioning or clear guidelines for indicating whether the results are optimal. As long as the person appears well motivated and the intervention is not obviously inappropriate, like attempting to teach manual signing to an individual without motor control of the hands or graphic signs to a severely visually impaired person, poor acquisition of the alternative communication form will usually be attributed to the learning difficulties of the person. This attribution may well be correct since some people are profoundly impaired in all areas of functioning. Others may have an impairment that is particularly detrimental to the processes underlying acquisition of language and communication skills or, on the contrary, have an impairment that, given appropriate conditions, allows language and communication to develop as a particularly strong area of functioning.

The result of this may be that it is the background and experience of each professional that determine the choice of intervention strategies instead of the particular limitations and possibilities of the intervention for the individual in its context. Professionals tend to base practice on what they *can* rather than on what they *should* (Bourdieu, 1977; Jensen, 1992), and since they often have their main experience with one alternative communication form, they may also tend to limit intervention to this form. It is thus important to gain insight into traditions, reflections and evaluations of professionals and the processes underlying their decisions, decisions which in fact may serve to hinder as well as to promote the achievements of communication impaired individuals.

The present study concerns the alternative language intervention for a 42-year-old woman with severe intellectual impairment and no

249

functional speech. All intervention took place within a conversational context. The foci of the study are her achievements, from mainly non-verbal communication and idiosyncratic gestures to multi-mode communication with manual and graphic signs and photographs, and the process of the intervention taking place in 1994 and 1995. It is based on earlier reports and notes, and observations and video recordings made during the intervention that started in 1994. Parts of the 64 intervention sessions of the school year 1994–95 were recorded on video tape. The average length was 9½ minutes (range 3–30 minutes), totalling 10 hours and 9 minutes. In the last part of the intervention presented here, conversations between the woman, a disabled man and a member of the staff at their residence were also recorded. The video recordings have served as clinical documentation of the 'dialogue games' as well as of the woman's spontaneous use of pointing, manual and graphic signs and photographs. In addition, three staff members were consulted and interviewed at the end of the project period about her communicative functioning at home.

## Background

'Bodil' was born in 1952. Since the age of three years, she has lived in various institutions, mostly sharing a room with three other persons and having few personal belongings. At present she lives in her own room in a sheltered housing together with 20 other people with intellectual impairment, divided into three groups. Only one of the other residents lacks spoken language. The house functions in many ways as a mini-institution, with a staff consisting mainly of social care educators and a few people without professional background.

Bodil's medical records show that from birth on, she has spent several periods in hospital. Her diagnoses during the years have included imbecility, short stature, and both too many and too few chromosomes have been suggested but no diagnosis has been verified. She started to have epileptic seizures in 1984 and has received various forms of medication, at present Tegretol.

Development has been slow: she learned to walk (on her toes) at four years. She can move her arms freely but they are short and the arm and leg movements appear inflexible and stiff, almost like a mechanical doll. Reflexes are normal. She has some fine motor skills and finger dexterity, points without any difficulties and can for example sew and thread beads. She has never liked walking and physical exercise. Until the age of 18 she actively resisted imitation. However, she has always enjoyed household activities and seemed to imitate such activities spontaneously from an early age. In the early descriptions she appears easily distractible and as having problems finishing tasks she had started, particularly if they were not self-initiated. However, this is not typical of her present functioning. Assessments have been rare. At three years, her developmental quotient (unspecified) was reported to be around 40. At a recent assessment with *The Leiter International Performance Scale* (Arthur, 1952) she obtained an age equivalent score of 3;9.

Reports through the years have generally characterised her as social, easy-going, interested in people, helpful in most situations and having good relations with children and adults. In periods, she has been emotionally unstable and withdrawn, taking little contact with other people. She did not babble or develop any form of speech. From an early age, gestures and vocalisations, often loud appeared to be her main forms of expressive communication. She was described as making herself well understood in this manner. However, because of her tendency to shout when using gestures, and a remarkable persistence in making herself understood, other people could find her noisy and difficult. Her speech comprehension has always been uncertain. Still, all reports from four years on to the present stage have explicitly or implicitly stated that 'she understood everything that was said to her' but there was no formal or systematic informal assessment. Recently, she obtained an age equivalent of 2;6 on the Danish version of *Reynell Developmental Language Scales* (Skovlund, 1983). It should be noted, however, that although the result may be indicative of her ability to understand complex sentences, her vocabulary and situational understanding differ significantly from that of a young child. Reynell was used in want of a more appropriate Danish test. The subtest Auditory reception of the *Illinois Test of Psycholinguistic Ability* (Gjessing and Nygaard, 1974) was attempted but even the first items were clearly too difficult for her.

She attended preschool and started school at the normal age, seven years, but according to the reports, education was dominated by preschool activities and activities of everyday life until in 1971 she was transferred to adult education. At present, she attends a sheltered workshop where she puts pencils and other items into plastic bags and performs similar jobs. One day a week she stays at home and helps clean her room together with another resident.

The environment Bodil used to live in may not appear particularly stimulating but was probably no different from that of other children and adolescents with intellectual impairment at that time. The staff acted according to common beliefs about intellectual impairment and language, and Bodil's development is also a result of the practices resulting from these beliefs.

## Alternative language intervention

All mention of language intervention had focused on sound production and speech. At least until she was 18 years old, occasional and unsystematic speech therapy consisted in attempts to make her blow out candles and in other ways strengthen muscles assumed important for speech production. Needless to say, without any success. At one stage, operation of the tongue tie was discussed; at another, it was hypothesised that she might learn to speak if she would relax the articulatory muscles more. There has been no mention of other approaches. She did not appear to have had any form of language and communication intervention in the period from leaving school in 1971 until manual sign instruction was initiated in 1983 (see below).

The alternative language intervention may be divided into three main phases. The first phase was not part of the present intervention but comprised Bodil's earlier manual sign training provided by other teachers. It is included because the intervention history of the individual should be considered an important basis of intervention decisions. The second phase comprised the reintroduction of manual signing and the use of structured 'dialogue games'. The third phase comprised the introduction of graphic signs and photographs, and the change from mainly structured to more free narrative-based interactions.

### Introduction of manual signs

In 1983, at the age of 31 years, Bodil was admitted to a new educational setting. During the next six years, except for holidays and leave due to illness, she received about three hours of language intervention every week but there was no systematic follow-up where she lived. The aim of the intervention was to teach her manual signs and alternatives seem not to have been discussed. According to reports, when the intervention was terminated in 1989, she could understand and use 16 of the 72 manual signs trained (Table 15.1), but this may have been inaccurate since she used seven of the alleged unlearned signs spontaneously several years later. She may even have known more signs but these were the ones she produced during video recordings. However, most of the manual signs taught were not learned, or were forgotten because they were not used. Although manual sign intervention for people with intellectual impairment has a fairly long history in Denmark (von Tetzchner and Jensen, this volume), manual signs were not used much by the staff in the residence where she lived. When the present intervention started in 1994, due to discontinuity of the intervention in 1989, she may not have been exposed to much signing for 4–5 years. As a result of her rigid arm movements and limited fine motor skills, Bodil's own manual signs were difficult to understand and their use had not been encouraged in the environment. In addition, her ability to distinguish and remember manual signs may have been limited. Thus, when alternative language intervention was initiated for this 42-year-old woman, it seemed almost like starting all over again.

Table 15.1 The manual signs introduced during intervention 1983-1989. The marked signs (*), Bodil has produced spontaneously during video recorded conversations in 1994 and 1995.

Manual signs learned and used:

| | | | | |
|---|---|---|---|---|
| TABLE | USE | BREAD | JACKET | CHRISTMAS |
| CAKE | BUY | *DRIVE | *MILK | SUMMER-HOLIDAY |
| FINISHED | DIRTY | POP | MAYBE | *COFFEE |
| BUTTER | | | | |

Manual signs trained:

| | | | | |
|---|---|---|---|---|
| *I | *BOOK | SWEETS | BUS | EVERYTHING |
| CITY | TAPE | BAG | COKE | WONDERFUL |
| YOURS | *DRINK | *YOU | COLOURS | BIRDS |
| TOGETHER | GET | *GLAD | GREEN | GOOD-MORNING |
| WALK | SHOP | HOME | HELP | EVERYBODY |
| *COME | PUT | LOCK/KEY | *FOOD | TELEPHONE |
| MINE | MUSIC | MONEY | SPREAD | DAY-AFTER-TOMORROW |
| RED | LATER | SELF | HURRY | TASTE-GOOD |
| MOMENT | SCHOOL | FOREST | SIT-DOWN | CHOCOLATE |
| LIGHT | TIME | TOMATO | WEATHER | WAIT |
| WE | TOILET | TIME | CEILING | ICE-CREAM |
| WORK | | | | |

## Reintroduction of manual signs

The staff where Bodil lives approached the school about communication intervention for her in the early spring of 1994. They thought that she would benefit from manual sign intervention and that this might reduce her tendency to be noisy when communicating, which disturbed both the other residents and the staff. She had great difficulties making herself understood and the staff believed this might be the cause of her behaviour.

Intervention for Bodil began in April 1994, consisting of three hours per week only, in a group with three other intellectually impaired adults. At the same time a signing course was arranged for the staff of Bodil's group. Some staff members were also included in the training sessions in order to increase the effect of the intervention. However, it was not until early 1995 that a sign language course was arranged for all the staff in the residence.

Food was the first language topic. It was chosen in order to provide the residents with an immediate means for controlling an important aspect of their environment. They would, it was argued, for example, be able to ask for juice or coffee without these drinks being present at the table. Intervention was integrated into several ordinary activities where food names might be useful. The following procedure was typical of these three-hour sessions:

1. The residents chose what they wanted to eat from pictures of the assortment of the local supermarket. Each resident chose 2–3 items.
2. The residents, staff and teachers drove to the supermarket. During the trip, the food items were rehearsed by the teachers who talked about them, using keyword signing.
3. In the supermarket, each resident had their own trolley and had to collect and pay for their food items themselves.
4. After returning to the house, the residents prepared the food and ate together.
5. Lastly, a diary page was made with pictures of the manual signs and food items used on that particular day.

This schedule appeared transparent, functional and motivating. The residents were active and signed spontaneously. At this stage it seemed obvious to the teachers that Bodil should learn manual signs. She seemed happy, active and interested in the signs. They thought it would be good if she could use her hands for communication without needing any boards or devices that might break or get lost.

### Increased intervention structure

For reasons unrelated to Bodil, the schedule described above was discontinued at the end of the school year, after only two months. Teaching was resumed in August after the summer holiday with three hours twice a week for Bodil and another resident, Ole, who could speak, but whose word-finding problems made it extremely difficult to understand what he meant. He might, for example, say *taxi* instead of *lighter*. The staff thought he would be easier to understand if his speech was augmented with manual signs.

Although Bodil seemed both happy and motivated during sessions, an evaluation of the efficiency of the intervention seemed warranted. New goals and activities were therefore introduced in order to monitor her comprehension and production of manual signs and to assess whether they were understood by the staff where she lived. The aim of the intervention was that Bodil should be more proficient in signing and that signing should be a more useful means of communication in the environment.

Central to these efforts was the development of dialogue games where members of staff participated. The staff member was asked to stay with Ole while Bodil and the teacher went into another room where they looked at a picture together while the teacher talked about it using key-word signing. Bodil would sometimes sign spontaneously, naming or commenting on something in the picture, or she pointed at the picture while vocalising. If she did not sign spontaneously, the teacher would show her the appropriate manual signs and help her to articulate them if necessary. Following this, the staff member entered and Bodil would try to explain the content of the picture without him having seen it. Afterwards, the staff member was given the target and two other pictures. Through communicating (speaking and signing) with Bodil, he had to guess which picture Bodil had looked at. Since it was an explicit goal that the situation should be successful, the two contrast pictures were rather different from the target but no cues beside the ones presented by Bodil were given. This part of the intervention was based on the principle that it should not be a game of pretence – it was Bodil's own communication that should succeed or fail. However, the teacher present knew both what Bodil was attempting to communicate and the contrast pictures, and was therefore able to evaluate the communication efforts of the two parties. The photographs contained objects, people, events and places that Bodil knew well and was assumed to need to refer to in everyday manual communication. The staff member had been taught in advance both to read and produce the necessary manual signs.

In addition to the dialogue games, a range of activities was used during intervention sessions to introduce different topics. Bodil was for example particularly interested in clothes, and looking at catalogues from warehouses and magazines, naming clothes and colours, was part of the sessions for a period. She and Ole also made coffee, listened to music, made pearl necklaces, looked at pictures, smoked, etc., themselves indicating with manual signs or otherwise what they wanted to do. Lotto was used to train and monitor comprehension of speech and manual signs.

Thirty conventional or idiosyncratic manual signs were used spontaneously by Bodil during the video recorded sessions without their having being taught (Table 15.2). Most of them made small demands on fine motor skills and many of them were correctly executed. Moreover, the majority were transparent and would usually have been understood without being taught, but the video recording showed that the staff still had problems reading them correctly.

Bodil also used some of the manual signs in a somewhat unexpected manner, for instance signing SMALL instead of CHILD. During a dialogue game, she corrected herself when the teacher used CHILD but forgot it and continued to use SMALL when she was telling the staff member about the picture. She also used the same sign for different meanings, for example FUN was used both for expressing that something was funny and that she was looking forward to something. Considering her limited number of expressive forms, this was a natural strategy but it contributed to making her difficult to understand.

Table 15.2 The manual signs of the reintroduction phase. The marked signs (*),. Bodil has produced spontaneously during video recorded conversations in 1994 and 1995.

---

Conventional and idiosyncratic manual signs used without being taught

| | | | | |
|---|---|---|---|---|
| *WORK | *CHILD | *BOOK | *SAD | *CAR/DRIVE |
| *DRINK | *TEASE | *YOU | *STUPID | *HAPPY |
| *NAUGHTY | *DOG | *I | *COFFEE | *CIGARETTE |
| *COME | *KISS | *CANDLE | *MILK | *CUT/SCISSORS |
| *SHAMPOO | *FUNNY | *SLEEP | *EAT | *KIND |
| *ANGRY | *YES | *NO | *WILL-NOT | *DON'T-KNOW |

Manual signs introduced or reintroduced by the teachers.

| | | | | |
|---|---|---|---|---|
| BABY | BAKE | PICTURE | FLOWERS | *NAME (of institution) |
| BLOUSE | BLUE | *TABLE | GLASSES | *BODIL |
| BREAD | TROUSERS | *WOMAN | DUVET | POTATOES |
| *COAT | GREEN | HOME | *HOUSE | TELEVISION |
| WHITE | *POUR | *BROKEN | CALENDAR | KITCHEN-PAPER |
| DRESS | POT | *KITCHEN | LAMP | *MAN |
| MOTHER | MUSIC | SKIRT | RED | CAKE-ROLL |
| JUICE | BED | SHOE | POP | PLAY-CARDS |
| *CHAIR | PLATE | BAG | APPLE | UNDERWEAR |
| EGG | PANCAKE | SHAMPOO | CAT | |

In addition to these, five names of students and staff were taught. She also used these spontaneously.

---

In the reintroduction phase, during video recordings, Bodil used 30 manual signs which had not been taught. Fifty-four new manual signs were introduced or reintroduced by the teachers (including five proper names). Eleven of these she produced independently, although often incorrectly, during video recordings. Some of the manual signs were fairly easy to understand while others were almost illegible. Some were correctly articulated and yet rarely understood, for example CIGARETTE and CAKE-ROLL.

Dialogue (1) is a typical example of her interactions in the dialogue games and demonstrates how difficult it could be for her to make herself understood. Due to the length of each dialogue, only excerpts are presented (For notation, see Table 0.1).

(1)      Bodil had looked at a picture of a child standing in front of an open refrigerator. Inside, there were, among other things, milk, pop and eggs. Bodil was very enthusiastic about this picture, in particular did she like to make the sign EGG. The partner was Tom. (The Danish manual signs EGG and WORK are shown in Figure 15.1).

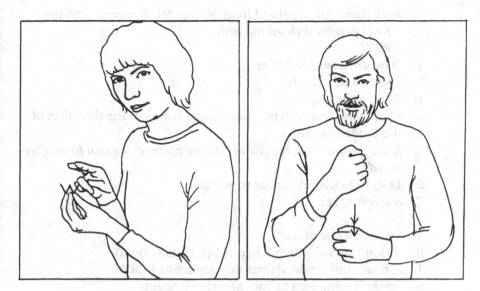

**Figure 15.1** The Danish manual signs EGG and WORK.

B: MILK.

T: *Milk, yes.*

B: DRINK.

B: EGG (articulated somewhat incorrectly).

T: *Coffee? Are you working?* (Misunderstanding the sign, first as COFFEE, then as WORK).

B: 'Yes' (nods, appearing somewhat puzzled – the work shop is usually called WORK).

T: *Are you working? Yes!*

B: EGG (modifying the manual sign: a flat hand on the fist, and repeating a short sound, *bum-bum*).

T: *Work. Yes?*

B: EGG (articulating it with the hands stretched out)

T: *Work.*

B: 'Yes' (small nod).

T: *What then?*

B: 'I don't know' (throws the hands up, indicates resignation).

T: *That's not much.*

B: EGG (this time articulated with two fists).

T: *Work.* 'Yes' (nods).

B: EGG (this time articulated with two fists).

T: *That is work.*

B: 'Yes' (nods).

    .....

T: *What about the milk?*

B: MILK.

T:   *Milk* (hand guides Bodil to articulate MILK more correctly).
T:   *A worker who is drinking milk?*
B:   DRINK.
T:   *Is he drinking milk? Yes.*
B:   Looks at her hands.
T:   *What more?*
B:   EGG (this time with two flat hands. Points in the direction of the hidden picture).
T:   *Bodil, you should tell me about the picture. We can look afterwards.*
B:   EGG (articulated similar to WORK).
T:   *A worker, yes.*
      .....
T:   {WHAT *What more?*}.
B:   'I don't know' (throws hands up. Looks down).
T:   *A book?* (misunderstands the gesture as BOOK).
B:   Looks down, then at Tom and down again.
T:   *No, no no. Don't look. Tell me.*
B:   EGG.
T:   *Work.*
B:   EGG (vocalises).
      (Time elapsed 2:00).

After six minutes, Tom's interpretation was that the picture contained 'a worker who is drinking milk'. At that stage, he gave up and turned to the teacher for the answer. Bodil modified the articulation of EGG in several ways, still failing to make herself understood. It should also be noted that Tom was very dedicated to the task but unable to read EGG into her manual sign in spite of the fact that he had been shown EGG beforehand. It seems as if Bodil had to articulate manual signs absolutely correctly in order to be understood. Still, although they usually took a long time, not all the dialogue games failed:

(2)   Bodil had seen a picture of a woman with ragged trousers pouring coffee into an elegant cup. Sten was the partner.
      S:   *What is on the picture?*
      B:   (Smiles) BROKEN (articulated over her knee).
      S:   *Is something broken?*
      B:   Points in the direction of the pictures.
      S:   *Tell me what you saw on the picture.*
      B:   BROKEN (articulated over her knee).
            .....
            (Bodil gets help from the teacher to understand 'who' and answer WOMAN).
      B:   DRINK.

S: *Was she drinking from a cup?*
B: POUR.
S: *Was she pouring something?*
B: 'Yes' (nods).
S: *What did she pour?*
B: DRINK.
S: *What did she drink?*
B: DRINK.
S: *Did she drink coffee?*
B: COFFEE (hits the table and vocalises noisily).
S: *Oh!!*
B: Hits the knee.
S: *Did she have trousers on?*
B: BROKEN.
S: *Was there a hole in the trousers? Were the trousers broken?*
B: 'Yes' (nods).
(Time elapsed 5:25).

Sten was then able to interpret the content of the picture as 'A woman with a hole in her trousers is pouring coffee' and picked out the right picture.

In this type of interaction, typical not only of the dialogue games but of all Bodil's interactions, the partners focused more on getting answers to questions than encouraging Bodil's use of independent relational expressions. Bodil rarely produced utterances that contained two or more manual signs, and typically without any preferred sign order, signing PANCAKE MAN instead of MAN PANCAKE to express 'The man is making pancakes' (see also Grove, Dockrell and Woll, this volume). What may also be considered multi-sign utterances, were utterances with a scaffolded form of vertical structure (cf. von Tetzchner and Martinsen, this volume) usually constructed in collaboration with the partner. In (3), the scaffold did not work:

(3) Bodil had seen a picture of a woman with a coat on who was smoking and drinking coffee by a table. She was supposed to express this to Anne by using WOMAN, SHOE, MUSIC, TABLE and COAT but paid particular attention to the smoking.
A: *Well, Bodil, what did you see?*
B: BOOK
A: {*Was it a book? BOOK*}.
B: BOOK. 'Yes' (nods).
B: Points towards the pictures. COFFEE.
A: *Was there coffee on the picture?*
B: 'Yes' (nods. Looks thoughtful and touches the table).
A: *And a table?*

B:(Touches the table, nods) 'Yes'.

.....

A:  *Can you tell me what else there was on the picture?*

B:  SMOKE (blows air while signing).

A:  Looks likes she does not understand, thoughtful, tries to imitate Bodil's sign, but makes it too large.

B:  SMOKE (looks at teacher).

A:  *A picture of a trip in the .... forest? A picture of a trip in the forest, and they are sitting eating?*

B:  'Yes' (small nod) WOMAN. WOMAN (somewhat incorrect). COAT (somewhat incorrect).

A:  (Tries to imitate WOMAN, does not understand). *Should I really guess what that means? Was it music?*

B:  COAT. (Teacher says *coat,* and Bodil looks happy).

A:  *Coat on, yes. It is a picture with different things on, coffee, table, coat ... and some food.*

B:  Vocalises loudly, puts the hands on the table. (Time elapsed 3:30).

After 6 months of intervention, it had been realised that physical limitations made it impossible for Bodil to learn the number of different manual signs that would have been needed for what she wanted to express. Observations and analyses of the video recordings made it evident that it took her a long time to master a manual sign. Moreover, she failed to use the signs spontaneously and her articulation of many manual signs was so poor that even when using them, she did not make herself understood. The many misunderstandings and the lack of appropriate strategies apparent in (1) and (3) were typical of the dialogue games as well as her interactions with the staff at home. Nevertheless, in spite of her forty years of unsuccessful communication, there was no doubt about her motivation or about the fact that she had a lot she wanted to communicate. In conclusion, it was decided to reduce the traditional manual signing intervention and to introduce also a graphic system.

## Introduction of graphic signs

In November 1994, the first communication board was ready, consisting of PIC, PCS and photographs (see Introduction). The dialogue games were retained as the central element of training sessions. In the first dialogue game after having got her communication board, Bodil had been shown a picture of a man, a woman and a dog in a kitchen. Tom was the communication partner and found the right picture in 37 seconds. In (4), communication is both faster and more diverse than in the dialogues above:

(4)    Bodil had been shown a picture of a woman who was looking sad, reading and drinking coffee. Allen was the partner.

A:  *Have you seen a picture?*
B:  *WOMAN* (graphic).
A:  *It is a picture of a woman. Is it a woman I know?*
B:  'Yes' (vocalises). *BOOK.*
A:  *The woman is reading a book?*
B:  'Yes' (nods).
A:  *Yes.*
B:  *SAD.*
A:  *Is she sad?*
B:  'Yes' (nods)
A:  *A woman who is sad. Is it a boring book?*
B:  'No' (shakes head).
A:  *No. Can you point to more signs?*
B:  *COFFEE.*
A:  *She is drinking coffee?*
B:  'Yes'! (nods and shouts).
A:  *She is drinking coffee and reading a book. Is it you, Bodil? Is it Bodil?*
B:  'Yes' (nods and shouts).
A:  *Is it right?* (addressing the teacher).
     (Looking at Bodil) *Are you sad?*
     (Time elapsed, 1:06).

Bodil had become easier to understand and communicated more effi-ciently. She could usually remember 3–4 items with more items the communication task would take longer, often 3–4 minutes. Also when the picture showed somebody she knew well, the task would take longer because she wanted to tell something else about the person.

The vocabulary was built up slowly in close collaboration with Bodil. The communication aid had two pages with a total of 216 locations of which 150 were occupied in June 1995 (Table 15.3). Forty-eight of these had been used for photographs of residents, staff and other acquain-tances. Thirty-eight graphic signs were used spontaneously 90 times during video recordings. In addition Bodil used 24 names of residents, staff and teachers 103 times, demonstrating her great interest in commu-nicating about people.

Realising that her language environment would mainly be spoken language, and only to a limited extent would include the use of manual and graphic signs, great care was taken to link the graphic signs with her comprehension of speech. Moreover, she was shown the PIC and PCS versions, for example of *CAR,* and asked which one she would prefer to be glued on the communication board. She also decided which people to have on the board. They were placed on the left side of the board in

Table 15.3 The graphic signs introduced. The signs marked (*), Bodil has produced spontaneously during video recorded conversations in 1994 and 1995.

| | | | | |
|---|---|---|---|---|
| BIRD | SCHOOL | COOKING | MUSIC | *NAME (of institution) |
| *HAT | WATCH | *DOG | *CAT | *WORK-SHOP |
| RED | GREEN | YELLOW | BLACK | BLUE |
| WHITE | BROWN | *HAPPY | *SAD | *SURPRISED |
| TEASE | *TIRED | ILL | MONEY | ANGRY/STUPID |
| PURSE | *BUY | POP | *JUICE | *WRITE/PENCIL |
| *CAKE | *TEA | *COFFEE | MILK | *CAR/DRIVE |
| *GOODIES | PLANT | *ROOM/KEY | TABLE | BIRTHDAY |
| *BATH | TOILET | *LIGHT | *EAT | SLEEP/BED |
| SOFA | LETTER | CALENDAR | VISIT | *TELEPHONE |
| A-WALK | SUGAR | BUS | *BOOK | SUITCASE/TRIP |
| PICTURE | MAGAZINE | CUT | CARDS | PAPER-COVER |
| HOSPITAL | DOCTOR | NURSE | BRUSH | *FISHING-TRIP |
| SHOE | *GLASSES | *NECKLACE | MAKE-UP | HAIR-DRESSER |
| TOWEL | LONGS | TROUSERS | SHORTS | TOOTH-BRUSH |
| SHIRT | BLOUSE | WEST | DIRTY | *HAIR-DRYER |
| *ORGAN | COMPUTER | CAMERA | DANCE | UNDERWEAR |
| TAPE-DECK | DRESS | SKIRT | *GIFT | FILM-CAMERA |
| PARTY | *MAN | *WOMAN | *FLAG | *TELEVISION |
| CAMERA | CHAIR | *KITCHEN | *BOY | *BRACELET |
| *GIRL | *TALK-BOX | | | |

In addition, there were 48 names (photographs) of residents, staff and other acquaintances. Twenty-four of these were used spontaneously.

order to encourage a 'natural' left-right agent-action or agent-object sequence.

Many graphic signs corresponded to more than one spoken word and had no clear word class allocation. For instance, *CAR was used to express both* 'car' and 'drive'. So far Bodil has neither seemed to understand nor be interested in attributes like 'big' and 'small', 'pretty' and 'ugly', etc. She expressed denial by shaking the head and did so only when asked simple questions about participation in a well-known activity. She did not appear to understand relational terms like 'similar'.

In the early phase of the current intervention, Lotto had been used to train and monitor comprehension of speech. At that stage she seemed able to point to pictures corresponding to spoken object words but had more difficulties with action words and locative prepositions like 'over' and 'under'. Lotto was also used for training and monitoring manual sign comprehension, and she seemed to have relatively more problems with manual object signs than action signs. This may be related to manual action signs being more transparent than object signs (at least for normal language users). Konstantareas, Oxman and Webster (1978) found transparency effects for manual signs denoting actions and attributes, but not for those denoting object categories.

Bodil's development demonstrates that she profited from getting access to a graphic sign system. Manual signing was still encouraged and she continued to use her limited repertoire of manual signs spontaneously, for example WORK, CAR/DRIVE, COFFEE, COME, STUPID, KIND and I were often used. However, new manual signs were not systematically taught. The teacher has continued to use manual signs because these were assumed to support comprehension. At times she has showed evidence of bilingualism, first pointing to *CAT*, and later, after communicating about something else, returning to the topic by signing CAT. She has also combined graphic and manual signs, for example by pointing to *GIFT* and signing I by pointing at herself.

In spite of the fact that she has the largest expressive (and probably receptive as well) vocabulary ever in her 43 years, we believe her vocabulary development is still at an initial stage. She often appeared to lack words, for example when pointing to a person or a photograph and vocalising, and the partner had to guess what she wanted to communicate about the person. There were also graphic signs she had not yet used during teaching sessions, such as *CHAIR, TABLE* and *SOFA*. The inclusion of these may have been the result of wrong guesses about what she is interested in communicating about. On the other hand, such items are necessary if the vocabulary is to be expanded and more topics addressed.

## Narratives

In March 1995, the dialogue games were abandoned. These had served as a means for teaching and monitoring development, but had also restricted the choice of topics because most of the time the teacher had decided the topics of the conversations. Bodil had become easier to understand and it was no longer necessary to use communication assignments and know beforehand what she wanted to communicate in order to evaluate the communication process. In fact, she had several times initiated conversations about 'free' topics in the sessions.

The new objective of the intervention was that *Bodil* should communicate about previous experiences and coming events chosen by herself, but photographs were occasionally used by the teacher for introducing topics. Her general knowledge about Bodil's activities and daily life of course aided the teacher's understanding but no attempt was made to get information beforehand in order to ask her about known events. Bodil's vocabulary selection and communication during sessions had demonstrated that people were her major field of interest and she seemed to have a genuine need for sharing experiences with others and for putting into words and getting a hold on her own positive and negative

emotional encounters with people. This is hardly surprising, considering her life space. Most events were collective or related to particular
people. During sessions, she has often named people to indicate some
kind of problem in her home. Once she told the teacher that a person
had hit her on the back. She did this by pointing to the person's photograph and making a fist, hitting herself on the back making loud noises.
Although she did have manual signs for some people, these were not
easily understood, and she had never been reported to express similar
meanings without graphic means.

When the more narrative-oriented approach was initiated, part of the
direct teaching and video recording was moved to her residence. These
conversations were supposed to be open, but most staff members
tended to start with: *What did you do in school today?* This question
was not easy to answer when nothing special had happened. In such a
conversation she might indicate *COFFEE* whereupon the enthusiastic
partner would ask whether she had coffee, as if this was very surprising.
These initiations are probably typical of professionals' interactions with
intellectually impaired people.

As a means for both her and the communication partners to place
events in the right time frame, in January 1995, Bodil got a calendar.
Although the calendar also functioned as a cognitive aid, supporting
acquisition of temporal categories and memory (most people at her age
need such a cognitive aid), its main function was to facilitate communication about past and present events until she eventually might be able
to use the grammatical graphic sign indicators of past, present and
future. At the time of writing, the calendar fulfilled this function, as
evident in the following example.

> One day in June 1995, Bodil told the teacher about a fishing trip
> she had been on the day before. She found the PCS sign *FISHING-
> TRIP* and glued it into the right day (Sunday) in the calendar. She
> also told the teacher who had been with her on the trip that they
> had coffee and cakes. This conversation took more than half an
> hour.
>
> A little later, Bodil and the teacher went to her home to video
> record a conversation with one of the staff members. Bodil imme-
> diately pointed to *FISHING-TRIP* and began to tell about the trip.
> The staff member, however, began talking about a fishing trip they
> were planning for the following Tuesday. He also mentioned
> different people and said they were going to have juice and cakes.
> But while he stuck to his story, Bodil did not. She was the first to
> realise that they were actually communicating about two different
> trips. She began to smile, manually signed FUN and pointed to
> the Tuesday in the calender, indicating that she was looking
> forward to the trip.

During this last conversation, which lasted 13 minutes, Bodil produced 17 different manual signs and gestures 34 times. Thirty-three times she pointed at 16 different graphic signs on the board and 14 times at eight photographs of people. The calendar was used three times. The staff member repeated what she expressed, took his own dialogue turns and pointed at the board 14 times, the latter probably indicating that he took the matter seriously and wanted to convince her that she was wrong.

This conversation was important because it demonstrated that Bodil was able to discover such an advanced misunderstanding as well as being able to repair it. The staff member did not know about the fishing trip Bodil had been on and did not believe her. He needed confirmation from a more authoritative source (i.e. colleagues). The teacher also thought Bodil had mixed up the two trips, which, given her limited comprehension of spoken language, did not seem unlikely. However, it was later confirmed by others that she really had been on the fishing trip. It was Bodil who first gave evidence of understanding that there were two trips and it is not likely this would have been possible for her without a calendar as part of her communication aid. Digressing, one may note that although Bodil would have been unable to understand the complex instructions of the tasks used in 'theory of mind' experiments (cf. Baron-Cohen, Tager-Flusberg and Cohen, 1993; Benson et al., 1993; Wellman, 1990), an understanding of somebody else's false belief seems evident.

## Staff

The staff played an important role in facilitating transfer of communication skills from the educational setting to Bodil's everyday life. Most importantly, they realised that she was able to communicate. Participation in the dialogue games was probably the major ingredient in giving them insights into her abilities and problems alike, but they also expressed concern that they were giving too much time to Bodil compared to the other residents. On the other hand, they realised that the improvements would not have been possible without such involvement.

In the interviews, all three staff members reported that Bodil used the communication aid daily to tell them something. They also found her less noisy and her temper tantrums had become rare. However, there were still occasions where her communicative means were insufficient for expressing what she wanted to tell, and such situations sometimes escalated into loud disagreements if she did not manage to get her meaning across.

With regard to communication with the other residents, there was little change. Although her relations with the other residents were good, the staff have not seen Bodil attempt to use the aid for communicating with them. Still, the staff thought that her standing had been raised. She had become more accepted among the other residents. They became less easily irritated and found it interesting that she attended school. Increased direct communication with the other residents is a major goal for the school year starting August 1995.

## Discussion

With hindsight one might ask why it took such a long time since the first manual sign intervention was initiated in 1983 until a new approach was attempted. There seem to have been several reasons for this. Firstly, the signing intervention was not totally unsuccessful. Intellectually impaired people vary greatly with regard to the number of manual signs they learn (cf. Bonvillian and Blackburn, 1991; Bryen and Joyce, 1985; Kiernan, Reid and Jones, 1982). Since one usually does not know how many signs to expect a person to learn, any progress could be regarded as a success. Failures to learn manual signs could be attributed to constraints on the individual's ability to learn caused by the underlying biological impairment. Bodil did learn some manual signs and within the structure of the training sessions the signs were always understood since the teachers generally knew what she was supposed to express. Secondly, she always appeared motivated and happy during training sessions. In fact, she would probably be happy to participate in any activity outside the ordinary. Thirdly, as in the other Scandinavian countries, the signing tradition is strong in Denmark. Manual signing is usually the first choice for alternative communication intervention, as in this case, typically argued for on the basis of an expressed desire for the person to be independent of devices. In many cases, the manual signing tradition will lead to appropriate intervention, but professional traditions may lead to people doing what they can instead of what is best (Bourdieu, 1977), such as using one form of intervention only. Changing to a system the professional is less familiar with may be laborious and take a long time (cf. Kalman and Pajor, this volume; von Tetzchner, 1995).

When the present intervention was initiated, it was clear that Bodil must have had some manual sign intervention earlier but the content of it was not known and it did not appear to have been very successful. It was, however, a possibility that poor sign teaching and follow-up had been responsible for Bodil's lack of progress. Further, the staff had explicitly asked for manual sign intervention and were motivated to try this, and changing language form would not be done lightly. It therefore took some time from alternatives to manual signs being first discussed until a graphic communication system was introduced.

Even with hindsight, the decision to start with manual signing seems correct. It was important to assess Bodil's signing skills and the nature of her difficulties in order to adapt new strategies and language forms to her abilities and interests. It would probably have been difficult to persuade the staff to use graphic communication without having been able to demonstrate both her ability to communicate and her difficulties in doing so with manual signs. We also believe that because Bodil knew the purpose of signing, the initial manual sign intervention created continuity and functioned as a 'bridge' that helped her to relate the functions of manual and graphic signs. In addition, it probably revived some forgotten skills and ensured that existing skills were retained, laying the foundation for true *total communication* (in the Scandinavian sense of the term, where all communication modes are included, not only simultaneous use of speech and manual signs only). Because her various expressive means contributed together in creating a more specific communicative context, less intelligible manual signs were more likely to be understood. In this way, the use of graphic signs actually increased the functionality of her manual signs.

The video recordings have been an invaluable source for analysing and understanding the conversational processes during the intervention sessions. Somewhat unexpectedly, Bodil took great interest in the recordings and spent many hours looking at them at home. It is not clear whether this has contributed to her development and understanding of the communication situations. However, she often watched the videos in the common television room and this seemed to have had an impact on the other residents' attitude towards her 'school work', as being on television implies a certain amount of celebrity. On the other hand, it could be somewhat irritating for the others having to watch her *all* the time.

Everyday communication with Bodil was based on an assumption of speech comprehension. This was also true for the graphic sign teaching, although supported with manual signs, pictures and photographs. It took a long time before the teacher realised how limited Bodil's comprehension of spoken language was. During the dialogue games it became evident that she did not understand many of the words used in questions asked her. For instance, she was unable to understand *who, what* and *where* outside ritualistic situations where the response expected of her was given by the immediate context. Only once during a video recording before June 1995 did she seem immediately to understand a question containing *who*.

On the other hand, she did understand some spoken words and sentences, at least in a restricted manner. One could ask her to find a dress in the catalogue whereupon she would turn the pages until she saw one. Clothes and hats were her great passions, and she would spend a long time shopping for a new item. She had clear colour preferences, demonstrated by her pointing at colour samples (graphic signs). She could also point at particular colours named vocally but had great difficulties both comprehending and producing the manual colour signs

RED, YELLOW, BLUE and GREEN. She seemed to learn them during teaching sessions, but did not appear to remember them. She could point to most body parts named, which is not surprising given her interest in clothes and the time usually spent on naming body parts in special education.

As a result of the new insights into her comprehension of spoken language gained from the alternative communication intervention, speech comprehension has become more actively integrated into the intervention. Comprehension and use of manual and graphic signs and comprehension of spoken words were explicitly related to each other. Greatly improved dialogue skills seem to have been the result, due to both functional alternative language modes and a better understanding of the language spoken by the communication partners.

## Conclusions

A number of lessons can be learned from the present study. Firstly, motivation and happy appearance are not sufficient indications of either speech comprehension or programme efficiency. A motivated student does not exclude the possibility that another intervention strategy, in this case, an additional form of communication, might gain better results. Assessment should be based on the student's performance in communication situations where he or she has true communicative responsibility.

Secondly, it demonstrates the importance of taking the collective history, that is, the professional tradition, into consideration. Professional traditions may lead people to do what they can instead of what is best, and habit may often be the most decisive determinant of intervention programmes.

Thirdly, it has become almost embarrassingly evident that for Bodil, in spite of her intellectual limitations, communication was not only a means for expressing needs and gaining control of her environment, but also for other forms of talk. She seemed to have a genuine need for sharing experiences with others and for putting into words her own positive and negative emotional encounters with other people, as well as for 'presenting' herself (cf. Goffman, 1959). The degree to which she began to manage this in the course of the intervention has been the true measure of success. It also emphasises the need for setting the language intervention within a conversational frame.

Lastly, in spite of her relatively advanced age and the earlier professional blind alleys, Bodil made remarkable progress during one year of intervention. At the beginning of the intervention, the problem was to make a few individual manual signs understood by the people in the environment. After just over a year, she used 84 manual and graphic signs and pointed to the calendar in a single conversation, and the problem was a misunderstanding needing the negotiations typical of ordinary conversations. This demonstrates that acquisition of linguistic and communicative skills may be expected even for people with a long negative learning history. However, it may also be noted that at the time of writing this, Bodil still rarely initiates communication but waits until somebody else starts a conversation. She will rather walk away than try to break in if another person holds the floor. This learned pragmatic passivity is a scar from the time without proper means of communication which may be visible for a long time or never disappear totally.

# Chapter 16
# Supporting graphic language acquisition by a girl with multiple impairments

CARMEN BASIL AND EMILI SORO-CAMATS

Augmentative and alternative communication systems first began to receive attention in Spain just over ten years ago. Since then they have been increasingly used in special schools and have gradually made their way, though to a lesser extent, into habilitation services, occupational centres, hospitals, residential centres, and the like. However, their use is still fairly restricted and training of professionals within this field is limited. A need was felt for a centre for assessment, training and supervision to provide guidance for practitioners in this area. The authors of the present study, in conjunction with other professionals, have set up a pilot service which has operated for four years through co-operation between the Catalan government and the University of Barcelona. The aim of the service is to enhance the competence of disabled individuals, their families and professionals in the use and teaching of manual and graphic signs, as well as technical aids for communication and writing, although emphasis is on communication and interaction rather than the technology. A major goal is that once an assessment has been made, it is followed up by an intervention process designed to bring about a real improvement in the disabled person's communicative skills and quality of life. This chapter presents a case study concerning one child dealt with by the service.

Providing suitable training for professionals and families of children with severe multiple impairments presents a specially difficult challenge. In Spain, the notion that many of these children are not ready for communication and that 'prerequisite skills' have to be taught first is still firmly entrenched. However, Kangas and Lloyd (1988) and von Tetzchner and Martinsen (1992) have shown that the idea of such prerequisite conditions has little empirical basis, often leads to inefficient teaching and has hindered promotion of communicative skills. The latter authors suggest basing early intervention on the theory of overinterpretation

(Lock, 1980) according to which care-givers' tendency to attribute communicative meaning to their children's actions over and above that which they actually have is an important propelling force in the language acquisition process. Children with severe motor disabilities have very few 'legible' activities which the people around them can overinterpret and respond to (Martinsen, 1980; Ryan, 1977). One of the aims of the centre's intervention is therefore to provide children with *action resources* capable of producing contingent effects on their physical environment and eliciting natural communication reactions in the social environment. To meet this end, several different switch-operated toys and simple systems for controlling the environment (Björck-Åkesson, 1986; Musselwhite, 1986) have been employed and graphic communication signs have been gradually introduced.

Empirical studies have shown that the discourse patterns and the symmetry of the dialogues between children using graphic communication systems and the people they usually interact with are disturbed (Glennen and Calculator, 1985; Kraat, 1985; Light, Collier and Parnes, 1985a). This makes it difficult for the children to play an active role and may lead to passivity and learned helplessness (Basil, 1992; von Tetzchner, 1993b). Thus, the interventions of the centre direct special attention to coaching parents and teachers in appropriate interaction patterns, in particular to the need for pausing in order to give the children time to intervene and initiate communication themselves (cf. Glennen and Calculator, 1985; Light, 1985; Light and Collier, 1986; Soro and Basil, 1993), and reacting systematically to the children's behaviours and attributing communicative value to them (von Tetzchner and Martinsen, 1992).

Professionals teaching communication to children with severe multiple impairments often find it difficult to choose appropriate strategies and adapt them to the characteristics of each individual. Children with different levels of understanding and action resources need different goals and strategies. Specially designed interaction strategies are required to facilitate the initial development of communication in children with multiple impairments and making the most of their natural environments for language teaching (cf. Beukelman and Mirenda, 1992; Reichle, York and Sigafoos, 1991; Siegel-Causey and Ernst, 1989; Soro-Camats and Basil, in press; von Tetzchner and Martinsen, 1992). Often the real level of functioning of children who lack reliable response forms cannot be determined to begin with (Goossens', 1989). This means that in some cases where progress appears satisfactory, more ambitious goals and more advanced intervention strategies should be introduced (Møller and von Tetzchner, this volume; von Tetzchner and Martinsen, 1992).

Family members are usually children's main interlocutors and thus play a crucial role in the progress they make in acquiring alternative language skills. Nevertheless, collaboration between parents and professionals is generally insufficient. In this study, both direct parent training and facilitation of interaction between parents and teacher were provided in order to make co-operation more efficient and satisfactory (cf. McConachie, 1991). The model employed for training parents is based on the use of direct intervention techniques in the family environment, allowing the parents to observe professionals interacting with the child and thereby furnishing opportunity for influencing the parents' interaction patterns. Other techniques employed include interviews and discussions of video recordings of interactions between the child and the parents or the professionals. These discussions – bringing together parents, teachers and researchers – have made it possible to interpret co-operatively some of the interaction sequences and have served as a way of educating teachers in skills they need for giving appropriate training to parents.

The aim of the present chapter is to describe the centre's approach, to report changes in a girl's communication and the adults' competence in communicating with her, and to discuss the assessment and intervention model used. This is done by presenting a case study. An attempt is made to determine how, and to what extent, the parents and the teacher were progressively enabled to create a more language-supportive environment with regard to their communication styles and skills in arranging activities and situations that might foster the child's communication. Particular consideration is given to the adults' self-perceived competence, that is, the way the parents viewed their child, what they and the teachers expected, and how the outcomes were valued. Showing how and why this came to change during the intervention process is one of the major goals of this chapter.

# Method

### Subjects and settings

Magda is an intellectually impaired girl with severe motor impairment due to athetoid cerebral palsy, aged 7;3. She has no voluntary control over any part of her body and is unable to use her hands functionally or move about independently. Prior to starting school, intervention consisted solely of two hours of physiotherapy per week, during which she usually cried continuously. When Magda started school at age 3;9, which was also the start of the present project, she cried frequently. The family reported that at home, unless she received direct attention or slept with her parents, she would cry incessantly.

The parents and the teacher felt that Magda understood a lot but could hardly make herself understood, and attributed her crying to wanting something they could not understand. In fact, she got most things by crying or moaning. She was capable of uttering some undifferentiated sounds, but did not use this or any other discernible response to express 'yes' and 'no' reliably. She looked intently at people and objects around her, but severe problems in controlling her head and posture made it difficult for her to fix her gaze accurately and hard for those who wanted to share her attention to see what she was looking at. Probably because of this, people did not tend to attribute communicative value to her gaze and Magda did not use it to communicate.

The family lives in a flat in Barcelona. Magda is an only child, the father is a mechanic, often working late. The mother makes clothes and does most of her work at home to be able to look after her daughter. However, this has also been a source of friction since the girl was continually demanding her mother's attention by crying if she did not pick her up or interact with her in watching television, listening to music or playing, making it impossible for the mother to get on with her work. Throughout the study the parents took an active part in the sessions and agreed to have interactions in the home recorded on videotape. The mother participated more than the father but he took part in the training sessions with the researchers and the teacher and in some of the interaction sessions.

Magda attended a small special school for children with severe motor disabilities. Due to legislation introduced in 1984, most disabled children in Catalonia go to mainstream schools. However, integration of children with severe motor impairments, particularly those needing augmentative and alternative communication, has proved difficult. As a result, Magda's school is attended by children with normal intellectual function as well as children with various degrees of intellectual impairment.

The school is quite well equipped with adapted toys, simple switch-operated environmental control systems, and computers with adapted software and access. Most of the students are taught manual signs and/or to use communication boards with graphic signs, and, occasionally, letters and written words. Some have electronic aids with digitised speech output. Magda's teacher had experience with these devices but it was a new challenge for her to use them for children whose range of action and expressive abilities were extremely limited. She also said that she found it hard to get communication skills acquired by the children at school accepted and used at home, and integrating skills learned at home in the classroom. This was the background for the intervention process described here. The teacher acceded to the conditions required by this type of study (the researcher's presence in the classroom, video recording, etc.), collaborated enthusiastically and tried to follow the researchers' guidelines scrupulously. She also kept a record of whatever facts or events were considered of significance in the process.

## Procedure

The study consists of two parts: an intervention phase lasting 15 months and a follow-up phase lasting 27 months. Initial observations were made in the first month of the project, during the intervention process, and at the end of the intervention. Follow-up observations were made 27 months after the intervention phase was terminated.

During the intervention phase, about every two months, one of the present authors observed and video-recorded several interaction situations with the girl and her teacher at school, and the girl and her parents at home. Each video recording contained two interaction situations at school and one or two such situations at home, lasting roughly fifteen minutes each. The interactions consisted mainly in playing with toys, story reading and conversation. Immediately following each situation, the researcher would discuss it with the parents or the teacher and make suggestions for improving various aspects, such as positioning, organisation of the board space, adaptation of materials, and, above all, the adults' and girl's communication patterns. During intervention sessions the researcher also interacted with Magda to illustrate points that had been discussed and to provide a model. Parents and teacher were given opportunities for guidance when practising new suggestions. This part of the intervention was also usually video recorded.

Except for holiday periods, between every two sessions at school and at home, a joint meeting was organised. At these sessions parents and teacher watched and analysed episodes selected by the researcher from the video recordings of the previous sessions and discussed issues related to the intervention. These sessions also provided an opportunity for parents and teacher to exchange opinions and gradually work towards a congruous approach.

During the follow-up phase, the researcher halted the sessions with the family but continued to train the teacher and gather data on interaction in the school setting. This was done in order to ensure continuity and hand over the responsibility for parent training to the teacher. After 31 months, the intervention sessions at school were also interrupted. After 42 months, a final follow-up session was held at the school along the same lines as before.

The analysis is based on qualitative interpretations of the video-recorded communication sequences, the teacher's records and diaries of daily teaching practice, and interviews with the teacher and the parents.

# Intervention

### Initial intervention at school

When she began school, Magda went through a period characterised by anxiety and frequent crying, often lasting up to $1^{1}/_{2}$ hours, without the teacher being able to pacify her. During the first session she was seated in an adapted chair with a strap across her chest to hold her in and supports for feet, head and shoulders. Attached to the chair was a tray large enough for the things she needed. The teacher sat facing her on a low chair so that their eyes were at the same level.

The girl and teacher were video-recorded while looking at a storybook and playing a game with objects. The teacher held up the book so that Magda could see the pictures without losing control of her head, but this meant that the teacher's hands were occupied. Throughout the 15-minute session, Magda paid attention to the pictures in the storybook and what the teacher said. The teacher spoke slowly, using clear and simple language, making her actions run parallel to those of the girl to obtain mutual attention (cf. Björck-Åkesson, 1990; Schaffer, Collis and Parson, 1977; Snyder-McLean, Solomonson, McLean and Sack, 1984) but clear turn-taking occurred only when the page was turned. Fifteen times the teacher asked Magda to turn the page, waited for a small movement of her right arm, and helped her complete the action. Occasionally, the girl moved her arm spontaneously and the teacher interpreted this as a request to turn the page, stopped telling the story, and helped her do so. In this way she ascribed meaning to arm movements which were practically involuntary and with a poor prognosis of eventually becoming functional for such fine-tuned activities as turning pages. On the other hand, though, she did not respond in any specific manner to the way Magda attentively looked at the pictures in the book.

On two occasions the teacher interpreted sounds made by Magda. After the teacher had asked her to turn over the page, the girl moaned and the teacher took this as meaning 'Oh, you want me to do it!'. The second instance occurred when the teacher said that the wolf knocked at the door. The girl made a noise which the teacher corroborated by replying *Yes, he knocked at the door* with an intonation indicating that Magda had meant that the wolf was frightening. This was the only time something the girl did was interpreted as a comment on the story.

Once the story was over she started to cry. The teacher unsuccessfully tried to comfort her until she saw that Magda was looking at a shelf with a jug of water. Interpreting this as a request, she gave her some water to drink. Magda drank the water and began to cry again, making the teacher explain: *If you want more water, look at the glass.* The girl did so and got more water. This interaction was repeated twice before the girl calmed down and the session came to an end. Magda was able to ask for water in her classroom by pointing to it with her eyes because five objects (a toy car, a storybook, a ball, a comb and water) were set on a shelf for this purpose and arranged to be both within range of the children's gaze and sufficiently separate for the teacher to distinguish clearly which one they were looking at. Beside each object was a large PCS sign (see Introduction).

Following this first observation, the researcher interacted with Magda for about eight minutes, telling the story while commenting on possible strategies that might be applied. After rehearsing the decisions they had agreed on, the teacher intervened again, guided by the researcher. It had been decided to put the storybook on a book rest which would leave the teacher's hands free, enabling her to point to the drawings as she told the story and react to the girl's eye-pointing. She should pause every so often while telling the story to give the girl time to contribute with vocalisations or gazes, and react to these, interpreting them as though Magda was pointing to, or commenting on, the pictures, as she had already done on one occasion. Less emphasis should be put on turning pages, and it was agreed that when Magda looked at the bottom right-hand corner of the book or made the movement with her arm, provided it was rapid and clear, this should be taken as a request to have the page turned. The teacher should turn the pages herself, rather than insisting on Magda doing it.

The second part consisted of an object game. When it was initiated, Magda started to cry. The teacher removed the objects and waited for the crying to stop. When Magda had calmed down the activity was recommenced but she started to cry again. This was repeated five times within a period of four minutes until she eventually accepted the game without crying. The teacher piled up some building blocks and encouraged Magda to knock them down with her hand, acting and speaking slowly with the girl watching attentively. However, they acted in parallel rather than in synchrony. Turn-taking was again related to arm movements, that is, the girl knocking over the tower. This sweeping arm movement, however, was potentially useful and might later be used, for example, for operating a switch to activate toys.

The intervention following the object game concentrated on Magda's crying. It was pointed out that the strategy of withdrawing the objects and waiting for her to calm down before going on with the game could sometimes be appropriate, as crying is often disruptive and prevents real interaction. However, notice was taken of the fact that, except for crying, Magda had very few resources for controlling situations in which she was involved, and that one major aim of the intervention was precisely to enhance such control. It was recalled that when Magda cried, the teacher had adroitly taken advantage of a gaze directed at the water jug to interpret it as a request. This had showed Magda that she could ask for water by looking at the jug instead of crying. Since few such opportunities arose spontaneously, the teacher should manufacture them by offering the girl the opportunity to choose between two activities by looking at one of two objects denoting what she wanted to do. The aim of this was to convey the idea to Magda that if she was not satisfied with something she could show this without crying and the teacher would try to understand her. In addition, this strategy would allow new communication experiences using eye-pointing, which at the time was her most useful resource. As in book reading, the teacher should introduce pauses in her activity to facilitate vocalisations and eye-movements that could be interpreted as requests or comments on what was going on. For instance, the teacher learned to wait until Magda looked at one of the blocks before placing it on top of the tower while saying: *Oh, you want me to put this block on.*

## Initial intervention at home

The video recording consisted of 25 minutes of interaction between the girl and her mother while the girl was eating, followed by a game with a doll. The girl was sitting in a low pushchair without any anatomical supports or tray to put things on. The mother was sitting on an ordinary chair, and it was impossible for her to see many of the girl's expressions and eye-movements. She said that Magda had very particular interests, always wanting the same toys, storybooks or videos, items that were kept where she could not see them.

During the observation the girl smiled and vocalised far more often than at school and she looked a lot happier. The mother almost always reacted to these manifestations with comments such as *Are you happy?*, *Do you want some more?*, *My, what a cough!* or *What do you want?*, establishing good interaction and turn-taking. However, she did not attribute any communicative content to the vocalisations and facial expressions. She often asked Magda a question and, when the girl responded with a smile and vocalisation that could be interpreted as 'yes', ignored it and went on with the previous activity or asked her another question which she also failed to react to, as in these examples:

(1)     Magda was having her tea and had been eating for five minutes.
        Ma: Makes a sound.
        M:   *What?* (Trying to give her a spoonful of food).
        Ma: Keeps her mouth closed.
        M:   *Don't you want any more?*
        Ma: Makes a sound and smiles.
        M:   *Come on, here we go, have some more!* (Giving her another spoonful).

(2)     The meal was over. The mother and the researcher were talking.
        Ma: Makes a loud sound and looks at her mother.
        M:   *What do you want? Shall we watch the tele?*
        Ma: Tenses her body and makes as though to lower her head.
        M:   *Hey, what do you want? Do you want a doll? Shall we play with the doll? Hey, how does the doll go? It's not here. It's not here. Mummy always puts it here, doesn't she? It's not here. How does the doll go? It goes 'oooooooh'. This ice cream is*

*lovely! Is that what the doll says? Wait. Shall mummy go and fetch the doll? You do want the doll?*

Ma: Smiles and looks at her mother.

M: *Yes, it's in here, in your room. Do you want it? Do you? I'll go and get it.*

Ma: Turns her head and clearly looks backwards, towards the television.

M: *Do you want to watch the tele? She wants to watch the tele. Shall we put it on?* (She turns Magda round to face the television set and switches it on).

Ma: Watches the television attentively.

M: (Stands in front of the girl, blocking her view of the television) *Do you want a doll?*

The game with the doll consisted essentially in asking Magda to do things with it that were too difficult for her, such as feeding it or stroking it, and helping her to do them by guiding her hand, although it was highly unlikely she would ever be able to perform these actions unaided. The happy tone and the exchange of smiles and sounds followed by the mother's comments continued, but without any specific consequences for the particular activity being pursued. Several times throughout the session the girl lost head control as the chair did not support an adequate posture. Each time the mother had to position her properly again.

In the intervention that followed, it was suggested that a few objects Magda was interested in – a video and a couple of toys – be placed where she could ask for them by looking at them. The importance of having control over the situation, being able to ask for things, and experiencing being understood by others, was discussed. Particular emphasis was placed on the need for adults to attribute meaning to her eye-movements and vocalisations and to react to them in keeping with these interpretations, thereby allowing themselves to be guided by the girl and do what they thought she was asking them to do. The mother objected that the girl already understood such things – referring to the objects – and that she did not see the need to have them in the view of Magda. She found it hard to grasp that the problem was not so much Magda's comprehension as her lack of ability to express herself in such a way that others could understand her, and that this was the reason for establishing a clear link between the girl's behaviours and the adults' reactions to them.

The mother was greatly concerned with the fact that Magda often cried to get her attention on occasions when she did not have time to be at the girl's beck and call. However, if the crying went on for a long time, she would try to make her stop. It was suggested that she should react to Magda's crying right away whenever she could, interpreting it as a request, and try to find out what she wanted by allowing her to indicate with her eyes or affirmative or negative expressions. She should then play with Magda for a short while and tell her: *That is enough now. Mummy has got to get on with her work.* If she could not attend to her at that time, she should say so from the very beginning. The reason given was that it was better to attend to the crying straight away and try to establish some rules on this basis rather than letting her go on crying for a long time, eventually attending to her just the same. The mother mentioned that the same suggestion had been put to her at school. It works there, but Magda does not take any notice of what she says to her.

**Intervention process**

Eight two-hour intervention sessions were held at school and six at home. There were also four joint meetings. During the first few months, the recommendations of the initial sessions were followed up. New strategies were gradually introduced, adapting the adults' interaction behaviour to the slow progress made by Magda. The reasons behind the strategies and the importance of persistence were underlined, especially with the family. If adults give up too soon, the child may fail to learn and the parents may have insufficient time to become aware of the effects they actually have on the child's development despite the multiple impairments. This vicious circle may confirm what they in some way had thought from the very beginning: that nothing could be done. Joint sessions allowed the parents to observe Magda at school and see that the teacher was persevering, confident in what she was doing, and achieved results. This helped them to understand and put into practice the suggestions made to them.

The family was recommended a chair with a table, necessary supports to provide postural control, and room for the communication frame the girl would be using, as well as storybooks, toys and objects of various kinds. However, it took eight months before the chair was available. It was too expensive for the family and the father made it himself, a slow and laborious process. Other simple technical aids were introduced both at home and school in order to provide Magda with improved action resources (adapted toys and small, switch-operated environmental control devices) and teaching and interaction strategies were recommended for activities with these aids. At school, single-switch programmes and elementary preschool computer activities were introduced.

Two months after the initial observation, a number of PCS signs were put on an acrylate eye-gaze frame attached to her table at school. At this time, the major focus of the intervention was teaching and practising appropriate interaction strategies for Magda's acquisition of graphic language. The vocabulary, *BREAKFAST, PLAY, LUNCH, REST* and *HOME,* was first used as signal signs, that is, the teacher pointed to them to announce activities in which the girl should take part. Shortly afterwards, two supplemental displays of clear vinyl were built, containing three and five graphic signs related to these activities. In situations indicated by *BREAKFAST* and *PLAY*, Magda was taught to use a display with *YOGHURT, BOOK* and *BUILDING-BLOCKS* while in situations designated by *LUNCH* and *REST*, she could choose who she wanted to be with by pointing to (photographs of) *CLASSROOM-ASSISTANT, PHYSIOTHERAPIST* or *SPEECH THERAPIST*, and to *MARIA* or *JUAN*, two other children in her class.

After three months, the displays were expanded and new displays made, gradually building up new vocabulary as Magda's communication progressed. A similar process went on at home, though at a slower pace, since it took six months before the displays were used at home. The researchers provided general criteria for selecting vocabulary, taking Magda's level of comprehension and, above all, her wishes, as the starting point. It was recommended that the words chosen should be ones that could be used frequently in a wide range of everyday contexts, thereby creating ample opportunities for her to learn them. It was also suggested that the vocabulary should be fairly specific, that is, related to particular activities to do with her education, leisure or daily routine in which Magda was involved. The teacher chose signs, discussed them with the researchers, and recommended some to the family. In view of the importance of the vocabulary available and the complex task it is to select an appropriate vocabulary, in retrospect even more attention should probably have been given to this process.

**Final intervention at school**

On the video recording Magda was having her clothes changed, a mid-morning snack with the rest of the class, and activities requested by her (language work, toy game, using a switch-operated cassette player and looking at a storybook). Magda had far greater control over the situations than before. Although her means of expression were limited and many problems still remained, she had become able to formulate specific requests, guide activities and make comments. In addition to communicating with vocalisations, facial expressions and indication of objects by looking at them, she was also using PCS signs on a three-sided eye-gaze frame with a core vocabulary attached to her table and seven supplemental topical displays (Figure 16.1). She also used a wall communication board and several graphic signs distributed around the classroom. Altogether, she had access to a vocabulary of 70 graphic signs (Table 16.1).

While having her clothes changed, Magda was on the floor and could see the wall communication board with the signs relevant to this activity.

Table 16.1 Vocabulary available to Magda at school at the time of the final observation

Graphic signs on the eye-gaze frame

| CHAIR | COMPUTER | DRINK | EAT | FLOOR |
|---|---|---|---|---|
| THAT'S IT | KISS | MORE | NO | HAPPY |
| PLAY | WORK | YES | TOILET | PHYSIOTHERAPY |

Graphic signs distributed about the classroom beside various objects

| BALL | BIRTHDAY | CAR | COLOURS | DOOR |
|---|---|---|---|---|
| PAPER | TABLE | TOYS | WINDOW | TOILET-BAG |
| TELEPHONE | BOOK | MAGAZINES | | |

Graphic signs on the wall communication board.

| BAG | COAT | CHRISTINA | CUPBOARD | HANG UP |
|---|---|---|---|---|
| JUAN | LOLITA | MARIA | NAPPIES | RICARDO |
| TROUSERS | WAIT | | | |

Graphic signs on the seven supplemental displays.

| Storybooks and music: | Game activities: | |
|---|---|---|
| MIGUEL BOSÉ TAPE | BUILDING BLOCKS | |
| MOZART TAPE | DOLL | |
| LITTLE RED RIDING HOOD | RADIO | |
| POPULAR MUSIC TAPE | STORY | |
| SNOW WHITE | | |

| Eating implements: | Food: | Animal game: |
|---|---|---|
| GLASS | BISCUITS | BEAR |
| PLATE | JUICE | CAT |
| BIB-SERVIETTE | MILK | MONKEY |
| SPOON | YOGHURT | CHICKEN |
| | | OWL |

| Little Red Ridinghood story: | Places to go: |
|---|---|
| BIG | HOME |
| EARS | CLASSROOM |
| ILL | PLAYGROUND/STREET |
| MOUTH | SCHOOL |

As she changed Magda's clothes, the teacher paused every now and then to give the girl a chance to look at the communication board. After each pause the teacher named the article of clothing she was changing, speaking while pointing to the corresponding graphic sign on the board (COAT, NAPPIES, TROUSERS, etc.). The teacher took advantage of every opportunity that came up to point to signs on the communication aid while she was talking in order to help the girl understand the signs and provide models for their use.

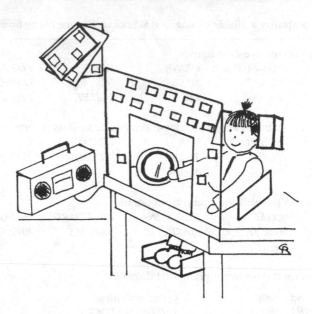

**Figure 16.1** The seating arrangement, switch, gaze frame, and supplemental displays. The small shoulder rest designed to prevent involuntary arm extension movements had been enlarged to support the whole arm.

For the mid-morning snack, there was a table where all the children could see milk, fruit juice, yoghurt and biscuits. They had to call the teacher and ask for what they wanted to eat and drink. On several occasions, Magda attracted the teacher's attention with vocalisation and was told to wait for a moment. Twice the teacher went over to her, and she expressed *YOGHURT* by looking at the sign on her eye-gaze frame. After ten minutes, Magda started to cry, as she still did occasionally, but this was turned into a communicative exchange. The teacher replaced the snack display with the core vocabulary frame and asked Magda what she wanted. Magda said *PLAY* and the teacher answered that they were going to play when they had finished eating. The girl indicated *KISS* and the teacher gave her a kiss. Another girl in the class, who could speak, also asked for a kiss and the teacher gave her one. Thus, Magda's request has led to another child entering the conversation.

The next situation began by Magda saying *WORK*. The teacher removed the eye-gaze frame and set up a language teaching situation by placing three pictures on a stand which the girl should look at as the teacher named them. However, Magda immediately started crying and this was interpreted to mean 'That wasn't it'. Magda looked at the communication frame and the teacher said: *No, now we are going to do some work. I will put the frame back for you after that.* For the next three minutes she tried to get the activity going without any result. Finally, the teacher agreed to put her communication frame back, giving rise to this exchange:

(3) T: {*WORK We said we had do some work for a bit*}.
Ma: Cries.
T: *What do you want to do?*
Ma: Looks at the frame without fixing her gaze on any particular sign and goes on crying.
T: *Nothing? When you want something you'll tell me.*
Ma: Looks at the frame without fixing her gaze on any particular sign and continues to cry.
T: (Waits for a while) *What do you want?*
Ma: Looks at the single-topic displays to her right (Figure 16.1) and continues to cry.
T: *Do you want another display?* (Puts one up) *Is this the one?*
Ma: Protest vocalisation.
T: (Puts up another one) *Is this the one you want?*
Ma: Stops crying and relaxes.
T: *OK, we'll do this for a while and then get back to some work.* (Starts playing with the talking toy indicated by Magda).

Despite the difficulties, Magda managed to control the situation, persisting with her crying until she was given the opportunity to express what she wanted. Thus, when she cries, adults can no longer say: *There is nothing we can do.*

During play, Magda looked at the pictograms of animals and the teacher worked the toy to have it make the sound of the animal chosen by Magda. The teacher was now paying less attention to the manipulative activity involved and more to communication. Like other non-speaking motor impaired children, Magda had such great difficulties handling things and getting about that, paradoxically, her expressive language proved to be, in spite of everything, her best action strategy. She will have to use it for common linguistic functions as well as for taking part in games which involve handling things, instructing others to perform the different actions she wants to get done (cf. von Tetzchner, 1993b). However, this was something the teacher found particularly difficult to adhere to. In the session two months earlier, she had still tried to get Magda to manipulate this complicated toy by guiding her hand and had been advised to carry out the activity in the way it was performed in this final session.

After three minutes play with the talking toy, the teacher gave Magda another opportunity to choose and this time she indicated *CASSETTE-PLAYER*. She turned on the time-controlled cassette player with the help of a large switch (Figure 16.1) several times. When she stopped, a girl in the class said: *Play, Magda.* Later, the same girl encouraged her again saying: *Come on, Magda!* Broadening her range of action possibilities, in this case by making adaptations to a cassette player, allowed her to play more independently but also opened up far more interaction with adults and children because they tended to comment on what she was doing. This focus on her actions and interests is similar to the way adults interact with normally developing children, and many researchers have singled it out as essential for acquiring concepts and words (Schaffer, 1992).

Finally Magda chose to look at a book, and the teacher let her select one by looking at it, as had been recommended in the initial session. The reading was structured as a dialogue. The teacher pointed at the pictures while she told the story, paused so that Magda could indicate a picture with her eyes, and said something about the picture she had focused on. During three minutes of story reading, the teacher made 25 comments, of which 15 were responses to vocalisations or picture indications made by Magda. Six comments were initiated by the teacher. Four of Magda's expressions were interpreted as requests to turn the page and the teacher reacted to them by doing so herself without trying to get the girl to do it. Thus, the interaction pattern had changed a good deal since the initial session where almost all the comments on the story were initiated by the teacher. During the first session, the teacher interpreted 17 of Magda's actions as attempts to communicate in the space of 15 minutes. During these three minutes of story reading, she interpreted 19 expressions as attempts at communication. In the first session, only one of the expressions was taken as a comment on the story while 16 were interpreted as requests to turn the page. This time there were 15 comments and four requests for page-turning.

**Final intervention at home**

The girl was sitting in an adapted chair with a table, similar to the one at school but lighter and easier to move. There was a core vocabulary frame with a vocabulary similar to the one at school and several topic displays related to activities taking place at home, such as places to go, things to buy, clothes, and things to play with. The parents had only recently begun to use the communication displays and said they had a number of difficulties with them. The researcher therefore started by interacting with the girl to show the parents, both of whom were present, how to use the eye-gaze frame and the displays and see which signs the girl was looking at.

The interaction with the mother began with Magda choosing BOOK by eye-pointing to it on the communication frame. The mother had already learned to do what her daughter indicated and read the story using most of the recommended strategies. She pointed to the pictures in the storybook, saying something about them. When Magda looked at a particular picture, the mother commented on it, allowing herself to be guided by her daughter. She also attributed meaning to some of the vocalisations made by the girl and the way she looked at objects in the environment, and reacted accordingly. This hardly happened during the initial session. She no longer tried to get Magda to turn the pages but interpreted the relevant signals as instructions to do it herself. This is the first minute of the interaction:

(4)   Magda had just used the cassette player while interacting with the researcher.

   M:  *What do you want?*
   Ma:  *CASSETTE-PLAYER.*
   M:  *The cassette-player again? Again the cassette-player?*
   Ma:  *STORYBOOK.*
   M:  *Oh, you want a story! You want a story, do you? Yes, you want a story. Come on then!* (Picks up a storybook). *Here goes then, a story.* (Opens the storybook in front of the girl). *Oh, what a story! Look, can you see, a daddy sitting on the sofa* (pointing to the picture). *He's sitting on the sofa reading a book.*
   Ma:  Following what her mother is doing very attentively. Looks at one of the pictures in the storybook.
   M:  *What is that? The fridge.*
   Ma:  Vocalises and looks at her mother.
   M:  *That's right, the fridge, for putting food in. Yes.*
   Ma:  Vocalises and looks at her father.
   M:  *Ah, what? You are telling daddy that you are looking at a story.*
   Ma:  Looks at the bottom right-hand corner of the storybook.
   M:  *Shall we turn the page?*
   Ma:  Vocalises and smiles.
   M:  *Yes, come on then, another page. Good!!* (Turns the page).

Following this the parents and the researcher talked about the communication displays. The mother said: *They are useful sometimes, but we don't need them much as we understand her very well ... with gazes, and 'yes' and 'no'.* The father added: *When we put it in front of her she laughs at it ... and for us it is a barrier.* On the other hand, they often used the topic displays. These allowed the girl to make specific decisions in situations such as playing, getting dressed and going out.

Thus, at this stage, Magda had the eye-gaze frame in front of her most of the time at school, while at home the communication displays were used only in specific situations where the parents felt that they needed them. However, the teacher would continue to help the parents – without forcing them – to integrate the aid into their communication habits in a natural way. Relying exclusively on pointing to objects in the environment, vocalisations and facial expressions would restrict Magda's range of expressions to subjects in the immediate context and not allow her to learn to refer to new situations, express opinions or make interesting comments. A situation that enabled her to express herself with only these resources would be a poor language environment. The parents' frequent use of *yes no* questions would leave little leeway for Magda's initiative (cf. Light, 1985) and possibly lead to learned helplessness since it would place her in a passive role, teaching her that she had to wait until asked before being able to express anything (cf. von Tetzchner and Martinsen, 1992).

It was emphasised that progress in the development of expressive skills is very slow for children like Magda but that it may lead to considerable enhancement of the quality of life. The parents stated that Magda was generally happier than before. They felt more satisfied and experienced less often that she was frustrated because they did not understand what she wanted to express. Nevertheless, when trying to implement the strategies suggested to them, the parents still tended to get discouraged fairly rapidly and think that such strategies are all very well at school but not at home, since Magda does not take notice of them when they try to modify their usual style of interaction – with which they also felt more comfortable. The researcher argued at great length for the need to persevere in order to achieve results and underscored the importance of such results for themselves and their daughter.


## Follow-up

Training continued at school for 15 more months and a follow-up observation was made 42 months after the initial session. Magda had a productive vocabulary of 151 graphic signs (Table 16.2) and used a four-sided eye-gaze frame with 32 PCS signs compared to 15 signs on the earlier, three-sided one. She and the teacher appeared to have maintained the skills they had acquired and had made considerable progress in some areas. In particular, the girl was now able to point to the signs on the frame by looking at them in a less ambiguous and more deliberate fashion. She sometimes systematically scanned the different signs until she found the one she was looking for. The language level and the complexity of the concepts involved were more advanced, although still limited. She appeared happy, willing to collaborate, smiled frequently and did not moan much. The teacher was very proud of Magda's progress.

Magda and the teacher were video-recorded dressing and undressing a doll, and reading a story. As in the situation recorded more than two years earlier, when Magda had played with the talking animal toy, she told the teacher what to do with the doll by looking at the signs on the communication frame. The teacher sometimes let Magda handle the doll herself as she appeared to like to touch the doll, the towel, etc. However, in spite of the similarities, significant differences could be observed. In the animal game, the graphic sign chosen was always right, that is, she knew the sound made by any of the animals. The point of that situation

Table 16.2 The 82 new graphic signs Magda had available to her at school at the time of the follow-up observation. They are on an acrylate eye-gaze frame with a core vocabulary, several supplemental displays and a wall communication board. This list, taken together with Table 16.1, constitutes a vocabulary of 152 items.

| | |
|---|---|
| ALEX | HOLIDAY/PARTY |
| ALSO | HOW ARE YOU? |
| ANOTHER/SOMETHING ELSE | I |
| BATH/SHOWER | I DON'T KNOW |
| BEER | I LIKE (IT) |
| BOOKREST | IT'S RAINING |
| BOTTOM | LIGHT |
| BOY | LOOK |
| BUS | MIRROR |
| BUY | MORNING/TOMORROW |
| CALL | MUMMY |
| CARLOS | PAGETURNER |
| CHANGE | PLEASE |
| CLEAN | PLUG |
| CLEAN TEETH | PUT |
| CLOTHES | RUN |
| COFFEE | SECRETARY |
| COFFEE MAKER | SHOP |
| COMB (NOUN) | SOFT DRINK |
| COMB (VERB) | SPONGE |
| DADDY | STORY OF `TEO' |
| DIRTY | STORY OF THE THREE LITTLE PIGGIES |
| DOCTOR | STREET |
| DRY | SUGAR |
| EXPLAIN | SUN |
| EYES | SUPPER |
| FAMILY | SWITCH |
| FILTER | THANK YOU |
| FRIEND | THEATRE |
| FRIGHTENED | THE WOLF |
| GIRL | TIRED |
| GO | TRICYCLE |
| GO FOR A WALK | VISIT |
| GOOD/WELL | WASH HAIR |
| GOODBYE | WATER |
| NICE/PRETTY | WET |
| GRANDMOTHER | WHAT? |
| GRANDFATHER | WHEN? |
| HAIR | WHERE? |
| HEAR | WHO? |
| HELLO | WOODCUTTER |

had been to teach her to use signs for directing the activities of the person interacting with her. This lesson had been well learned and the teacher had gone a little further, for example asking *wh*-questions to which Magda usually gave relevant answers. *After* was used to establish activity sequences:

(5)    Magda was drying the doll with the towel after having given it a shower and washed its hair.
       Ma: *SHOWER.*
       T:   *Yes, we have given her a shower. And what did you do after the shower?*
       Ma: *WASH HAIR.*
       T:   *Washed her hair. And after that?*
       Ma: *COMB* (noun).
       T:   *Do you want a comb? Why do you want the comb?*
       Ma: *COMB* (verb).
       T:   *To comb her, of course!*

In this dialogue, the teacher's interventions are turnabouts (cf. Kaye, 1982): She confirmed what the girl had said and added a question or comment that led to a new turn in the dialogue. This is a natural strategy for facilitating conversation skills and is commonly observed in interactions between children who are developing speech and their more competent communication partners (Kaye and Charney, 1981). When Magda indicated *COMB* in her attempt to reconstruct the activity sequence, she was missing out a step. After the shower and hair wash, they had dried the doll with a towel and it was only then that her hair had to be combed. However, the teacher did not correct her. She had been advised to proceed in this way due to the need to invest Magda's communicative acts with credibility and had kept this up to encourage the girl to take a more active part. By this stage, though, Magda's skills and attitude were sufficient to allow corrections, and this would have been a good opportunity. Whereas previously the pragmatic side had been given virtually exclusive priority, it had now become both possible and necessary to foster the development of more formal aspects of linguistic acts as well. The teacher had recently begun to teach her to ask questions and use social terms:

(6)    Ma: *MIRROR.*
       T:   *Do you want to look at yourself in the mirror? Where is the mirror?*
       Ma: Looks at the shelf where the mirror is.
       T:   *The mirror. Look at it.* (Goes to get the mirror and lets the girl look at herself). *Oh, Magda is pretty today.* (Takes the mirror away).

Ma: *PRETTY.*

T: *Yes, you are pretty, that's right.* (Long, expectant pause, i.e., structured waiting).

Ma: *THANK-YOU.*

T: Thank you. You're welcome, Magda. (New pause or structured waiting).

Ma: *HELLO.*

T: *Hello. You have already said hello to me this morning.*

Ma: Looks at Laura (who is video recording).

T: *Ah, Laura. Haven't you said it to her already? Haven't you said hello to her?*

L: *Hello. How are you?*

Ma: *BIG.*

T: *Are you big? Yes, you are getting to be a big girl.*

L: *But you were a bit poorly yesterday. How are you today?*

Ma: Looks at Laura and smiles. *WELL.* (Follows with her eyes the direction the teacher is pointing in order to help Magda produce this sign).

T: *Today you are well.*

L: *Well!!* (At the same time as the teacher).

The teacher employed strategies such as structured waiting and gaze guidance to teach Magda new graphic signs during conversations which, although planned to some extent with specific educational goals in mind, turned out to be quite natural. The girl also revealed a number of important skills. For example, following the second structured wait she could have said anything, such as asking for another activity. But she said *HELLO.* She appeared somehow to have grasped the idea that the social terms she was being taught were expected of her. If this interpretation is correct, Magda demonstrated an ability to establish fairly abstract linguistic categories. It is also worth noting that the reply *BIG* in response to *How are you?* may be regarded as part of a social routine. When adults see a child of her age, they are certain at some point to exclaim: *Look how big you are!*

A new development in the storybook activity, compared to two years earlier, was that Magda made comments on the story by looking at signs on the communication frame, that is, with words instead of only indicating pictures in the storybook. Furthermore, she referred to the plot of the story, not just to particular pictures:

(7) T: *Her mother said: Go to....*

Ma: *GRANDMOTHER.*

T: *... grandma's house because she is ...*

Ma: *ILL.*

Joining in telling a story may be a first step towards learning to structure a story, although for Magda such a complex linguistic skill still seems quite a long way off.

## Conclusions

The intervention carried out in collaboration with Magda's family and school achieved positive results, although progress was slow and probably could have been improved. Both the girl and her adult communication partners gradually acquired new and increasingly complex skills which enhanced their ability to interact and communicate with each other. The adults were successfully taught to foster language development naturally in that they acquired improved interaction abilities and learned to prepare suitable materials and richer and more appropriate activities for her. This led to increased satisfaction, gave them confidence in their own ability to introduce changes capable of having an effect on the child's development, and helped them to appreciate the utility of such changes. The parents' initial reluctance to make changes, due to lack of confidence in their effectiveness, together with their limited understanding of the benefits aided communication could bring their child, led us to the conclusion that in the early stages, family training should be very intensive. The difficulties encountered by the family in obtaining communication aids and suitably adapting materials also point to the need for continued family support.

In spite of the difficulties, it became evident that it is possible to create an environment which enhances the development of communication in children with multiple impairments even if they seem to lack skills considered to be prerequisites for language learning. The strategy of overinterpreting signals produced to some extent by all such children, and attributing communicative credibility to them, is a good starting point from which it may be possible to move towards acquisition of increasingly complex language skills. This finding supports the theoretical approach underlying this idea (Lock, 1980; Ryan, 1977) and shows that useful educational strategies can be derived from these theories (von Tetzchner and Martinsen, 1992). The present study illustrates that strategies should be continually modified to match the child's level of competence to help it make further progress. Initially, the main focus had to be on the pragmatic aspects of communication, while at a later stage, due significance was also given to the conceptual and linguistic aspects of language. The difficulties the adults had in introducing new contents and strategies in order to maintain progress when the approach with which they were already familiar had rendered good results, were quite apparent. This has led us to the conclusion that specialist participation in intervention should continue over a long time span, although the frequency of sessions and meetings may gradually be reduced.

The adults adopted some of the interaction and teaching patterns that are typical of adults' interaction with developmentally normal children who are learning to speak (Lock, 1980; Moerk, 1992; Schaffer, 1992) as well as strategies which were more suited to the specific characteristics and needs of a child with multiple impairments acquiring a graphic language. The extent to which the natural strategies observed in the language environment of developmentally normal children were appropriate for children who need aided forms of communication is an important issue requiring further attention from researchers (cf. Beukelman and Ansel, 1995). More research also remains to be done on the special interaction strategies and styles needed to create a 'natural' supportive language environment for graphic language acquisition.

# Chapter 17
# Cleaning ladies and broken buses: A case study on the use of Blissymbols and traditional orthography

MANFRED H. GANGKOFER AND STEPHEN VON TETZCHNER

Augmentative and alternative communication is still a young, although growing, field in Germany (Braun, 1994). Many children who might benefit from intervention with alternative forms of communication have not received it, due both to limited knowledge about these forms of communication and to negative attitudes toward them. The history of 'Rudi' presented here, with a late onset of alternative language intervention focused mainly on text processing, illustrates the possibilities that are emerging as well as the barriers that exist to this kind of intervention in the German school system. Rudi did not develop speech, and traditional speech therapy did not prove effective. He attended a special school for intellectually impaired children in a small town in Germany, where his teachers during the first school years attempted to teach him reading and writing with very limited success. When he was 13;5, an intervention programme was introduced, designed to teach him Blissymbols simultaneously with traditional orthography. The present chapter describes the intervention and his achievements over 14 months until the age of 14;7, and the environmental barriers to making full use of these achievements.

## Background

The pregnancy and Rudi's birth had been normal. Immediately after birth, he had breathing difficulties, and his medical diagnosis was brain damage due to lack of oxygen during and after birth. A number of medical examinations were performed in the neonatal period, without any particular abnormal conditions being diagnosed. Rudi's motor development was delayed. He began to stand at 13 months and to walk at 18–20 months. At 13 years he still walked somewhat clumsily. If he ran, his movement would become increasingly uncoordinated. His mother reported that around his first birthday he used ordinary gestures like waving and clapping hands. He also used his hands for playing with keys and music boxes. However, when the project was initiated, he had considerable problems with fine motor skills like drawing and writing, indicating a disorder of motor planning and coordination. He is of small stature; at the age of 13, he had the height of a 10-year-old. His short-sightedness was diagnosed at an early age and he has been wearing glasses for many years.

## Assessment

At the age of ten years, Rudi had been assessed with *The Columbia Mental Maturity Scale* (Burgemeister, Blum and Lorge, 1972) and *The Progressive Coloured Matrices* (Raven, 1965). On both of these tests, he obtained an age-equivalent average of five years. Rudi attended a school for intellectually impaired children (Sonderschule für geistig Behinderte). His test scores were average for the population attending this kind of school. Still, in most subjects, he performed far above the average of students in such schools. Based on reports from his classroom teacher, Rudi was able to ascertain the number of elements in a set up to five elements; and add and subtract with numbers up to 20. At the age of 13 years on tasks which implied learning of artificial concepts, Rudi performed at a level described as 'thinking in complexes' (Vygotsky, 1962), or 'pre-operational' (Piaget, 1952). Rudi's overall performance at 14 years of age indicated that he had left the stage of pre-operational reasoning and reached the stage of concrete-operational thinking. Children usually enter this stage around the age of 6–7 years (Piaget, 1952).

Rudi's general development was also assessed with the *Heidelberger Kompetenz-Inventar* (Holtz, Eberle, Hillig and Marker, 1984) by the staff at the beginning (1989) and end (1990) of the programme. This is a check-list comprising everyday skills, cognitive skills and social skills, each of which is divided into different areas. Performance on each item is scored on a scale from 1 (does not have the skill) to 4 (complete mastery). However, the results of this assessment were found to depend on the persons who rated. Rudi's classroom staff changed entirely between 1989 and 1990. Although the members of the staff in 1990 were certain that Rudi had developed positively during the preceding year, their ratings were, with two exceptions, lower than the ratings of the 1989 staff. These differences in the evaluation of Rudi were not caused by any major changes in his performance, but rather by different points of view of the professionals involved.

The results on the Heidelberger Kompetenz-Inventar demonstrate the difficulties with using this kind of check-list for children who lack the ability to express themselves, and the variation that may exist with regard to how the competence of a disabled child is perceived.

## Speech

Rudi did not develop speech normally. He received speech therapy in preschool, without much success. At the age of 13, he was able to articulate the vowels and some consonants in isolation, but he was unable to articulate sequences of speech sounds, that is, words. *Manfred,* for example, was articulated: *mmmm ... ei ... ea.* People who did not know Rudi would be unable to understand such utterances. Even for the staff working with Rudi and his parents, Rudi's speech was mainly unintelligible. However, he had a large receptive vocabulary and his comprehension of grammatical and syntactic structures was well developed. At the age of 10 years, his score on *The Peabody Picture Vocabulary Test* was above the 75th percentile according to norms for the population attending schools for intellectually impaired children in Germany (Bondy, Cohen, Eggert and Lüer, 1975).

## Reading and writing

Rudi had received individually based education in reading and writing in the three years prior to the project. The teacher who taught reading reported that Rudi could point at the following letters and graphemes when the corresponding speech sound was articulated by the teacher: a, b, c, e, f, g, i, j, k, l, m, n, o, p, r, s, t, u, v, w, ch, sch, au, ei and ä. Moreover, Rudi was able to articulate most of the sounds corresponding to these letters individually. Though they comprised nearly all of the German alphabet, Rudi was hardly able to produce any words from their constituents. When he tried to read a word, he articulated the individual sounds, but was unable to pronounce the whole word or provide the meaning of the word he had spelled. However, he was able to recognise a few well-known words. He could for example find <u>Mama</u>, <u>Heidi</u>, <u>Papa</u> and his own name on a printed book page without any problems. Thus, his speech problems and his writing problems seemed to reflect similar underlying problems related to analysing word constituents and sequencing (cf. Mann and Brady, 1988).

In spite of his negative learning experiences with reading and writing, Rudi was very motivated to participate in activities with written characters. For example, though he needed a great deal of help to write a letter, he very much enjoyed doing this. He liked to use a typewriter. He could also write most of the letters mentioned above by hand, but due to his coordination problems, the characters he produced were very large. In order to write his own name, he needed an entire A4 sheet of paper. His good motivation was probably a result of his understanding of the functions of written language and the status assigned to writing through the school's and the parents' emphasis on this activity.

## Non-vocal communication skills

Obviously, neither speech nor writing was Rudi's primary mode of communication. Before the present project, Rudi had not received any alternative communication intervention. He communicated mostly with body posture, idiosyncratic signs and gestures. For example, Rudi articulated the name of his friend Larry like *LlII ... ei... ee.* Those who were not familiar with Rudi's speech would not understand this. Rudi might then point at his belly (Larry was quite fat), an idiosyncratic sign that most of the staff had come to know. If Rudi was still not understood, he pointed to his glasses, indicating that the person he wanted to say something about was wearing glasses. Finally, he used his fingers to indicate the number of Larry's classroom.

Rudi displayed his feelings clearly. If he was happy, nothing could stop him. If he was angry or disappointed, he became very reserved. He expressed 'yes' and 'no' with head movements, and people in his environment tended to communicate with him by asking *yes/no* questions. It often took a long time for them to understand what he wanted to express. Dialogue (1) is typical of Rudi's communication before the alternative communication intervention was implemented.

(1)   Rudi had entered the room together with his classroom teacher (CT). He wanted to ask the special education teacher (ST) something.

      R:   Points at his belly.

      ST:  *Do you want to eat something?*

      R:   'No' (shakes head).

      ST:  *Do you have a stomach ache?* (Rudi had not been attending school the last few days).

      R:   'No'.

      CT:  *You can say what you want!*

      R:   Vocalises with some effort.

      ST:  Does not understand. Rudi's speech was too loud and unintelligible.

      R:   Points at his stomach again.

      CT:  *Rudi wants to communicate about a particular person.*

      ST:  *Do you think of a round belly?*

      R:   'Yes' (nods).

      ST:  *Is somebody pregnant?* (Rudi's former teacher was on leave because she was pregnant).

R:     'No!'

ST:    *Do you think of a fat person?*

R:     'Yes!'

ST:    *Do you want to talk about Larry?* (Larry came every morning with Rudi in the same school bus).

R:     'Yes!'

ST:    *Larry is ill, he didn't come today.*

R:     Looks very angry. (He had known of Larry's illness since early the same morning because Larry had not been on the school bus).

ST:    *Do you want to know when Larry will attend school again?*

R:     'Yes, yes, yes!'

ST:    *I don't know, Rudi. His parents did not call. You must wait till tomorrow. You will be the first to know.*

R:     Appears satisfied with this answer.

Rudi addressed adults only, never his classmates. He was sometimes surprisingly persistent when he was not understood. The *yes/no* questions functioned well with familiar topics, but the conversation tended to break down when Rudi wanted to communicate about something new. His speaking partners were usually willing to break off the communication without any result much earlier than he would. If Rudi wanted to communicate something, it was difficult to make him concentrate on another subject. If nobody understood his message, a disturbance would develop which had to be cleared up or all work in the classroom would stop. Rudi's insistence was a strength because it showed that he had not developed the learned passivity of many children with speech and language problems. His motivation provided a good foundation for intervention. However, his insistence was also a problem because the staff, other students and his family might regard him as 'difficult'.

The reason alternative communication intervention had not been initiated earlier might have been related to the fact that Rudi could vocalise and both read individual letters and articulate the speech sounds corresponding to them. However, the perseverance of the teachers and the continued focus on speech therapy and writing in spite of Rudi's use of non-verbal skills and motivation to communicate probably also mirrored the fact that in most German special schools, non-vocal modes of communication were not yet part of the educators' repertoire. It was not until 1989, when Rudi was 13 years old, that a new approach was suggested.

## Intervention

It was the first author, working as a special education teacher in Rudi's school, who raised the possibility of attempting alternative communication for Rudi. The fact that Rudi communicated with body posture and idiosyncratic gestures indicated that manual signs might be the system of choice. His difficulties in face-to-face communication and his interest in producing text in the form of letters indicated that he needed both a means for direct communication and a written language, and the possibility of combining manual signs and Blissymbols was raised. This led to long discussions among the educational staff. The general advantages and disadvantages of a graphic system (Blissymbolics) and a manual system (German Sign Language) were considered, as well as which system would be the more appropriate for Rudi's communication. It was argued that there was no reason to assume that simultaneous use of manual and graphic signs would interfere negatively with each other. On the contrary, research had shown that simultaneous use of different systems might enhance learning (Gangkofer, 1989,1993). The opponents of a multimodal approach feared that having to learn both systems would be too difficult for Rudi and might confuse him. In particular the speech pathologist did not agree with teaching Rudi manual signs. She argued that nobody could learn three languages at the same time (Blissymbols, manual signs, and spoken and written German). However, this debate was not sincere because at that time, nobody was able to or willing to teach manual signs. Only later a teacher was hired who for a short period taught manual signs to Rudi a few hours per week in the classroom setting. This teaching was terminated due to shortage of staff, and it was not integrated with the teaching of Blissymbols.

Some of the teachers thought Blissymbolics was a too difficult and complex system for Rudi to learn. However, Rudi played *Memory* with trade marks, mostly knowing what kind of objects the trade mark referred to. Trade marks represent a form of logographic writing, similar to Blissymbols. It was also argued that using Blissymbols together with traditional orthography on a computer might possibly improve Rudi's acquisition of reading and writing.

It was typical of the situation that most of the staff members were indifferent, considering alternative communication as a subject for which they were not responsible and which would have no implications for their own teaching of Rudi. It was probably this indifference that led to the decision to attempt multimodal communication intervention, namely, to begin teaching Blissymbols and implement manual signs when a teacher became available. However, when the alternative communication was initiated, it was as an isolated activity. Neither the use of Blissymbols, nor the use of manual signs later, was followed up outside the intervention sessions. Therefore, the use of Blissymbols as a means for writing was emphasised. This would take advantage of Rudi's interest in producing letters, and it was hypothesised that focus on text processing would increase Rudi's understanding of both Blissymbols and written and spoken German (cf. Koppenhaver and Yoder, 1992;

Olson, 1993), and thus would also improve his face-to-face communication. Provided it was successful in individual intervention sessions, the use of Blissymbols could later be extended to the environment in general.

Thus, the teaching of Blissymbols had two aims: firstly, to provide Rudi with better means for communicating in text and face to face; and, secondly, to demonstrate the efficiency of alternative modes of communication for the staff and the parents in order to convince them to use these in the environment at large.

## Introducing Blissymbols

The teaching strategies used were based on Rudi's comprehension of spoken language, usually in the form of definitions and explanations of Blissymbols, that is, explicit teaching similar to second-language teaching (cf. Martinsen and von Tetzchner, this volume). This entailed a number of activities. The guideline for selecting vocabulary was that all Blissymbols should fill a defined need in Rudi's communication. They should be wanted by him, not only by the special education teacher. For example, in the first intervention session with Blissymbols, a recipe for making soap bubbles had been prepared, and a vocabulary including SOAP-BUBBLE. Rudi turned out to be less interested in the soap bubbles than the fact that the cleaning ladies would have to clean the floor because of all the soap. He had a lot of fun with this idea. In order to communicate about this, a Blissymbol for 'cleaning lady' was needed. Similar to many other words Rudi needed, there was no ready-made Blissymbol in the dictionary, and it was necessary to create one. CLEANING-LADY (Putzfrau) became very complex (Figure 17.1). In spite of this, it was presented to Rudi without explaining its constituents until later. This procedure proved effective. Rudi remembered this Blissymbol many weeks later without any problems. In fact, Rudi did not usually appear to have difficulties remembering the Blissymbols as they were introduced. It was sufficient to show him a Blissymbol once in a meaningful context, sometimes accompanied by an explanation of its meaning, and he would store it for later use. He was able to recall most Blissymbols after a single intervention session. Pictographic Blissymbols like WINDOW, CUP and CLOCK he often understood without any explanation.

At the end of the first half year, the special education teacher started to read stories to him in which some words were omitted. Rudi had to listen to the story and fill in the gaps with Blissymbols or words. He was able to select the appropriate Blissymbol from a sample of all the Blissymbols needed for the empty slots in the text. Though some Blissymbols had only been mentioned once and displayed shortly 1–2 weeks before, Rudi usually filled the slots correctly.

| Auto | Bild | blasen | Brief | Bruder | Buch |
|---|---|---|---|---|---|
| Bus | Computer | Du | fahren | Fisch | fischen |
| Fluß | Frau | Freund/in | Frühstück | gehen | glücklich |
| Hund | Ich | in, innerhalb | Junge | Kaffee | Kamera |
| kaputt | Klassenzimmer | Kleister | kochen | kommen | krank |
| küssen | Liebe,r | Löffel | Mädchen | Mann | mein |
| mit | mitbringen | mögen | Mutter | nicht | Oma |
| Opa | Person | Putzfrau* | regnen | sagen | Scheiße! |
| Schnee | schreiben | Schule | Schüssel | See | Seife |
| Seifenblasen* | sein | Stadt | Sturm | Tasse | Taxi |
| ticken* | Toilette | Topf | tot | Uhr | Vater |
| Wasser | Weihnachten | Wind | wollen | Zeitung | Zimmer |
| Zucker | Zuhause | | | | |

* nicht standardisiert

**Figure 17.1** Blissymbols used in the intervention. Those marked (*) are not standard forms, that is, they are not listed in the dictionary of the Blissymbolics Communication Institute.

**Traditional orthography**

The gloss of the Blissymbol was always written above the graphic sign. Rudi never seemed to confound printed words and Blissymbols, or to be confused because both forms were presented together. On the contrary, he could be observed trying to make the best out of the information provided. This required that the Blissymbols, and sometimes the written words as well, could be discriminated visually. For example, the Blissymbols *MIT* (with), *MEIN* (my) and *MARCUS* were mixed up by Rudi several times. These glosses started with an M̲ and two of them comprised a big plus sign (Figure 17.1).

However, Rudi did not seem to combine the two graphic representations either. He used either the graphic sign or the letters when recognising a Blissymbol.

> Rudi and the special education teacher were gluing cards with Blissymbols and written words on the doors of the school. Rudi was shown the correct Blissymbol on a list and had to find the matching card. He did this correctly even with complex Blissymbols and Blissymbols he had not yet learned. Suddenly, he chose *SCHULHOF* (school yard) instead of *SCHAUKEL* (swing). He was prompted to change his choice but was very confident that he was right, pointing at the word printed at the card. Both words began with S̲c̲h̲ and Rudi had paid attention only to the letters.

For 'mama' and 'papa', Rudi preferred written words, which was not surprising since these words were well known to him. On the other hand, he could not find the written word c̲l̲e̲a̲n̲i̲n̲g̲ ̲l̲a̲d̲y̲, although he could easily find *CLEANING-LADY*.

In September 1989, the school had got an IBM compatible computer, and Rudi used *Personal Bliss* for writing letters. This programme's library contained 1400 Blissymbols, and the accompanying glosses could be written in any language or style. There could be up to 25 Blissymbols on each screen page, and the programme included 20 pages. Each screen page could be given a specific colour. Blissymbols could be selected by moving the cursor with the arrow keys or a joystick and pressing <enter> or the fire button (Schulte-Sasse, 1994). A concept keyboard was also used to select Blissymbols, words and letters.

Rudi had no problems handling the computer though it was the first time he had worked with this medium. It took him some time to learn the function of the arrow keys because he looked at the keys when pressing them, and therefore did not see the changes he made on the screen. A joystick appeared easier for him to use; he mastered it almost perfectly after five minutes. After a few weeks with the joystick, Rudi wanted to switch to the standard keyboard and has used this successfully since then.

As cues for finding a particular Blissymbol on the computer screen, Rudi used not only the gestalt of the Blissymbol and the shape of the word, but also the individual colours of the screen pages and the Blissymbol's location on the screen. On the screen page, the Blissymbols were placed in a ɔ x 5 grid, while the manual board and paper concept keyboard had a 4 x 6 grid. Therefore the location of most Blissymbols on paper and the concept keyboard did not correspond to the location on the screen. At first Rudi seemed confused by this, but he found the Blissymbols he needed. He thereby demonstrated both his strategy for finding Blissymbols and his knowledge of them.

The Blissymbols were used for writing short letters since this was an activity Rudi liked, and production of text was a main focus of the intervention. It was Rudi who decided what he should write. The screen pages were not prepared by the teacher in advance, and the creation of new Blissymbols on the screen when needed was part of the joint work.

> SNOW was needed for a letter. The teacher found the code number for SNOW in the manual and started the programme. Rudi typed the four-digit code number, and SNOW appeared on the screen. The special education teacher explained its components and Rudi wrote <u>snow</u> above the Blissymbol by copying the word letter by letter from the teacher's note pad. Then they communicated about SNOW before Rudi moved the new Blissymbol to the square where he wanted it to be located. The new screen page was saved and Rudi started to write his letter using the new Blissymbol.

The contents of Rudi's letters were typically influenced by recent experiences, but for a long time he insisted on writing the same basic letter again and again in different variations. Only after several months did he start to expand his topics. He even wrote a letter to his younger brother. Before this he had refused to take any Blissymbols home or use them with his family. Another time he wrote about his father having taken him fishing. After one year of intervention Rudi still tended to write the stereotyped letter but had begun to introduce some new contents. This provided opportunities for teaching him new Blissymbols in a natural context.

The special education teacher and Rudi usually communicated for about 15 minutes about the content of the letter before Rudi started to write, using manual signs, speech and Blissymbols. This conversation functioned better as Rudi learned more Blissymbols. The special education teacher formulated the text and Rudi corrected it if he did not agree with the formulations.

Rudi occasionally switched between Blissymbols and traditional orthography, which was possible because he used the standard keyboard. Most of the time he wrote his own name with letters instead of using *BOY* with his name written above it. If he wrote spontaneously, he wrote the way he spoke.

> Rudi wanted to write <u>Klaudia.</u> He started several times with an <u>a,</u> which was the first sound in his pronunciation of *Klaudia*. He was unable to say k. The special education teacher brought a set of Blissymbols and Rudi found *FRAU* (woman). Copying the word from the special education teacher's note pad, he wrote <u>Klaudia</u> above *FRAU*. However, he started by typing <u>l</u> because he wanted his letter to begin as usual with <u>Liebe Klaudia</u> (dear Klaudia). He then typed the word correctly, but had difficulties finding <u>d</u> because the model on the keyboard was <u>D</u>. On the screen, Rudi's text read: <u>aaa l lklaudia.</u>

When Rudi worked with word processing, it was often difficult for him to find the letters he typed on the screen. Though he had some experience with typewriting, he had to look for each letter on the keyboard. This kind of work was both confusing and exhausting for him.

To facilitate his search for letters, a concept keyboard was introduced, containing known letters only, and in alphabetical order, and with some letters combined to graphemes (e.g. <u>sch</u> and <u>ch</u>). This was easier but still arduous for Rudi. On the other hand, if he used Blissymbols as input on the concept keyboard and only the printed word occurred on the screen, Rudi, having selected a Blissymbol, was often uncertain whether his choice was correct. He had to compare the word on the screen with the gloss above the Blissymbol. This might have been a good educational exercise but bothered Rudi who wanted to write a letter, not to do exercises.

These problems did not exist with Personal Bliss. Although the graphics resolution of this programme was not very good and Rudi was visually impaired, he handled the programme well. Traditional orthography and Blissymbols were often related to each other in a natural manner, for instance in editing and writing the glosses of new Blissymbols, and in writing various names above the Blissymbols *WOMAN*, *MAN*, *GIRL* and *BOY*. Thus, names mainly differed in their spelling.

## Syntax

The syntax used by Rudi reflected his communication modes and his comprehension of spoken language. The following observation illustrates this:

> Rudi wrote alone on the computer: *ALEX (TO)SWIM BUS (TO)DRIVE ALEX SHIT! BROKEN-DOWN BUS.* Thus, he

constructed his messages in the same manner as he communicated face to face with manual signs, written words, vocalisations and Blissymbols. The special education teacher accepted this form of writing, but Rudi did not like his own writing when it was read aloud to him. He wanted a syntactically correct text and was satisfied only when it was interpreted and read as: *Alex drives the bus for swimming. Alex says: 'Shit! The bus is broken-down'.* Thus, Rudi knew the syntactic forms of spoken language but was not able to follow the same syntax in his own writing.

The teacher would sometimes add words that seemed important for Rudi's message and which were not accessible on the screen, such as the words to and for in the following letter. Another time, with a little help from the special education teacher, he had written:

> *DEAR LARRY*
> *(TO)RIDE BY BUS to CITY for BREAKFAST*
> *WIND (TO)BLOW (TO)RAIN LARRY (TO)SAY SHIT!*
> *I (TO)WRITE LETTER WITH COMPUTER*
> *RUDI*

(Due to the different syntax rules of English and German it is not possible to translate the peculiar style of this letter). When the letter had been written, the special education teacher read it aloud to Rudi. If it was read exactly as he had written it, Rudi would become very angry and insist it should be read properly. Thus, when reading the letter above, the teacher had to say *the wind blows* instead of *wind to blow*, and *I write this letter with a computer* instead of *I to write letter with computer*. This demonstrated his relatively advanced comprehension of speech, syntactic awareness and an ability to distinguish grammatically correct and incorrect sentences.

The syntax of Rudi's productions should not be regarded as only reduced or delayed but also as following different linguistic rules than spoken German, in particular with regard to word order. He did not use any articles, and sometimes began his communication with a word as a clue to the topic or context of his sentence. He very often began a message by telling the subject and the object of the sentence in the beginning, followed by a verb. Similar constructions have been reported for other users of communication aids (e.g. Collins, this volume; Smith, this volume; von Tetzchner and Martinsen, this volume). For example, indicating *RAY* (the Blissymbol *MAN* with the gloss Ray above) and laying his arm over the teacher's shoulder would literally be translated with 'Ray friend'. However, Rudi's statement was equivalent to the sentence: 'Ray is my friend'. If the special education teacher in direct communication used a telegraphic form when communicating with Rudi, saying only one word or showing only one Blissymbol to ask a question, Rudi usually accepted this. This indicates that Rudi understood that there was a difference between his own syntax and the syntax of a spoken utterance, as well as there being differences between writing and speech.

**Face-to-face communication**

Rudi used Blissymbols as a means of communication with his special education teacher, together with manual signs, gestures, spoken words and sometimes pictures. He often used Blissymbols to confirm already negotiated facts if these had been unclear, but he rarely used manual signs to verify Blissymbols. Thus, Blissymbols seemed to be his highest level of communication. They were the least ambiguous forms but always functioned in combination with the other modes.

Dialogue (2) demonstrates that Rudi had understood that Blissymbols could be used for establishing topics for communication but that he had problems with providing comments to the topic (cf. von Tetzchner and Martinsen, this volume).

(2)     Rudi and the special education teacher were gluing Blissymbols on a piece of paper. By chance, Rudi found *CLOCK* in the Blissymbol book. The special education teacher wanted Rudi to glue this on paper together with the others.

R:     'No'. He seems to want to tell something about a clock.
S:     *Do you want to know the time?*
R:     'No'.
S:     *Do you want to know when this lesson ends?*
R:     'No'.

The special education teacher asked several questions without success. He therefore asked Rudi to continue his work, but Rudi insisted. After many more questions without success, the special education teacher gave up, and Rudi absolutely refused to work.

R:     Makes several gestures and points at the big clock on the wall of the classroom again and again.
S:     *You mean that the clock ticks?*
R:     'Yes'.

The clock had ticked all through this conversation, and half an hour had passed.

Multimodal communication and pragmatic functions were given priority before the structure of the educational programme by the special education teacher. Without the alternative modes of communication Rudi would not have been able to make himself understood fast enough, and sometimes his message would not have been understood at all.

Rudi was able to use Blissymbols for communicative purposes outside the educational setting. For example, he once brought *LETTER* to the school's office in order to get an envelope. However, he used the Blissymbols in this manner only when explicitly instructed to do so. It was part of the intervention plan that Rudi was provided with a book containing all Blissymbols trained after each session. This would enable him to communicate in other settings about the topics of the sessions. It was a particular goal that he should be able to tell his mother what he had done in school during the day. This did not work because Rudi refused to take this book home and show it to his mother.

After the initial period, communication between Rudi and the special education teacher had improved because they had developed a lot of common activities. The special education teacher had learned to understand Rudi's idiosyncratic gestures, and Rudi had learned to combine his communication modes; Blissymbols, manual signs, gestures and some speech. Rudi was easier to understand when he provided redundant information. However, at a later stage, communication became worse.

> Rudi wanted to communicate with the special education teacher. He was sitting in front of the special education teacher without looking at him or moving, only producing some unintelligible speech sounds. His arms were hanging down, and he did not use any gestures, not even his body, for communication. Several times he was encouraged to use manual signs or point at Blissymbols and objects in order for the special education teacher to understand him.

Rudi's behaviour appeared to reflect the attitudes towards non-speech communication displayed by the educational staff and significant people in his environment.

# The environment

As a rule, Rudi used Blissymbols only in intervention sessions. Moreover, he seemed to associate the use of Blissymbols with the computer. He always pointed at the Blissymbols on the computer screen though they were provided on paper too. He did not want to take his book with Blissymbols into his classroom, and, as it happened, the staff did not want him to use it. His reluctance to use Blissymbols outside the intervention setting was probably related to the derogatory attitude of the classroom staff, but also demonstrated the problem with teaching communication skills in an isolated setting which hardly allowed transfer to his other everyday contexts. This isolation was not an intended feature of the intervention; it had been hoped that the skills he demonstrated would soon make the staff adopt all his modes of communicating.

Neither did his few lessons with manual signs have much impact. One reason was a change in the staff caused by a lack of teachers in the school. However, probably more important, the classroom staff, led by the speech pathologist, had started to encourage Rudi to use only speech. A class conference was arranged where the special education teacher argued against this oral strategy, emphasising its former poor results and the improbability of a fundamental change in Rudi's spoken language as a result of traditional speech therapy. However, a few days after this meeting, Rudi again wanted to talk about Larry in the classroom, and pointed at his belly. This was immediately understood by his classroom teacher, who told Rudi to say *Larry* instead of signing.

## Conclusions

From one point of view, the teaching was successful: Rudi significantly increased his repertoire of expressive forms. Blissymbols appeared to be a real alternative to alphabetical writing for him, and an important supplement to his mainly unintelligible speech. It was not clear whether the Blissymbols would function as a precursor to traditional orthography, or as a parallel system augmenting or substituting for traditional orthography. At the end of the intervention period, the latter seemed to be the case. On the other hand, he had not learned to read traditional orthography with other instructional methods either.

Rudi seemed to learn Blissymbols as gestalts, a strategy that circumvented his problems with analytic and synthetic processing. When new Blissymbols were introduced, the meaning of their components was usually explained but whether these explanations had any influence on Rudi's learning is not known. He seemed to learn most Blissymbols as they were introduced and named in the intervention sessions. However, teaching had intentionally been kept at a slow pace. Thus, at the end of the programme Rudi had 74 Blissymbols on five computer screen pages (cf. Figure 17.1). In addition, he was able to recognise some pictographic Blissymbols which were not on the screen pages.

Rudi appeared to be aware of the difference between traditional orthography and Blissymbolics, and was never observed mixing them up. On the other hand, neither did he seem to relate them to each other. When using *Personal Bliss*, he could get his messages printed in Blissymbols and traditional orthography, or in traditional orthography only. Rudi sometimes favoured the written words and sometimes the Blissymbols. On the screen, however, he looked more at the Blissymbols than at the words. This may have been caused by the fact that the Blissymbols were much larger than the written glosses in Personal Bliss, or that letters were generally more difficult to recognise. Rudi chose to use the standard keyboard after working for some time with a joystick and concept keyboard, and though mainly selecting Blissymbols and whole words with the arrow keys, he sometimes switched to typing for well-known words.

Due to the circumstances, the focus of the intervention had become text production, and this may be considered successful. Rudi wrote letters of his own choice, and seemed to enjoy this activity more and more as he became more proficient in the use of Blissymbols. His letters were comprehensible to the staff and some of the other students, and he usually received positive responses when he showed or 'sent' his letters. By using Blissymbols and the computer, Rudi was encouraged to write, thereby increasing his understanding of text production and the importance of literacy.

Moreover, Rudi was very concerned about expressing himself in correct grammar and syntax. Writing in a whole-word mode relieved him of unfunctional spelling, and he was able to focus on the content and structure of his text. It was not necessary to encourage Rudi to write correctly because it was he, and not the special education teacher, who wanted the text to be 'correct'. This focus on structure was reinforced by the fact that only the special education teacher encouraged Rudi's use of alternative communication. In spite of his lack of progress in expressive spoken language, the speech pathologist and the rest of the staff had actively counteracted Rudi's use of non-speech modes of communication. Rudi was probably influenced by these attitudes and therefore did not want to bring Blissymbols to other situations. He seemed to have adopted the belief that Blissymbols belonged to training situations only. Maybe he also associated Blissymbols with writing text and use of the computer, which was also only available during intervention sessions. Transfer to other settings might have been easier if use of Blissymbols had not been so strongly associated with the computer.

With regard to the use of Blissymbols as a means for face-to-face communication, this was achieved within the context of the intervention sessions. The second goal had been to make the educational staff start to use Blissymbols with Rudi outside the special intervention sessions. This goal was not easy to achieve. The staff argued that using Blissymbols would make Rudi less familiar with traditional orthography, and that this might reduce his ability to build up written language by synthetic and analytic processing. This view had not been supported by Rudi's development, and considering his advanced age and lack of such skills in both spoken and written language, this argument did not appear valid. His achievements with Blissymbols indicated that he had a potential for learning more Blissymbols, and, if properly implemented in his everyday communication, they might greatly expand his communicative means. Considering his achievements during the year of intervention, with the use limited to intervention sessions only, it is likely that Rudi could have expanded his vocabulary and the applications of the Blissymbols. Even the Blissymbols already learned would have led to a manifold increase in his expressive vocabulary, and decreased the number of problematic situations related to his communication difficulties. However, Rudi's development demonstrated that optimal results might only be obtained if all the educational staff become involved.

The fact that alternative communication intervention was not initiated until the age of 13 years might be related to the fact that Rudi could vocalise, and both read and articulate individual speech sounds. However, it also reflected the state of this field at the time in Germany. The attitudes displayed by the educational staff in Rudi's school were not unique. They reflect a widespread, although gradually declining, view that still bars a wider application of augmentative and alternative communication in many places. The intervention decisions have been ideological rather than professional, being based on folk theories instead of analyses of the children's development and cognitive and linguistic processing. Similar attitudes may be found to a greater or lesser degree in other countries (cf. Martinsen and von Tetzchner, this volume). An overriding aim of presenting Rudi and other case studies has been to create more awareness and insight into alternative communication forms, and thereby accelerate the processes of change that are already taking place.

# Chapter 18
# Improving communication and language skills of children with developmental disorders: Family involvement in graphic language intervention

LOURDES LOURENÇO, JOAQUIM FAIAS, ROSA AFONSO, ANA MOREIRA AND JOSÉ M. FERREIRA

Although Portugal has a rather short history of augmentative and alternative communication intervention (cf. Mendes and Rato, this volume), it has already become apparent that there is a need to change strategies. There are three major reasons for this: changes in the educational system, a lack of family orientation, and, in the case of graphic language, a need for competence created by technological developments. The present chapter presents the background, issues that relate to the introduction of the new methodologies, and examples that illustrate them.

## Background

At the moment, the education of disabled children in Portugal is going through significant changes. Recent legislation requires full inclusion of students with special education needs in the regular school system. However, the training options for professionals working with augmentative and alternative communication are limited, and insufficient for developing the systematic work necessary to achieve successful integration of motor impaired children with speech and language impairment.

The change from specialised institutions to socio-educative integration implies that any teacher may have a student who needs augmentative and alternative communication intervention. Consequently there is a need, not only for educating specialists, but also for training and supervising ordinary teachers in the use of augmentative and alternative communication systems and strategies. And professionals used to the security of their own special schools will have to adapt to working in regular school contexts, a change that may not always be easy (Chueca y Mora, 1988; Cruickshank, Morse and Grant, 1990).

In addition to educational segregation in Portugal, language intervention has traditionally been performed without much concern for the child's patterns of communication at home. Parents were given a passive role. It was the professionals who defined the goals of the intervention and implemented the strategies they deemed necessary. There was often a large gap between the programme developed by the professionals and the real needs of the child in its family context.

Related to this, we have experienced a lack of generalisation of augmentative and alternative communication skills taught in preschool and school. In spite of the endless difficulties non-speaking children have in expressing themselves, we have found that parents and other significant people in the environment are satisfied with the children's use of pointing and 'home signs', that is, idiosyncratic gestures whose meanings have developed in an interactive process within the family.

However, although functional in some situations at home, this mode of communication is not functional outside the home. In order to attribute meaning to the idiosyncratic forms, it is necessary to have family-based information, which in most potential communication partners is lacking. In addition, even within the home, there will be restrictions in the children's ability to communicate. The limited efficiency of the communicative behaviours both at home and in broader environments has made it necessary to increase the awareness of people in the environment about communication opportunities, in order for more generally understood alternative ways of communication to be established.

Realising that the importance of communication at home for the child's social and communicative development had been neglected was a result both of influences from recent literature on augmentative and alternative communication (e.g. Basil, 1992; Beukelman and Mirenda, 1992; von Tetzchner and Martinsen, 1992) and clinical observations creating doubts with regard to the efficiency of the intervention that was being performed. It was felt that there was a real need to develop a new intervention methodology which focused more on the role of the family and the child's social participation than on particular training activities. The aim of this methodology was to make the family more competent, participative and active in every part of the decision process concerning their own child.

Lastly, the use of assistive technologies in habilitation has increased greatly during the last years. This has created a need for helping professionals to get a better understanding of the methodology, the process and the results of their work. An important distinction is between 'hard' and 'soft' technologies. The hard technologies include communication aids and graphic communication systems. The soft technologies include human skills in decision making, strategy use, training and concept formation (Cook and Hussey, 1995). The soft technologies may be crucial for making the hard technologies useful for the child at home and in school and the larger community, and with family and friends, as well as alone with strangers.

## The challenges

Oporto Cerebral Palsy Habilitation Centre was established in 1975. Oporto is the second biggest city in Portugal, and the Centre serves a population of 1.2 million. Clients comprise young children with developmental disorders, usually cerebral palsy, most of whom live in the Oporto district. The children's need for augmentative and alternative communication is largely due to difficulties in speaking caused by their motor impairment.

During the school year 1994–95, 117 children (aged 0–16 years) attended the speech therapy department of the Centre. Seventy-four of them (63 per cent) needed augmentative and alternative communication intervention. Fifty of the children were 6 years old or younger. The high proportion of young children reflects a focus on early assessment and intervention, an emphasis which is in line with international trends. Early intervention is assumed to prevent developmental delay and secondary impairments, as well as problems in the family, thereby contributing to better interaction between parents and child and a more balanced emotional relationship (cf. Meisels and Shonkoff, 1990).

Von Tetzchner and Martinsen (1992) describe three main groups of augmentative and alternative communication users. The *expressive language group* includes children with a significant gap between speech comprehension and the ability to speak. The aim is to provide them with an alternative means to express themselves. Of the 117 children described above, 28 (24 per cent) belonged to this group.

*The supportive language group* comprises children who need a supporting language. Part of this group compromises children with delayed language development, and the function of the alternative communication mode is to promote comprehension and use of speech as a temporary supporting language, a help to language development. The supportive group also includes children whose speech is insufficient to make themselves understood with some partners and in some situations. Thus, the augmentative communication functions as a supplement to the speech. Twenty-six children (22 per cent) belonged to the supportive language group.

Those who belong to the *alternative language group* need an alternative language. They include children with reduced abilities to use and understand the speech. The alternative communication is, at the same time, a way for the children to express themselves and for the partners to communicate with them. A majority, 63 children (54 per cent), belonged to the alternative language group.

Many children with motor impairments are in unfavourable conditions for sustaining interaction and communication with their environment. Basil and Puig de la Bellacasa (1988) distinguish four main problems that severely affect the interaction of these children:

- A reduced capacity to interact with and explore the environment.
- A reduced capacity to play and interact with other people through movements and vocalisations.
- A reduced capacity to express emotions, needs and thoughts, and to exchange information with other people.
- A reduced capacity to control the speech mechanism and fine movements.

Difficulties in walking and manipulating objects, lack of mobility and limited ability to explore various environments and objects provide few opportunities for interaction with the environment, and may create learned passivity (von Tetzchner and Martinsen, 1992). Margarida is a typical example of the earlier situation of many severely motor impaired children in Portugal.

Margarida was severely dystonic. She had no speech and was unable to produce vocalisations loud enough to be heard. Until she was eight years old, she did not have the opportunity to show her basic needs, wants and feelings in an efficient way. When she arrived from school, she was seated on the sofa with the television in front of her, her parents occupying themselves with their daily duties. Unable to walk and vocalise she could not move away or even get the station changed of her own volition. The parents said that she loved to watch television because she stayed still for two or three hours without giving them trouble.

Also primitive and pathological motor reactions may limit the possibilities for interaction between the child and its parents, and thereby also influence attachment processes and the child's relationships to other people (von Tetzchner, 1993b), as in the case of Marta.

Marta was two years old and had facial hypersensibility. When the mother wanted to give her a kiss, a hyperextension pattern made Marta's head move away from the mother's face. The mother interpreted the movement as a sign of displeasure, and consequently avoided kissing or getting close to her own daughter.

Communicative development starts early in life and problems of interaction may already be apparent in infancy. Early communication depends on social and affective involvement that forms a basis for a balanced and harmonious development. Affective communication between parents and infants may be at risk or damaged when a child has severe motor impairment (Basil and Puig de la Bellacasa, 1988; Kent, 1983; Leitão, 1994; Rondal, 1983).

Parents often have little knowledge about how to stimulate and communicate with disabled children, or about the communicative possibilities open to children who do not speak naturally. Caring and child-rearing tasks usually take more time when the child is disabled, leaving little time for play and interaction. In addition, due to the economic situation in Portugal, in a majority of families, both parents are working . The time they are at home with the child is spent mostly on basic needs and caring activities. There may be little time for activities that can promote communication and interaction.

Thus, the problems of communicative interaction experienced by children with motor impairment are related to the styles and characteristics of the children as well as the styles and characteristics of the communication partners. Clinical observations documented in the reports of the children at the Centre indicate that the children typically displayed a passive communicative style and reduced ability to participate in dialogues, in particular due to:

- absence of legible signs which adults can interpret or overinterpret to promote communication;
- the child's difficulties in initiating and maintaining communicative interactions;
- the child's difficulties in participating in new social and communicative situations;
- the child's difficulties in adapting to new communication partners;
- the child's difficulties in producing speech or making preferences known due to limited motor control, leading to expression of one-word utterances only;
- the child's dependence on the attention of adult communication partners and interpretations made by them during conversations;
- the child's lack of opportunity for varying vocabulary due to reliance on *yes/no* questions by adults;
- the child's lack of opportunities for maintaining a conversation with peers without the help of an interpreter.

We believe that these difficulties result from the paucity of successful conversational experiences. Non-speaking children may achieve communicative success rarely and only when communicating with the parents or others who know them well.

Clinical observations (both direct and video recorded) of the communicative styles and abilities of various communication partners of the children showed that:

- adult communication partners tended to initiate and maintain control of the conversation all the time;
- adults tended to use *yes/no* questions, requiring closed answers only for the child's turn;
- adults tended to have long conversational turns, turning dialogues into monologues;
- adults tended to increase voice volume;
- adults tended to ask questions in cascade without giving the child time to prepare an answer;
- adults tended not to use communication aids or used them only infrequently.

In addition to problems with the communicative interaction itself, many parents expressed fears that the use of alternative language intervention might inhibit the child's development of speech. Due to the difficulties in maintaining a dialogue, they tended to avoid communication exchanges which they perceived as potentially embarrassing situations or failures. Rather, they anticipated or guessed the desires of the children without giving them an opportunity to express themselves. Some parents gave little attention to communication, being more concerned with the development of motor skills, in particular independent mobility.

These observations are in accordance with others reported in the literature (e.g. Basil, 1992; Harris, 1982; von Tetzchner, 1993b). We believed that many of the difficulties were a result of poor or insufficient intervention methodology, in particular the tendency among clinicians to focus mainly on the communication system (form) and to give less attention to the development of language skills (function) in augmentative and alternative communication intervention. Further, the traditional practice of not involving parents in the assessment and intervention process had led to a dissociation between the goals established by the professional staff and the needs felt by parents in their daily lives.

## Change of intervention methodology

In Portugal, assessment and intervention in augmentative and alternative communication have customarily been carried out mainly in therapy rooms which are usually quite different from the child's ordinary environment. Recent legislation requires full integration of all disabled children in the regular school system, foreseeing that all the supporting services necessary to fulfil the specific needs of each child will be part of the general system. As a response to these new circumstances, a multi-disciplinary habilitation team for children with developmental disorders including speech and language impairment, allowing more activities outside the Centre itself, was established in 1992 at the Centre in Oporto.

A broad concept of augmentative and alternative communication includes not only sign systems and communication aids but also the range of teaching strategies, as well as the support methodologies (e.g. teaching, supervision and modelling) that build up and shape the skills and transdisciplinary practices of professionals and parents. Thus, an overall aim of the team was to function as a source of support for these groups.

In a population of children with severe speech and language problems, there will be a range of special needs in education that go far beyond communication. These needs also have to be taken into consideration in the planning of language intervention. 'Language and communication training that does not take into account the total life situation of the person concerned, and does not contribute to an overall improvement, is inadequate in terms of the individual's interests, and will probably be poor training as well' (von Tetzchner and Martinsen, 1992, p. 77). Hence, the team did not only address communication but all relevant intervention matters.

### Including the natural environment

In the habilitation and education of children with motor impairments, parents have traditionally been given a passive role. The professional defined the goals and took care of the intervention. However, no attempt to communicate is functional unless the usual communication partners perceive the message and respond in an appropriate manner. The performance of the communication partners in the interaction process may in fact either enhance or inhibit communication. We had become aware that the traditional form of intervention was inadequate, making it difficult to motivate the children and their families and harder for them to accept intervention with an alternative communication system. The new methodology was based on integration and participation of the local teachers and the family. Margarida, described above, and Pedro reflect the changes:

> Margarida had received three years of graphic communication
> intervention and had a vocabulary of 200 graphic signs, a mixture
> of Blissymbols and PCS. She eye pointed to indicate the signs on
> the board at home, and in addition, she had a computer with digi-
> tised output at school. The parents reported that she had become
> more active and assertive, choosing television programmes and

other activities. She used movements to get attention and then used the communication board to express what she wanted to say.

Pedro had spastic diplegia and language delay. When he first came to the Centre at the age of four, he rarely initiated interaction and was unable to sustain a conversation. At home he was given few opportunities for establishing interaction and he usually stayed alone for long periods during the day. As part of the intervention process, he started to attend a regular kindergarten, and the environment and activities were organised in such a way that they facilitated interaction. Because he was living alone with his mother, and she was working, it was difficult to influence his communication in the home except for regular talks with the mother. The intervention therefore focused on the school setting.

Wheelchair training was initiated. This allowed him to move around more freely, explore the environment and get more varied experiences. He got thematic communication boards with PIC signs to augment language acquisition. Both the teachers and the other students in the class were taught to use the graphic signs, as well as strategies for interpreting and responding to his vocal and graphic expressions. A set of teaching strategies were planned, including structured waiting, overinterpretation and expansion of his vocal and graphic utterances. For example, while he looked at a picture book, the interlocutor started: *The little boy wants...*, and waited until Pedro said ... *ter* (water) or pointed to *WATER*. At other times, Pedro said *anth,* which the interlocutor interpreted and expanded: *Bath? Yes, the little boy is taking a bath.* Or, looking in the same picture book, Pedro might point at *BICYCLE,* expanded by the teacher as: *Yes, now the little boy is bicycling* while at the same time pointing at *BOY* and *BICYCLE.*

After six months, Pedro spontaneously addressed his friends, proposed changes of activity, worked and played in group activities, and showed a great desire and persistence to be understood. He often wanted to use his communication boards when he could not make himself clear with speech on its own. Although the home situation had received limited attention, the mother reported that communication had been improved and that she now understood his speech and supportive communicative behaviours better.

Vocabulary selection often proved the most important part of adapting a communication aid to the user. It was often not an easy task, neither for professional nor parents. For example, the adults tended to be too concerned about basic needs and cleanliness. The vocabulary on a communication board might be more efficient and appropriate in a wider range of situations when siblings and friends at the same age actively participate in its selection.

André was 8 years old. He had good comprehension of spoken language and age appropriate non-verbal cognitive skills. He was social and got easily along with other people. He used a communication board with 150 Blissymbols and 20 written words, and during the school year 1994–95 he had learned to use a Macaw II (a communication aid with digitised voice output). Assessment and intervention were developed together with André's family, and the digitised sentences were selected according to what the parents found most useful for his daily activities after school. However, sentences like *'I'm hungry'*, *'I want to watch television'* and *'I need to go to the bathroom'* proved rather useless to André, and he never used them spontaneously. André and his teenage sister therefore proposed a new set of sentences, such as: *'Mother, these clothes are out of fashion!'*, *'Now it is my turn to speak!'*, *'The Football Club of Oporto is the best'* and *'Change the television channel'*. A few days after the new sentences had been read into the communication aid, the mother called the Centre:

*He does not shut up for a minute. He does not allow me to see my favourite television programmes, telling me to change the channel. At family meetings he never stops saying 'Now it is my turn to speak!'. After such a long time of silence, I now realise the lack of opportunities my son has had to initiate a conversation.*

Even non-verbal expression may be part of the aided vocabulary.

Miguel was seven years old with severe dystonic cerebral palsy, and good language comprehension and cognitive development. He used eye pointing and coding to select graphic signs on a board, and had recently been given a Macaw with 16 messages and scanning. After a few weeks, an aunt who usually assisted during training sessions asked the speech therapist to record the whistle that older boys do when they see a beautiful girl. Later the same afternoon, Paulo went to a coffee shop near his home with a cousin and he found whistling more important than asking for ice cream.

However, not all attempts at introducing the new intervention methodology were successful, as demonstrated in the cases of Andreia and Susana.

Andreia was 15 and Susana 16 years old. Both had a severe form of cerebral palsy and were unable to speak. Systematic informal assessment indicated good speech comprehension and cognitive function within the normal range. Both had had training since the age of seven in the use of communication aids with Blissymbols. They accessed the communication board directly with head pointers. They managed the communication aids proficiently and could have made good use of them, except for the fact that these were used only during training at the Centre. Neither of the families felt a need to use the aided systems because they considered the idiosyncratic gestures of the children sufficient to meet the family needs of interaction.

At the time the intervention was initiated, in 1984, the professionals regarded the intervention not only as adequate but as the best available. Following the ideas of the new methodology, it was decided to change the intervention for Andreia and Susana, and the families were made partners in the intervention. The vocabulary was revised with the participation of Andreia and Susana, their families and the professionals in order to be more useful in daily activities, such as having a meal or refreshments in the school bar. Andreia and Susana were given communication aids with digitised voice output for making conversation in natural environments possible (e.g. *'I want some cold juice', 'I want a lunch ticket, please'* and *'How much does it cost?'*). The parents, the teachers and the other professionals were taught about language and communication, and the possibilities created by the communication aids, and were made aware of the importance of using the aids.

However, in spite of the fact that the communication aids were portable, easy to use and with voice output, and Andreia and Susana learned to use them, generalisation to contexts outside training sessions failed. At the evaluation, Andreia, Susana and their parents and teachers refused to use the aids. They considered it unnecessary to change the form of communication that they were used to (idiosyncratic gestures).

We believe a major reason for the failure of the intervention was that Andreia, Susana and their parents were brought into the decision process too late. Throughout the years, alternative communication had been established as a domain belonging to the school, outside the sphere of family and leisure life, a non-functional ritual without real-world value. Parents and children had created a state of interdependent communication where the children had adopted a passive style of communication, adapted to the limitations of their communication partner's skills. This failure emphasises the need for an early start, not only for developing the skills of the child, but, equally important, in order to prevent less optimal communication strategies and interaction forms becoming established and difficult to change.

**Technological development**

There are two main reasons for the need to make adaptations to standard systems of aided communication. Firstly, the standard techniques may not be comprehensive enough to meet the full range of an individual's communication needs. Secondly, an individual may be unable to use standard augmentative and alternative communication techniques due to severe physical, sensory or cognitive impairments. The work presented here concerns mainly the latter group.

In intervention of children with severe motor impairments, assistive technologies may be used both to increase functionality of the communication as an orthosis and as an aid in the habilitation and education process. In each case, supportive technology can go from a low to a high price, or from low to high technology. In general, inexpensive low technology aids are usually chosen, such as head pointers and manual communication boards. However, there may be different reasons for introducing voice output.

> Paulo was a 10-year-old boy who for five years had used a simple communication board with Blissymbols. He indicated a code of four colours and clusters of four Blissymbols by moving his shoulders and looking at the corner of the board where the colour corresponding to the Blissymbol he wanted to select was located. This was a very slow and laborious method of communicating. The teacher therefore did not encourage use of the communication board, and Paulo did not appear motivated to use it. With digitised voice output, however, even when the same method of selection was used, Paulo became more efficient in using the aid and more interactive both in the classroom and at home. His movements became more precise so that in a short time he could select one of the message fields of the device more precisely.

At the Centre, appliances and tools that may be adapted to the needs of each individual are preferred to ready-made commercial tools that may fulfil the needs of only a small group of individuals. This preference means that the professionals in the team and the parents need to know the goals in order to prepare multiple components in a way that can optimise the child's potential to communicate and interact in all relevant contexts. Most early software appliances contained one graphic sign system only (Blissymbols, PIC, PCS, etc.), did not allow adaptation with regard to type of voice output (if they had the option of voice output), and the number of messages was limited. It was only when tools appeared on the market which allowed a wider range of functions that true adaptation became a reality; that is, individualised communications aids with graphic signs that meet the immediate needs and current skills, and are prepared to meet the needs and skills of the future (cf. Beukelman and Mirenda, 1992).

Luis was five years old, lived in Matosinhos, a town near Oporto, and attended a regular kindergarten. He had severe dystonic cerebral palsy. When he was three years old, he got a portable computer (Apple Powerbook 180C) with special software for communication, writing, drawing and computer control (Ke:nx), and was taught to use scanning and single-switch input for selecting Blissymbols. Initially the system and the training were focused on communication of basic needs. As the vocabulary grew and he achieved greater skills in using the system, a hierarchal vocabulary structure was developed, linking thematic choices. For example, *SCHOOL-ACTIVITIES* was linked to a board set up with things to do: *PAINT, READ-BOOK, MUSIC, REST, DOLL-HOUSE, CARS,* etc.

In the classroom, opportunities for communication may depend on the imagination and motivation of the teacher and class mates. Reading, drawing, make believe and role play, singing and story telling are just a few examples of activities that may enhance communication skills and where access to assistive devices can make a difference between passive and active participation.

When learning to draw became an educational goal, Luis' computer-based system made it possible for him to control choice of colours, the direction of the mouse for moving the pencil and the control of the clicks and double clicks used to perform the drawing (using the KidPix software). When the music teacher found that Luis was not really participating in the music class, the same software was used for creating a way for him to play a 'piano', utilising the same colour system for tone indication as the other children in the class used for their xylophones. In the future, an environmental control will be incorporated in the same aid.

At the time of writing, Luis is beginning to learn the alphabet, starting with the letters of his own name, and numbers. Using the same software and the same portable computer he can see the characters on the screen in the sequence chosen by him to form his first words.

Synthetic speech has proved useful in reading instruction, but unfortunately this option is not yet available in Portugal. Attempts have been made to develop synthetic Portuguese but the results have not been very good. Low phonetic quality makes the speech unintelligible.

The assistive technology used for Luis has more functions than just providing a way to produce conventional communicative expression. It gives him access to various activities which will both give him a richer life and promote his development of language and communication skills. In fact, he and his peers have come closer to each other since he started to use the drawing and music software, which seems to have made him more interesting for the teacher and the other children to communicate with, thereby giving him more opportunities to initiate conversation and interact.

For Luis and his family, the new intervention strategies have proved successful. However, it should be noted that the description above does not reveal the full range of adaptations that have been necessary, such as:

- Positioning; he can use the aid while sitting in class, in the wheel-chair or lying down because he controls it with a single switch and head movements.
- It is usable in all environments: school, home, shopping centres, playgrounds, etc. However, he is limited by the two-hour life of the battery.
- It allows a range of topics for conversation reasonably quickly, and because of the voice output, he can communicate over a distance, and call and interrupt speaking turns.
- He can communicate with peers, family, friends, teachers and strangers with the digitised voice of a child of the same sex and age. The communication partner does not need to know how to operate with the aid.
- Attempts have been made to make the system the least tiring to use as possible, a feature of the individual adaptation which is very important considering the severe nature of his impairment. Fatigue may hinder the use of an otherwise functional system.

The fact that the system was portable and could be used in different environments, including with people who had no experience of computers, made it's durability, simplicity and security issues of great importance.

## Training parents and professionals

The complexity of presently available technology enables the development of more and more sophisticated devices which are able to meet a wide variety of user requirements. This also means that in order to adapt an aided communication system, a significant amount of engineering expertise may be needed. However, the role of the technician in the team is not only to make adaptations but, equally important, to ensure that the child, its parents and teachers have sufficient technical knowledge.

When Luis took his portable computer home for the first time, his sister and father, representing the whole family, had only attended two training sessions at the Centre. After this first week-end, the battery of the portable computer had run out and damage had been done to the operating system. The family had not been properly prepared to deal with such a sophisticated device. The computer was not plugged into the mains and battery life was short. After two hours of a joyful interaction with his family (recorded on video), Luis became frustrated because there was much more he wanted to say and his wonderful new communication device was already failing him.

A sophisticated device may not be the best solution if one fails to take the constraints of the environment into consideration. The family, teachers and peers will have to deal with the system because the natural contexts are where it will mainly be used. After making the choice of communication aid, most of the intervention time is now spent in the natural environment, leaving therapeutic sessions for introducing concepts and training, and for adjusting selection method and speed, switch delay, configuration of the communication board, positioning and body sites to control the access.

It was also the experience at the Centre that general advice was often difficult for parents to follow and therefore had little functional value. The new approach required that not only general strategies but specific goals had to be defined in collaboration with the parents. With clearly defined goals it seemed to be easier for parents to understand what needed to be done and whether it worked, and they became more likely to co-operate. As a result of this, the children got better opportunities for achieving proficiency in using their augmentative and alternative communication.

Fábio was a 5-year-old boy with Angelman syndrome, which includes severe intellectual impairment and limitations in comprehension and expression of spoken language (Angelman, 1965). Hyperactivity made him difficult to manage, and due to poor facial control he had very few expressions that might be interpreted as communicative. Strategies of overinterpretation had been discussed with the parents but the mother expressed concern about the absence of necessary cues and did not know how to proceed. It was therefore decided, in collaboration with the parents, to attempt teaching Fábio to choose between two activities which were present in his daily routine. PIC signs were used and training was made jointly by parents and therapists. In the first month, Fábio's hand was guided to one of two graphic signs on the board, whereupon the designated activity was started up. After two months, the mother reported that Fábio had started to point spontaneously at *MUSIC,* meaning 'I want to hear music' and *BUBBLES,* meaning 'Let us make some soap bubbles'.

Getting 'proof' that Fábio was able to learn to communicate (the literature is not very promising, cf. Pembrey, 1992) made the parents more enthusiastic and motivated to follow more general intervention strategies.

In the natural environments, training of the communication partners has become more important, because if they cannot deal with the system intervention will have limited use and may increase instead of lessen frustration, as in the case of Luis. However, environmental intervention is not restricted to technical issues only. Strategies have been developed for giving the families better knowledge of the real skills and needs of their disabled children. Video recordings have been made of the children in different contexts – at home, in school, in therapy sessions, in the playground, etc. – and watched and discussed by parents and professionals together. Several parent groups meet regularly to share ideas and experiences, giving each other new ways and situations to promote communication for their children. The use of notebooks where parents, teachers and habilitation staff write down daily observations and particular events has increased the knowledge among all parties about each child and its life. The notebooks also function as a tool for exchanging information between home and school.

## Conclusions

Recent developments have made it necessary to change some of the intervention strategies traditionally applied in Portugal. This chapter has focused on issues that deserve particular attention in the process of assessment and intervention for severely motor and language impaired children who need augmentative and alternative communication. These changes included a greater focus on integration and non-educational settings, family involvement and a need for increased knowledge and awareness outside the specialist environment. Positive results of the new methodologies have already become apparent, exemplified by individual children who have increased their proficiency in the use of communication systems, their motivation to use them, and their participation in social situations. However, in spite of the results that have been gained, we hope that progress in the field will continue to create new questions, doubts and challenges.

# Chapter 19
# Collaborative problem solving in communication intervention

EVA BJÖRCK-ÅKESSON, MATS GRANLUND AND
CECILIA OLSSON

Recent studies have shown positive effects of communication intervention involving both the disabled person and communication partners (Basil, 1994; Johansson, 1988; Jonker and Heim, 1994; Light, McNaughton and Parnes, 1986). However, intervention models involving both the person with a disability and partners are sparse. Such models need to focus not only on the forms of communication but also on the outcomes of communication in everyday life. It is an ultimate goal of intervention that possibilities should be increased for people with disabilities to make their 'voices' heard and to control their own environment (Blackstone and Williams, 1994).

In this chapter, a model for communication intervention is described, within the framework of empowerment. The essential feature of empowerment is that disabled people and significant people around them, for example family and group home staff, should gain increased control over the help-giving processes, through active participation in the planning and implementation of intervention.

Traditionally, a developmental or 'new skills' perspective has been adopted in communication intervention, focusing on increasing the complexity of the form and use of communication (Granlund, 1993). Interventions thus aim at increasing the person's future communicative behaviour (which may or may not be functional), without considering which desired outcomes of communication pose difficulties for the disabled person at the present time. Within this perspective, professionals have based intervention decisions mainly on their expertise in communication disability. An alternative way to approach intervention is to use an adaptation perspective (Granlund, 1993; Granlund, Björck-Åkesson, Brodin and Olsson, 1995) where the competence of the person is in focus, that is, the ability to obtain desired communicative outcomes. The person, the context and the tasks necessary to accomplish the mission in order to reach the desired outcome may then be regarded as possible intervention parameters. The person with disabilities and/or significant people will decide the desired outcomes of interventions.

## Theoretical perspective

In documenting the functional communicative status of a person, it is necessary to combine measures of the person's communicative behaviour, with information about what the disabled person and communication partners consider a desired outcome of communication in a particular context. For example, if a desired outcome for the person with disabilities is to experience social closeness, the frequency of behaviours leading to 'closeness behaviour' in partners is important to assess. The functional communicative status of an individual will vary according to the desired outcome of communication, the actions necessary for realising the outcome, the interaction partner, and the context of interaction. Hence, communication intervention is focused on problems that are dialectical by nature. Intervention will '... necessarily yield many divergent rather than one convergent solution, not only over time but even at the same moment of time' (Rappaport, 1981, p. 7).

Communication intervention will be less than optimal if professionals act as if communication problems were convergent rather than divergent. 'Most problems have a variety of solutions, some of which are contradictory, and both sides of the contradiction need to have attention paid to them. When we pay attention to paradox we are more likely to find ourselves being useful' (Rappaport, 1981, p. 7). For example, in teaching a person to use graphic signs, communication partners may be instructed to ignore less complex means for conveying identical messages and, paradoxically, thereby decrease the disabled individual's motivation for communicating. Paradoxes and contradictory solutions should be welcomed in order to avoid one-sided solutions. By identifying a wide range of communicative difficulties that are possible to solve and discussing how these problems are interrelated, the complexity of communication may be taken into consideration and one-sided solutions may be avoided.

The empowerment theory (Rappaport, 1981, 1987) addresses the complex realities of life. Empowerment is defined as 'a process of becoming able or allowed to do some unspecified thing because there is a condition of dominion or authority with regard to that specific thing, as opposed to all things' (Rappaport, 1987, p. 129). Expressed in simple words, this means being able to follow one's intentions. It requires an intervention model which allows for pursuing paradox and the consideration of many simultaneous, different and contradictory problems and answers. The empowerment theory implies that:

- many competencies are already present or at least possible, given niches and opportunities;
- what one sees as poor functioning may be a result of the social and physical structure of the environment as well as lack of personal resources which makes it impossible to use existing skills to reach desired outcomes;
- to increase an individual's competence, changes must be made in a context of real-life activities rather than in artificial settings.

Since both problems and solutions are divergent, it follows that people may work out different solutions. Thus, for one person with a disability, intervention solutions may be based on different assumptions. Context, interaction partners and desired outcome play a role in the creation of an intervention plan. Empowerment is a multi-system construct, and empowerment at one level of analysis influences other levels (Rappaport, 1987; Sameroff, 1987).

A model of communication intervention based on the theory of empowerment aims at obtaining desired outcomes on multiple levels simultaneously. The three implications of the empowerment model mentioned above may be used as organising principles for an intervention model based on collaborative problem solving. In a broader perspective, collaborative problem solving may be seen as a learning process, resulting in increased problem solving skills for the disabled person and the communication partners in the environment, as well as enhanced control of their own life for the disabled person.

## A model for collaborative problem solving

According to empowerment theory, it must be possible to apply intervention objectives and strategies in the everyday environment of the individual. In order to develop a functional intervention plan, it is crucial that the disabled person, as well as significant persons in the environment, participate actively in all steps of the intervention process (Björck-Åkesson and Granlund, 1995; Jones et al., 1987). Involvement of the family and other care-givers in the goal-setting process has been demonstrated to lead to positive developmental outcomes for children with disabilities (Shonkoff and Hauser-Cram, 1987). However, individuals with disabilities, parents and other care-givers are not usually given an active part in the intervention process. They are provided with information and then asked to give their consent to assessment and intervention suggested by professionals (Granlund, Steensson, Sundin and Olsson, 1992). In addition, parents seldom participate actively in decisions when assessment and intervention plans are being formulated (Björck-Åkesson and Granlund, 1995).

The process of intervention based on collaborative problem solving involves six steps that recur over time: problem description, explanation of the problem, problem ranking, goal setting, intervention design and process, and outcome evaluation (Granlund, 1988). Within each step, several factors add to the progress of the collaborative problem solving process. The intervention cycle is described in Figure 19.1. The checklist is used to guide the collaborative activity within each of the six steps.

---

**Problem description**
Use the four questions for generating problems.

**Explanation of problem**
* Are there divergent explanations to each problem?
* Do the various explanations sought to each problem add information to what is already known?
* What explanations do several problems have in common?
* Can problems be grouped according to their explanations?
* What explanations may point to possible intervention strategies?

**Ranking and evaluating**
* What is the hypothetical desired outcome for each problem?
* What other hypothetical outcomes are there?
* Does the desired outcome of any problem automatically reduce other problems?
* Is the desired outcome transient or enduring?

**Goals and objectives**
* Does the goal describe a state in positive terms?
* Is it possible to see the relation between the problems and the goal?
* Is it possible to categorise many objectives under the same goal?
* Is the objective formulated in terms of the behaviour of the disabled person and the effects of that behaviour on the immediate setting?
* Is there a clear relation between the goal and the objective?
* Is the objective possible to implement in daily life?
* Is the objective equal to the desired outcome?

**Intervention strategy design and implementation**
* Does the intervention strategy explain how each objective should be reached?
* Can all who will be working with the intervention recognise and explain the relation between the objective and strategies?
* Are the intervention strategies formulated on basis of the explanations of the problem?
* Is the intervention strategy intervening with everyday activities?
* Is the intervention strategy taking time from other activities?
* Is the intervention strategy possible to carry out in everyday situations?
* Does the intervention strategy take a short time to carry out each time?
* Is one named person responsible for the implementation of the intervention strategy?
* Is this person responsible for making everybody in the setting active in the implementation process?

---

**Figure 19.1** Checklist for the collaborative problem solving model

## Problem description

Within the model, a problem is defined as the perceived difference between the existing state and a desired state within a specific context. The desired outcome of the communication defines the problem to the same extent as the communicative behaviour itself. For example, gaining attention is the desired outcome of attention-seeking behaviour. In order to intervene in real-life problems, the person with disabilities and/or significant persons within the environment must perceive and be able to describe in what way the existing state is problematic. Test results, for example, may be used to explain real-life problems, but the test results cannot in themselves be considered a real-life problem. The problem is best described in the words of the person experiencing the difference between the existing and the desired state, or by using the description of significant people perceiving the problem.

In the collaborative problem solving model, the problem description is based on the paradox that existing behaviours may have the same desired outcome as new behaviours that need to be taught. It is necessary to address both sides of the paradox, that is, to discuss how existing communicative behaviours may be increased or decreased and what new behaviours should be developed in relation to the desired outcome. In order to reveal such contradictions, divergent problem solving is used. Four questions are used as the basis of the problem description:

- What skills within the existing communicative behaviour repertoire leading to desired outcomes are seldom used?
- What new skills leading to desired outcomes need to be developed?
- What skills within the existing communicative behaviour need to be used less often to obtain desired outcomes?
- What aberrant behaviours need to be replaced by communicative behaviours leading to desired outcomes?

## Explanation of the problem

Explanation of the problem is defined as information about factors that hypothetically explain the existence and maintenance of a communicative problem. Whether the explanations are 'true' or not can only be established after the intervention is implemented. Factors explaining a problem can be related to any of the three components in the competence construct, that is, the person, the context and the tasks necessary to be accomplished in order to reach desired outcomes. Communicative problems are diverse and as a rule have more than one explanation. In most instances it is difficult to establish the direction of a cause-effect relationship. Each explanatory factor influences the probability of solving a communicative problem. Since communication is a transactional process, it is more important to identify the factors that may be manipulated in intervention than to establish the direction of cause-effect relationships (Sameroff and Fiese, 1990).

Explanations of problems constitute the foundation of the intervention approach. Numerous and divergent explanations make it easier to design effective intervention methods. In the collaborative problem solving model the person with disabilities, significant people in the environment and the professionals are looking for a multitude of explanations for each identified problem. Finding factors by which various problems may be explained is important in order to ensure a broad focus in intervention. Intervention aspects are also inherent in the problem solving activity itself. By explaining the problem, both the disabled person and people in the environment learn about their own communicative skills and are given opportunities for redefining their perceptions of the problem (Granlund, Olsson, Andersson and von Dardel, 1990).

## Ranking and evaluating

Evaluating and ranking problems pertain to selecting from an array of possible problems and deciding the order in which the problems shall be solved. It thus requires prior identification of problems as well as multiple explanations. Each problem has several solutions, making it important to discuss the possible consequences of different choices from the perspectives of the disabled person, significant people in the environment and the professionals. Intervention specialists often give priority to other outcomes of intervention than do parents and other care-givers (Cadman, Goldsmith and Bashim, 1984). A Norwegian investigation of young children using communication aids (von Tetzchner, 1995) furthermore indicated that the rationale behind communication intervention decisions is often diffuse.

Ranking is focused on existing problems in relation to hypothetical outcomes of the intervention. It is furthermore important to make a distinction between problems to be solved and the need for solutions. People tend to express their need for a solution, without specifying what problems might be solved with the help of that solution. In ranking problems to solve, it is important to keep in mind the following four characteristics of need identification (Dunst, Trivette and Deal, 1988, p. 14):

• There must be a concern that something is not as it ought to be.
• The mere recognition of a discrepancy between what is and what ought to be is not sufficient to define a condition as problematic, unless the person or a significant person in the environment

makes a personal judgement that the discrepancy is currently, or will potentially, influence his or her behaviour.

- There must be some evaluation or awareness that there is a resource that will reduce the discrepancy between what is and what ought to be.
- There must be a recognition that there is a way of procuring a resource to meet the need, before a discrepancy is perceived as amenable to help.

The characteristics listed above do not necessarily evolve chronologically. Consequently, the first two are especially important to acknowledge. Failure to acknowledge these may lead to a situation where a person might, more or less routinely, procure a resource, without actually knowing what the problem is.

## Goals and objectives

The goals and objectives of communication intervention are defined as the desired outcome, as prescribed by the person with disabilities or significant people in relation to what is perceived as 'not as it ought to be'. The difference between a goal and an objective is a matter of generality and time frame (Nakken, 1993). The goal is a general description of the desired outcome, in which the generic communicative behaviour of the disabled person is emphasised more than the specific effect of that behaviour on the immediate setting. The goal is often described as an enduring state. The objective, on the other hand, is a description of a desired outcome, in which the specific effect of the communicative behaviour on the immediate setting is emphasised, to the same extent as the behaviour itself. The objective can be either a transient state or an enduring state. This definition implies that the objective should contain not only a description of the behaviour of the disabled person, but also a description of the desired effects of that behaviour on the immediate setting. For example, if Tom has problems with initiating interaction, the objective might be phrased as: 'Tom uses attention-seeking behaviour more than 15 times a day and is responded to in at least 12 of those instances'. Due to the specified quality of objectives, many objectives belong under the same goal.

In the collaborative problem solving model, the formulation of objectives is emphasised. Objectives should be phrased in terms used by the disabled person and/or significant people. According to empowerment theory, changes must be made in real-life situations. For this reason, the objective must be functional, that is, it must make a difference in how a person can achieve mastery over his or her own life (Sigafoss et al., 1991). A common problem in collaborative problem solving is that both goal and objective describe the implementation of the intervention method, rather than the desired outcome of implementing it (Granlund, Steensson, Sundin and Olsson, 1992). By formulating the goal and the objective in the third person and present tense (as in the example with Tom above), this problem is avoided.

## Intervention strategies and implementation

The intervention strategies are defined as the actions taken by people in the environment, or professionals, in order to assist the person with disabilities to reach the desired outcome. The intervention strategies encompass actions by people, adaptation of the physical environment and provision of assistive technology. The expertise of professionals is used to generate ideas about what the important elements of the strategy are. The person in question and/or significant people provide information about how and when the method can be implemented. Intervention strategies that people in the immediate setting perceive as easy to implement and requiring little time to carry through, are complied with to a greater degree than methods which are perceived as complicated and time consuming (Gresham, 1989).

In the present model, strategy design is focused on enhancing already existing competencies and resources in the immediate setting. Discussions and observations of the rare instances when the person with disabilities actually has reached desired outcomes, give information about the content of the intervention strategy. This information needs to be related to the explanations of the problem from which the basic components of the intervention strategy are generated. If possible, the intervention strategy should assimilate the explanations of the problem and extend the use of existing behaviour and resources in the environment rather than introducing 'new factors' (Witt and Martens, 1988).

## Evaluation of outcome

In order to estimate a time period for attaining the desired outcome, information is needed about the desired outcome and the intervention strategies. Information about the implementation of intervention is also necessary if any conclusions about the effects of intervention are to be drawn (Gresham, 1989). Discussing 'implementation behaviour' offers a learning opportunity for the individuals who implement the intervention, by allowing them to evaluate their own communicative behaviour toward the person with disabilities. In the meetings following intervention, the implementation of intervention is considered before the outcomes of intervention are discussed.

Outcome evaluation includes evaluation of the desired outcome as well as consideration of unexpected effects (Simeonsson, 1995). In the collaborative problem solving model, *Goal Attainment Scaling* (GAS;

Kiresuk, Smith and Cardello, 1994; Vriesema, Miedema and VanBlok-land, 1992) is used for evaluating desired outcomes of intervention. Using the GAS criteria, desired outcomes can be scaled as 'less than expected' (−1 or −2), 'expected' (0), and 'better than expected' (+1 or +2). Goal attainment scaling is the last step before implementation of the intervention strategies. When the scaling of possible outcomes is made, existing or initial performance is specified according to the scale. The extent to which the desired outcomes are attained is evaluated, by comparing initial performance with performance attained in the intervention period.

The GAS approach serves two purposes in the model. First, since the scaling activity includes speculations about consequences of the intervention, it is an opportunity to contemplate whether the projected outcome really is desired. Secondly, it is a means of documenting intervention effects (Ottenbacher and Cusick, 1993).

## Collaborative problem solving with families

Assessment and intervention for children with communication impairment is often made from a developmental or new skills perspective, with little consideration of the everyday communicative environment of the child (Björck-Åkesson, 1992, 1993). Parents and other care-givers, who constitute the child's daily communication partners, tend to be left out of the planning and implementation of the intervention. In the project described in this section, collaborative problem solving was used to involve parents of children with cerebral palsy and communication impairment in the intervention process. The general features of the programme and the collaborative problem solving process for a 2-year-old girl, Maria, is described.

Based on empowerment theory, the goal of the project was to create conditions for optimal communicative interaction between Maria and her care-givers. An adaptation perspective was used for implementing the intervention in Maria's everyday life. Significant people in her environment participated in the entire assessment and intervention process. Assessment and intervention were based on collaborative problem solving. Video recordings of the communicative interaction between the girl and her parents and other care-givers (e.g. preschool staff, grandparent) formed the basis of the intervention. Protocols for systematic observation of the communicative interaction were used. The professionals functioned mainly as consultants, using their expertise in handicapping conditions and collaborative problem solving.

Assessment had a threefold purpose: first, to give professionals information about child and family needs and characteristics; secondly, to give the parents first-hand influence over the intervention process; and thirdly, to create a common language of intervention. The first step in the intervention process consisted of screening the needs and resources of the child and the family with an emphasis on functional assessment. A number of formal and informal instruments were used, such as the *Abilities Index* (Simeonsson and Bailey, 1988) and the *Early Social Communication Scales* (Seibert and Hogan, 1982). Interviews with the parents and other care-givers about problems in everyday life were a major source of information. The results of the assessment were used for both problem description and problem explanation. The second step was video recording everyday interactions with the girl and her parents and other care-givers. One protocol was used for analysing the form and functions of the girl's communication, another for analysing the strategies of her communication partners (cf. Light et al., 1986). Collaboration in analysing the video recordings and filling out protocols served to establish common terms and a basis for intervention and implementation (cf. Launonen, this volume).

Following screening and assessment, problem description was initiated with Maria's parents. A number of problems were identified on the basis of the four questions of problem description presented above. Communicative skills which were available but seldom used by Maria were: initiating communication, asking for more of an activity, protesting, expressing 'yes' and 'no', pointing at things she wanted, and referring to non-present activities. New skills that needed to be developed were: the expression of wants and needs by the means of language ('yes' and 'no'), and choosing between objects and activities. A behaviour that needed to be used less often was fretfulness. Maria often became fretful when she received too little attention, for example when her mother was occupied in the kitchen and unable to pay attention to her.

In ranking problems, a common denominator seemed to be that Maria had problems initiating and maintaining interaction, and a number of explanations were suggested as to why Maria had these difficulties. These referred to Maria's motor impairment and her difficult behaviour, as well as the communication strategies of her communication partners. Examples of the former kind were:

> The motor impairment restricts Maria's options for expressing herself sufficiently clearly. When she is ready to initiate or required to respond, her spasticity increases. Maria does not need to initiate, since she often acquires what she wants anyhow. Maria cannot use her voice for communication and often surrenders to the interpretations of the communication partner.

Examples of the latter kind, that is, partner strategies were:

> People in the immediate surrounding do not require distinct expressions from Maria in order to understand her. They pretend

to understand her, even when they are not sure of the aim of her initiations. With too few and too short pauses in the interaction, partners do not give her enough time to take her turn in the interaction.

An explanation directed towards the physical context was that Maria had too few sitting positions which facilitated communicating. She often sat in positions where she needed a lot of energy to keep her head up, thus making it difficult to communicate at the same time. The partners also created few good situations for initiating, for example placing toys beyond Maria's reach, thereby requiring an initiation from her, in order to get a toy.

In setting priorities, both the problem description and the problem explanation were examined, resulting in two sets of problems being chosen as potentially fruitful: 'Maria seldom initiates the continuation of an activity', and 'she seldom initiates an activity'. The goal of the intervention was expressed as 'Maria expresses herself clearly and is understood by different persons and in different situations'. This long-term goal was agreed upon after a lengthy discussion about Maria's future communication possibilities. The parents first wanted to formulate a goal in terms of Maria's use of spoken language. However, considering her severe motor impairment, this possibility seemed unrealistic, hence it was formulated in more general terms. The objectives of the intervention were easy to formulate on the basis of the two goals that had been given priority. The desired outcome of the first objective was that Maria initiated the continuation of an activity, and this objective is the focus of the example below.

To arrive at strategies for implementation, the objectives and explanations of the problem were examined. The following suggestions ensued from the explanations of the problem: increase the pauses in the interaction; wait for Maria to express a distinct initiative with gaze, sound or movements before responding to her; and create situations which facilitated initiatives from Maria. It was decided that the parents should start an activity that Maria liked, stop doing it after a while, and wait until Maria initiated continuation of this activity by the use of gaze, sound or movement. The parents should wait for Maria's initiative longer than they usually did. Situations for implementing the method were discussed, resulting in the following 'good situations' for implementation: playing games, playing music or reading stories when Maria stood in a standing brace or sat in her adapted chair at the table or was lying on her back.

The time frame of the intervention was set to two months. The goal attainment scale for Maria was:

+2    Maria takes the initiative to continue an activity that is responded to, 5 times per day.

+1     Maria takes the initiative to continue an activity that is responded to, 4 times per day.

0      Maria takes the initiative to continue an activity that is responded to, 3 times per day.

−1     Maria takes the initiative to continue an activity that is responded to, 1–2 times per day.

−2     Maria takes no initiative to continue an activity that is responded to (function at start of intervention).

At the end of the intervention, Maria took the initiative to continue an activity four times a day, an attainment that was better than expected.

A number of other problems were addressed simultaneously in the problem solving process, without being accounted for in the goal attainment scale. For example, difficulties were discerned relating to attention-seeking behaviour, positioning and assistive technology, as well as to the staff situation at the preschool. When revising the intervention, new objectives were formulated by collaborative problem solving based on previous and repeated assessment.

# In-service training

A group home or a day centre often constitutes the main environment of adults with profound intellectual impairment and multiple disabilities. Care staff in these settings frequently implement communication intervention which has been planned and designed by external professionals. However, such interventions are often planned without considering the communicative environment (Granlund, Terneby and Olsson, 1992a). To increase the functional outcomes of intervention, staff can be trained to plan and implement communication intervention through collaboration with external professionals. An in-service training programme based on empowerment theory has been developed and evaluated with several groups of care staff (Granlund, Terneby and Olsson, 1992b). The programme had the following rationale:

- Communication involves not only the individual with disabilities but also the persons in the environment of the individual.
- An in-service training programme will lead to positive changes in the communicative environment only if the focus is on the actual environment that the participants are working in (Mittler, 1987).
- It is not only the degree of impairment but also the extent to which the person is using the remaining ability in different settings in daily life that affects the communication.
- The best persons for estimating how an individual with disabilities is functioning in daily life are those who share this daily life with that individual.

- Theoretical lectures and reading yield mainly theoretical knowledge about communication. If people are supposed to make changes, they need to apply their knowledge in practising new skills and receive feedback on the application of those skills (Granlund and Björck-Åkesson, in press; Granlund, Terneby and Olsson, 1992b).

The objectives of the in-service training programme were threefold: first, to provide care staff with the necessary knowledge and skills for planning and implementing communication intervention; secondly, to train participants to function as local supervisors collaborating with other staff members, parents and other significant individuals; and thirdly, to enhance functional communicative skills among the people with disabilities in the settings where the participating staff members worked. As already pointed out, empowerment is a multilevel construct. The first objective involved one person as a resource for the rest of the staff, while the second objective involved the staff as communication partners and implementors of interventions. Together, these two objectives formed the conditions aimed at facilitating collaboration between staff members and significant people. The third objective focused on the individuals with disabilities; in-service training was supposed to have a direct impact on their communicative competence.

### The in-service training programme

The purpose of the in-service training programme, attended by staff members from group homes and day centres, was to develop better functional communication for adults with profound intellectual impairment and multiple disabilities. Two months before the programme was implemented, a one-day lecture was presented to all staff members about communication intervention for people with profound impairments, providing a rationale for participation. After the lecture, the staff members of each working unit elected two staff members who should attend the full course. Through this design, staff members who did not participate in the training obtained a frame of reference for facilitating future collaboration. The reason for having two participants from each unit was that they could support each other in implementing new ideas at their work unit. They could also provide each other with continuous feedback on the implementation after the training course.

The programme started with 14 participants from nine working units; three staff members from two group homes, nine staff members from seven different day centres and two speech pathologists. Before the first course meeting, each participant selected an adult with profound intellectual impairment and multiple disabilities in need of communication intervention, whom they intended to work with during the course.

The course included seven full day meetings in a four-month period, and a one-day follow-up two months after the last meeting. During the 2–3 weeks between meetings, participants completed home assignments in collaboration with their non-participating colleagues. Preparatory work before the first course meeting included a brief description of the unit and the clients' disabilities and communicative abilities. There were two purposes to the preparatory work: to start the in-service training collaboration between the course participants and the rest of the staff, and to give the course leader information about the work units and the clients, in order to adapt the course format and the content to the settings where the intervention was to take place.

The themes covered in the course were the communication model, assessment methods and intervention programmes. These themes alternated during the course and were treated from a general knowledge perspective, a client perspective and a collaboration perspective. In Figure 19.2, the themes and different perspectives are structured in 'boxes' to summarise the course content. For example, a theoretical lecture about communicative functions was immediately followed by a viewing of the video recording of one the participants' selected clients, and collaboratively analysing the occurrence of communicative functions. At the working unit, the participant later assessed, together with one or two other staff members, the communicative functions of the selected client using an interview guide.

Each meeting had the same structure. It started with feedback on home assignments and discussions about the collaboration with the rest of the staff. A lecture on a topic related to the communication model or problem solving model then followed. The meeting ended with instructions on how to complete the next home assignment. Home assignments included assessment, and planning and implementing an intervention programme for the selected client.

The in-service training programme was evaluated with the help of GAS. Scales were made for 12 clients with 1–3 objectives per client, totalling 22 scales (see Figure 19.3). Eight of the clients attained all objectives with at least expected outcome. For client F, only one of the two objectives was attained. The staff attributed this to the methods being time consuming. They had preferred to concentrate on one of the objectives. Clients J and L showed no progress towards the objectives. The reason was that staff had not yet implemented the methods, in one case due to illness, in the other due to a delay in obtaining prescribed assistive technology.

The communicative environment was assessed for each client prior to and after two months of intervention. Assessments were made by staff with the help of the check-list *The Social and Physical Environment Survey* (Granlund and Karlan, 1985). This check-list was developed for measuring general qualities of the communicative environment of

| | General knowledge | Client perspective | Collaboration |
|---|---|---|---|
| Communcation model | Skills in communicative content, form and function. Cognitive level, perception, motor skills for communication. Social and physical environmental factors influencing the communication. | Group discussions with focus on present client and examples illustrating the general knowledge in some, but not all, cases. Video recordings of client as illustrations to theories. | No actual emphasis was put on collaboration concerning the general knowledge. The one-day introduction for all staff served as a common basis for information exchange. |
| Assessment | Different forms of assessment of the factors above. Instructions and guidance on why and how to assess. | Information collection on present client using a selection of relevant assessment instruments. Analysis of assessment results. | Assessment conducted as interviews with staff members who did not participate in course. Feedback from participant to informants on assessment results and analysis. |
| Intervention programe | Problem solving model: problem formulation and explanations, formulating goals and objectives, strategy design and implementation. Evaluation with goal attainment scaling. | Implementation of the intervention programme with present client. Communication intervention (strategies for reaching goals and objectives). Evaluation of effect of intervention on client. | Intervention programme developed together with staff members. Intervention together with staff members. Evaluation of intervention made together with staff members. |

Figure 19.2 In-service training programme

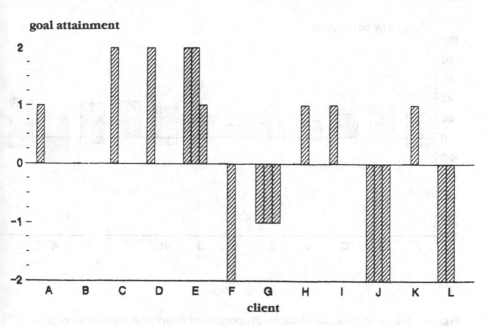

goal attainment

**Figure 19.3** Goal attainment for each client

people with profound multiple impairments. Figure 19.4 indicates that some positive environmental changes had occurred for each client, even for J and L where interventions had not yet been implemented.

Several causes for the changes are plausible. First, they may reflect improvement in communicative function on the part of the disabled person. An increase in active involvement in communication will yield higher scores on several of the ratings of the social environment. Secondly, they may represent an effect of the strategies implemented, for example giving more options and offering a variety of social activities. Finally, they may constitute a generalised effect of increased knowledge and awareness in staff of the importance of the communicative environment (in other words, unplanned interventions). There were also negative changes in communicative environment. Due to increased knowledge among staff, the environment might be evaluated as less accessible after training in communication intervention. An alternative explanation would be that positive changes in a disabled person's communicative functioning may lead to increased interaction within the setting. This might be expressed as negative changes in terms of how the environment is evaluated by the staff.

## Implications for intervention and research

It has been argued in this chapter that communication intervention should focus on dialectic problems demanding divergent solutions. The

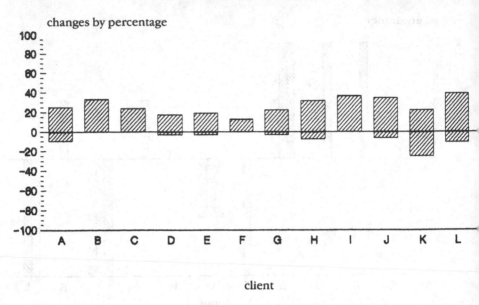

**Figure 19.4** Environmental changes. Proportion of items with positive or negative difference scores (N=64)

case of Maria is an example of identifying a number of diverse communicative problems with several explanations allowing for divergent solutions and multiple desired outcomes. What problems to solve and the order in which the problems should be solved are matters of priority among hypothetical outcomes. A critical issue in communication intervention is thus who decides the desired outcome of intervention. If an enduring effect of intervention is to be increased control over their own life for disabled people, outcome decisions must be made by these people and significant people in the environment. A communication intervention model based on empowerment theory is a means to this end.

The essential feature of empowerment is that people with disabilities and significant persons in their environment have control over the help-giving process. This process is basically a problem-solving activity. The form and content of the problem-solving process influence the degree of control over desired outcomes of intervention as perceived by the individual with disabilities and significant persons. The case of Maria demonstrates the collaborative problem-solving process. Maria's parents were active participants in all the steps of the intervention process. Assessment was formed as an opportunity for the parents to gain the knowledge and skills that were necessary for participating in decision-making. Problems and desired outcomes were described in everyday terms in order to secure the impact of intervention on everyday functioning. The use of goal attainment scaling, with desired outcomes formulated as everyday functioning, made it possible for the parents to evaluate the effects of the intervention.

In communication intervention research, information is needed about how the actual intervention process was accomplished, how assessment was performed, who decided what to assess and how to assess, who defined the desired outcomes of the intervention, and who evaluated whether or not desired outcomes had been reached.

Communicative competence is dependent on factors pertaining to the person with disabilities, the context in which the person is living, and the tasks needing to be accomplished in order to reach desired outcomes. Intervention can be directed towards any of these factors. A communication intervention model based on empowerment theory aims at reaching desired outcomes on multiple levels, for several factors simultaneously. The in-service training programme described here is an example of how desired outcomes of intervention on several levels are combined within one intervention package. On the individual level, increased communicative competence for the disabled person was the desired outcome. On the environmental level, increased competence in communication intervention among all staff members was a desired outcome, including changes in their own communication strategies. On the instructional level, improvement of the participants' skills and knowledge as supervisors was a desired outcome. The in-service training programme is focused on creating opportunities for using competence in everyday life and collaborative problem solving on all levels.

In most research in communication intervention, outcome is reported on one level only, typically on the individual level. In models based on empowerment theory, outcome effects need to be investigated on multiple levels, and for desired outcomes as well as unexpected effects. The in-service training described here is an example of effects reported on two levels (cf. Figures 19.3 and 19.4). Multilevel outcomes would have included outcomes on the instructional level, that is, outcomes related to the participants' skills and knowledge as supervisors. Ideally, outcome reports should include not only the behaviour of the disabled person, but also the effects of that behaviour on persons in the environment. Moreover, reports should include how the self-efficacy of the person with disabilities and significant persons affects the ability to solve problems in other contexts.

# Chapter 20
# From system to communication: Staff training for attitude change

ELISABETE MENDES AND JORGE RATO

The present chapter addresses the implementation of augmentative and alternative communication in Portugal, which took place through collaboration between governmental agencies, universities and institutions of habilitation and rehabilitation. Through this process, a need had become apparent for changing the professional views of those working with severely intellectually impaired individuals. The results of a project directed at staff training, attitude change and competence development among this group of professionals are discussed.

## Background

Augmentative and alternative communication is a rather new professional field in Portugal, particularly with regard to intervention for people with intellectual impairment and severe problems in spoken communication. The fact is that resources have been practically non-existent for this group, compared to many other countries in Europe. It is only in the last decade that any significant progress has been made within this field. Considering the prime importance of communication for the personal independence and social integration of people with intellectual impairment, there was clearly an urgent need for development in this area.

Although estimates of the population differ, a considerable number of people have severe speech and language difficulties and will need augmented communication or an alternative mode of communication. According to Beukelman and Ansel (1995), 10–12 persons in 1000 have severe communication problems. On the basis of various sources, von Tetzchner and Martinsen (1992) suggest an estimate of 0.5 per cent for developmental disorders. For Portugal, with a population of 10 million inhabitants, this implies that 50 –100 000 000 people may need augmentative and alternative communication. (A Portuguese survey of people with disabilities is in progress and will provide more detailed information about the group).

The first alternative communication system to be introduced in Portugal was Blissymbolics (see Introduction). This occurred in 1981, following several national training courses led by experts from Cardiff University in Wales. Blissymbols were used for children and adolescents with cerebral palsy and other forms of motor impairment. The habilitation centres for people with cerebral palsy had a pioneering role in introducing this new form of communication. A more widespread application of augmentative and alternative communication systems, particularly for people with intellectual impairment, followed a series of joint Portuguese and Swedish courses in 1983. These courses were organised under the auspices of an agreement between the Portuguese and Swedish governments in the area of special education. Among other initiatives, the co-operation established a resource and development centre for educational material for children with special educational needs, and provided in-service training for professionals working with individuals with different types of impairment. Augmentative and alternative communication was a component of the training course for those working with people with intellectual impairment, and in this context PIC was introduced (see Introduction). PIC was thought to be more adequate and efficient than Blissymbols for this population.

The first attempt to expand the use of augmentative and alternative communication systems to children and adolescents with intellectual impairments was thus a consequence of this initiative. A Portuguese version of PIC, adapted to Portuguese cultural references, was published in 1989 by the Ministry of Education's Integrated Education Resource Centre. A wider national implementation of PIC was the result of a cooperative venture between the National Federation of Cooperatives for the Education and Rehabilitation of People with Intellectual Impairment (FENACERCI) and the General Bureau for Elementary and Secondary Education. In 1991, training courses in the use of PIC were organised for professionals all over the country. More recently, in 1994, PCS (see Introduction) was also adapted and translated into Portuguese.

Many of the early studies of augmentative and alternative communication involved the use of manual signs (Kiernan, Reid and Jones, 1982), and the acceptance of the sign languages of deaf people as true languages has been an important basis for the development of augmentative and alternative communication. There has been a strong oralist current in the education of deaf children in Portugal and, due to political reasons, Portuguese society was for a long time very isolated and closed, including the scientific institutions. This limited the development and usage of manual signing for deaf children, as well as the use of manual and graphic sign systems for speech and language impaired

people without hearing impairments. Almost concurrent with the introduction of PIC, a Portuguese translation and adaptation of the Makaton
vocabulary (Walker, 1976), using Portuguese Sign Language, was carried
out by the Integrated Education Resource Centre. However the vocabulary strategies and the intervention methods of Makaton have mainly
been employed by the people who have been attempting to implement
them. In general, manual signs of the Makaton vocabulary have not
become widely used in Portugal.

Although the present volume is not concerned with the use of sign
language among deaf people, the work carried out in this field by the
Jacob Rodrigues Pereira Institute should nevertheless be mentioned, as
well as the publication of a Portuguese Sign Language dictionary by the
National Secretariat for Rehabilitation in 1991. These represented
important first steps toward using sign language with non-speaking
hearing populations.

Parallel to these initiatives, the Non-verbal Communication Commission was set up at the Technical University of Lisbon. This commission
has promoted thematic seminars and courses led by experts within the
field, aimed at creating awareness among professionals working within
this area of habilitation. This work has been carried on by the Centre for
the Analysis and Processing of Signs, with particular emphasis on training in the use of assistive technology (Azevedo, 1995).

During the last few years, there has been real progress within this
area and a growing interest among professionals in implementing intervention based on augmentative and alternative communication. This
began with research projects addressing intervention methodologies
and the development of technical aids, for example for people with
severe motor impairment (Ferreira, da Ponte, Azevedo and Carvalho,
1995), and for promoting integration (Soro-Camats, Duarte and
Mendes, 1995). Among the important technical developments was a
portable communication device (Ferreira, Teixeira, Ramalho and
Lourenço, 1994). The publication of these and other projects, together
with the translation into Portuguese of foreign articles and books, will
constitute a significant factor in encouraging the use of augmentative
and alternative communication systems and lead to a compilation of a
Portuguese bibliography on the application of augmentative and alternative communication. This is considered particularly important as the
professional literature in English and other foreign languages is inaccessible for the majority of the population. Progress within this area in
Portugal is also apparent in the fact that some universities have included
modules on augmentative and alternative communication in the curric-
ula of educators and teachers who will be working with populations
with special educational needs.

During the first 10–12 years of involvement, a number of professionals have emerged who have been pioneers within this field, attempting

to find solutions to the problems of children with severe speech communication difficulties. It has been a period characterised by a lack of resources and knowledge about the intervention procedures that should be used, and by difficulties in gaining access to existing systems. Moreover, up until this time, the focus of intervention had been solely on aided communication systems as such, that is, on their physical characteristics and technical features and problems. However, it became apparent that the mere provision of such systems often did not lead to improved communication, in particular for children with communication problems and intellectual impairment. The focus of intervention changed from the pure provision of systems to teaching communication functions and promoting a higher level of communicative interaction. In this process, knowledge was sought from professionals in other countries who had more experience in these matters. From these contacts and the joint reflections resulting from them, new branches of intervention have emerged, paralleling similar developments in other parts of Europe. At the end of the early stage of augmentative and alternative communication in Portugal, a need for greater methodological rigour had become apparent, particularly with regard to the theoretical basis and use of intervention strategies.

## Theoretical bases of intervention

The theoretical foundation of communication intervention in Portugal is increasingly developing into an interactionist approach (cf. del Rio, 1995; Soro-Camats et al., 1995; Vygotsky, 1962). According to this view, interaction implies active participation by the interlocutors, who are mutually affected by making use of their own communicative resources. All processes or actions involved in communicative development are essentially interactive and supported by processes of mutual adaptation. In this sense, adults have to feel that they can allow themselves to be influenced by the child and depend on it to develop its own educational assignments. However, despite the mutual influences in communicative interaction, adults have greater responsibility and control over events during these exchanges (Rondal, 1988a and b). They therefore have to pay attention to the signals of children, in order to follow the children's initiatives, wait and eventually respond to them. Adults have to structure dialogue situations as well as acknowledge and increase communication opportunities (Lock, 1980).

Atypical signals and reactions produced by disabled children and adolescents may alter the interactive exchange in significant ways. The signals of the children may not be understood by the adults, who in turn may become confused and consequently fail to produce appropriate strategies of interaction (Ryan, 1977). Children with intellectual impairment may find themselves in conditions which are not conducive to

maintaining interaction and communication with people in their immediate surroundings. These difficulties may have a negative effect on their
development of speech, making it necessary to create means to augment
their attempts at communicating, and provide them with the means to
produce readable signs which can engender, in a natural way, contingent
reactions from their interlocutors (del Rio, 1986; Gràcia and Urquía,
1994).

Adults have a crucial role in resolving this situation, and for that
reason they need means for improving interaction with disabled children and facilitating the children's acquisition of communication skills.
However, inefficiency in the normal interactive process has been
reported for parents and other adult interlocutors who have not learned
to respond to the attempts of interaction by the children (Soro-Camats
and Basil, and Soro and Basil, 1993; this volume). Thus it is not merely a
matter of providing intellectually impaired children with an effective
communicative code. For some children, owing to profound intellectual
impairment and specific characteristics, it may be necessary to encourage both emergent needs for communication and the actual use of
communication (Basil, 1992; von Tetzchner and Martinsen, 1992). The
intervention provided by professionals is therefore extremely important.
Their responsibility for establishing conditions for development of
communication makes it necessary to influence their behaviour in the
interactive process, and thereby to promote a change of attitude that
may advance the acquisition of communicative functions by children
and adolescents with communication problems. To achieve this aim,
professionals need to become aware of their own interactive behaviour,
and to apprehend and apply various strategies that may make it easier
for the children to take the initiative and maintain interactive communication (Soro and Basil, 1993; von Tetzchner, 1993b).

Interaction in relation to the development of language in natural
contexts, may be defined as an implicit educative process, in which
instruction is produced in a spontaneous form. This may have both positive and negative effects: positive because it concerns a natural, quasi-
spontaneous process which generates opportunities for learning and
interaction; negative if, for that reason, the importance and the worth of
this behaviour for the intervention process is not perceived. As interaction is a process of mutual influences which excludes the possibility of
attaching the responsibility to only one of the interlocutors, it is important that professionals become aware of their responsibility and change
their attitudes accordingly.

In a traditional sense, an attitude is 'positive or negative affective
reaction toward a denotable abstract or concrete object or proposition'
(Wrightsman, 1972, p. 216). In the present chapter, an attitude is understood as the disposition to use a set of strategies, which may or may not
enable the adult to teach and promote the acquisition of communication

skills. The attitude may be influenced and changed through training in intervention methodologies for supporting the development of communication and language. It was this form of attitude change that was the focus of the staff training project.

## Staff training

During 1991–1993, FENACERCI organised 22 courses addressing augmentative and alternative communication intervention. These courses, attended by 493 professionals, provided information about alternative communication systems and specific training in the use of PIC signs. However, in spite of the need for distributing information about different alternative communication systems and their utilisation, theoretical study and support for more effective intervention methodologies had emerged as more important priorities. It had been recognised that independently of the system used, the real challenge was the development of the individuals' communicative skills. According to reports from the instructors on the courses, a large number of the professionals who had attended them seemed to believe that the mere introduction of an alternative communication system would solve the children's communication difficulties. As a consequence of these reports, it was decided that more of the course time should be allocated to strategies for promoting communication functions in children with communication disorders, as well as to the skills the professionals themselves would need in order to be able to interact more efficiently with communication impaired individuals.

Due to these reflections, a project was initiated by FENACERCI, which focused on the following activities:

- Training of professionals to implement augmentative and alternative communication on the basis of an interactionist perspective.
- Investigations of methodologies aimed at improving the acquisition of communicative skills.
- Development of means for improving the communication abilities of people with intellectual and/or motor impairment and severe communication problems, with particular emphasis on the interaction strategies of professionals.

Twenty-two professionals (aged 30–55 years) from different parts of Portugal were invited to participate in the project, including five psychologists, seven teachers, four special teachers, five speech therapists and one occupational therapist. They represented varying degrees of experience in implementing augmentative and alternative communication intervention.

In the first phase of the project, from January to July 1993, the professionals involved received theoretical and practical training. This covered language and communication development from an interactionist perspective; augmentative and alternative communication systems; assessment of persons with intellectual and motor impairment; intervention strategies; and technical aids as auxiliary communication resources. This phase consisted of reading assignments directed by questions given by the instructor, production of written essays about theoretical issues, and seminars for analysing and discussing theoretical and practical issues related to each topic.

The second phase of the project, from September 1993 to July 1994, consisted of practical intervention work. Children and adolescents with communication problems appropriate for the purpose of the project were selected, and pairs of professionals from the same institution were responsible for each case. Initially, each individual was described with particular emphasis on communication skills, followed by a more comprehensive assessment, upon which an individual intervention plan was produced.

The intervention carried out by the professionals was regularly recorded on videotape (20–30 minutes every month) and shown at supervision meetings. The analyses of the video recordings focused on both the progress made by the child or adolescent and the achievements made by the professionals. These took place in individual sessions or small discussion groups with the supervisor every second month. The aims of the supervision sessions were to encourage the initiatives of the professionals and promote changes in their attitudes, particularly with regard to their own interaction strategies. In spite of the fact that they had participated in the training seminars and discussed the importance of their attitudes for the interaction, the video recordings did not bear evidence of much change in their behaviour. The professionals were not able to actually demonstrate their knowledge during the first sessions with the children and adolescents. This fact led to the conclusion that the behaviour of the professionals would have to be given priority in order to achieve adequate communicative interaction.

At the end of the training phase of the project, an evaluation of the work was carried out, based on analyses of video recordings and a questionnaire designed to elicit the professionals' opinions regarding augmentative and alternative communication intervention, and changes in their attitudes and communicative behaviours after the initiation of the project. The following areas were addressed in the evaluation:

- Assessment related to communication intervention.
- Adaptation of language used by the professionals to the characteristics of the disabled individuals.
- The role of interaction strategies in the development of intervention plans.

- Functional adaptation of augmentative and alternative communication use to different contexts.
- Organisation of space and location of materials in order to optimise communicative interaction.
- Planning of activities that may advance the development of communicative functions.

In addition, the professionals were asked how they perceived eventual changes in attitudes as a result of the project, and the nature of the most significative change they felt had occurred in their own communicative behaviour during their intervention project.

## Changes in attitudes

Some of the changes in the professionals' behaviours and attitudes were related to attempts to adapt the language to the individual characteristics of the disabled person:

*'I started to become aware of all the attempts, ways and possibilities used by the girl to communicate, allowing her time to take her turn, avoiding a situation where her every effort ended with the frustration of being misunderstood'.*

*'The most important factor was the development of my skills as an interlocutor. I learned to observe, to be attentive and to react better to the child's behaviour. I started to adapt my speech to my communication partner'.*

The professionals seemed to have understood that if the children's expressions even when atypical, were attributed meaning and replied to, communication could be fostered. Other changes concerned their promotion of developing communication skills, particularly with regard to acquisition of communicative functions:

*'There were lots of changes. Through the strategies I acquired, I became able to improve the communicative skills of the adolescent. Before this, I had essentially taught him how to use the system and the vocabulary. After the introduction of some interaction strategies, he learned and started to use communicative functions like initiating a dialogue, changing the topic, and finishing the conversation'.*

In a video sequence, a teacher was talking with an 18-year-old boy with Down syndrome, augmenting the speech with the use of PIC and manual signs. Both were sitting at a table, and the teacher started the dialogue by asking the boy about his participation in a programme on the local radio station. The boy gave short answers and changed the topic saying that he had been to see the physician, who had said that the boy had to wear glasses. The teacher said that she also had to wear glasses, and that she thought the boy would enjoy doing so. However, the boy concluded the conversation saying that he was unhappy with the glasses. In order to make the dialogue a motivating and gratifying activity for the boy, the teacher gave him the opportunity to take the initiative and chose the subject, and maintained the interaction by following his suggestions.

*'Before, when working with this child, I confused the teaching of graphic signs with the need for developing communicative functions. I thought that teaching the graphic signs would, by itself, improve his communicative abilities'.*

By taking the boy's abilities and interests as a starting point, the teacher found that she introduced more relevant elements into the conversation; and by considering graphic or manual signs as words, she found that the boy's acquisition of communicative skills, in terms of both content and function, was enhanced.

Another topic concerned the structuring of contexts and the organisation of the classroom and materials, an attempt being made to achieve optimal conditions for interaction and thereby stimulate the development of communication.

*'The space of the classroom was re-organised and the materials tagged with graphic signs in order to improve the communicative interaction'.*

In a video sequence, a speech therapist was working with a 7-year-old boy with intellectual impairment. All the cupboards and shelves in the room were tagged with PIC signs denoting their content, and the objects were placed in a way that made them accessible to the child. The boy chose activities by pointing to the appropriate graphic signs. When he chose to look in a book, he pointed first to *BOOK* and then to the shelf where the books were located. The speech therapist articulated his choice and helped him to take the book from the shelf. They then sat down at the table, looked at the book and communicated about it.

*'Before participating in the project, I chose the graphic signs without taking into account the different contexts of the child's everyday life; they were essentially centred on use in the class-*

*room. Afterwards, I have tried to expand their usage to all parts of the school, giving special attention to peer groups, and the home environment'.*

In a video sequence, a teacher was talking with a 12-year-old boy with Coffin-Lowry syndrome, augmenting her speech with written words and manual signs. The boy had just arrived at school and was showing the teacher the messages in the book used for communication between home and school. The teacher then involved a girl from the boy's class in the conversation. They talked about a trip they had made the week before. During the conversation the boy tried to interact with the girl with the help of the teacher. In order to enable the girl to communicate more efficiently, the boy reproduced the strategies the teacher had used with him, introduced manual signs, helped her with the ones she had started to use, and attempted to clarify her spoken messages.

The professionals' change in attitudes became apparent in their expectations of the communicative abilities of the children and adolescents:

*'To study the theoretical background and the research on intervention methodologies was essential for me in order to understand the disabled child. It made me regard and treat the child in a totally different way'.*

*'I felt less anxious in my relationship with the child; better knowledge of its abilities raised my expectations'.*

The professionals expressed the view that they had come to deal with the children in a different way, more accurately and with a higher level of communicative interaction. The professionals remarked that they had felt uncertain about what to do when they had to deal with children who had profound difficulties in expressing themselves. When they had been taught how to react and foresee the responses of the children, they had become more confident. Knowledge had reduced their anxiety.

The changes in attitudes were also reflected in a greater flexibility, with more effort directed at obtaining symmetry in turn-taking during conversations:

*'Before the project, I thought that difficulties and abilities lay only with the children. So there was not always a comparability between what I expected from the boy and what he was able to produce. During the project, I think I have changed my behaviour. I have started believing that the boy has specific abilities and that the adult has an important role in achieving synchrony and turn-taking'.*

In a video sequence, a speech therapist was working with an 8-year-old boy with Down syndrome. They were sitting at a table talking with the aid of PIC and manual signs. The boy told the teacher that he had had his hair cut and who had cut it. In the interaction, the boy was given opportunities for taking his turn. The teacher and the boy both attempted to simultaneously use speech and manual and graphic signs for expressing themselves, and for clarifying what they were communicating to each other.

*'I learned to wait, speak less, and attribute meaning to the initiatives of the child'.*

In a video sequence, a teacher and a 9-year-old boy with Down syndrome were sitting at a table, talking with the support of manual signs about pictures of the boy in different everyday situations, which had been taken by the teacher and organised into a book to be used in conversations. The teacher stopped talking for short periods, so that the boy might feel a need for communicating, encouraging him to initiate and maintain the interaction. The participation of the boy was also stimulated by the teacher beginning a sentence without finishing it, leaving it to the boy to complete it with a spoken word or a manual sign.

Awareness of the significance of their own roles as interlocutors was particularly apparent in the professionals' comments on the strategies they used in the interactions:

*'Through the effort of incorporating effectively the strategies in my intervention, I became aware of my own role as an interlocutor and of its significance for developing communication skills'.*

*'My intervention ceased to be a pure intuitive adaptation to the child's communicative performance, and became a deliberate application of adequate strategies for developing optimal communication abilities for the child'.*

To sum up, the explicit instruction in interaction strategies seemed to enable the teachers to use them in a natural manner and to develop positive attitudes towards the children. The implicit strategies reported by Rondal (1988a and b) and Moerk (1988) to support communication and lead to acquisition of language did not seem to develop spontaneously. Neither did intuitive adaptation to the children's characteristics appear. The communication partners had to learn how to use appropriate strategies in order to be able to interact in an adequate manner.

The opinions expressed by the professionals about the changes that occurred in their communicative interaction with the disabled children and adolescents as a result of their participation in the project were fully corroborated by their behaviour in the video recorded sessions of the last phase of the project. The results indicate that the professionals' development of communicative skills led to greater confidence in their intervention. Increased attention by the professionals to the signals of the children and adolescents made them attribute more intent and meaning to these signals. Having learned that it was not necessary to wait for the development of prerequisite skills before implementing alternative language modes increased the professionals' promotion of communication intervention. Finally, they had recognised that the difficulties of the communicative interactions did not rest only with the disabled individuals, but often came from the professionals themselves, or from other interlocutors.

## Conclusions

Several factors that may influence the development of effective interaction in communication had been identified in the staff courses held before the present project. Most important was the recognition of the fact that implementation of augmentative and alternative communication is not a matter of merely providing communication systems and aids, but of integrating this with an understanding of language development and the consequences of the altered communication processes. More critical than teaching particular language forms or a vocal or non-vocal code was teaching the children and adolescents to communicate, providing them with strategic actions which permitted them to operate in everyday contexts.

In the training project, priority was given to creating functional communication. The training course made the professionals more aware of the practical realities and alerted them to the fact that difficulties in the communication process do not rest solely with the individuals with language problems, but also with their interlocutors. When professionals, as part of the project, were taught to take the factors mentioned above into account, there was a positive effect on the acquisition and development of communication and language of the individuals with motor and intellectual impairment.

As a result of the training project, a network of professionals from different regions of the country has been established, enabling a dissemination of knowledge to the staff of their institutions, as well as to other professionals in the area. In the present project, parental involvement was not an explicit goal. The rationale for this was that it would be necessary to let professionals gain the necessary confidence in working with this kind of intervention before they would be prepared for collaboration with families. It is not known whether this is, in fact, the case and whether such a precaution was necessary. In any case, a closer relationship with families and the extension of augmentative and alternative communication intervention to other natural contexts are the next steps in the process.

## Acknowledgement

This chapter is a result of the participation in the project 'Alternative language and new technology in the promotion of integration', a collaborative venture of the National Federation of Cooperatives for the Education and Rehabilitation of People with Intellectual Impairment and the Calouste Gulbenkian Cerebral Palsy Rehabilitation Centre. We would like to thank Carmen Duarte and Emili Soro-Camats for their constructive ideas and suggestions regarding the project and this chapter.

# Chapter 21
# Some psychological and psychosocial aspects of introducing augmentative and alternative communication in Hungary: Tales, facts and numbers

SOPHIA L. KALMAN AND ANDRAS PAJOR

For intervention to be useful, it has to be applied with the appropriate clinical groups. However, new intervention approaches may meet considerable resistance from professionals, users and authorities, in particular if such approaches impact on fundamental aspects of daily life, such as language and communication. They will also usually be crucially influenced by local cultural conditions. The history of the introduction of augmentative and alternative communication in Hungary was probably similar to that in many other countries. However, changes – and the introduction of a new discipline is a real change – are always influenced by local conditions, history, complexity and individual commitment (Gale and Grant, 1990). In Hungary, the latter was particularly important because the process was based almost exclusively on personal interest and dedication rather than on official recognition of the need for these new approaches to communication intervention.

## Background

In 1981, the authors (a paediatrician and a psychologist) had two clients without functional speech, one with cerebral palsy and developmental delay and the other with autistic behaviour. The lack of communication was disturbing and depressing for everybody involved: therapists, families

355

and teachers. On the basis of some vague information, while on a visit to Canada in 1983, the authors made contact with the Blissymbolics Communication Institute in Toronto. The first author attended an elementary training course in the use of Blissymbols and in 1985 an advanced course. This was the start of augmentative and alternative communication in Hungary and also the reason why Blissymbols, until recently, was the sole focus of the field in Hungary.

Dissemination of information, consultation, publications, teaching and training have been organised and supported by the Hungarian Bliss Foundation, founded in 1987. In 1993, the Foundation opened the Helping Communication Methodological Centre, probably the first of its type in Eastern or Central-Eastern Europe. The programme of the Centre features teaching, training and dissemination of information. It also provides family and individual counselling, psychotherapy, assessment and social programmes, as well as opportunities for research.

From January 1993, when the regular diagnostic programme was opened, to June 1995, 160 assessments related to augmentative and alternative communication have been carried out at the Centre. During this period, 28 students have attended the Centre for shorter or longer periods (range 6 weeks to two years). Their average age was 12 years (range 2;6–30). Sixteen of them had cerebral palsy, four had an acquired disease of the central nervous system, three exhibited severe behaviour problems with autistic symptoms, and two had intellectual impairment of unknown origin. One student had multiple impairments caused by a car accident, one had a genetic disorder, and one student had multiple impairments due to complications related to extremely low birth weight. Nineteen of the students had normal intellectual abilities, four showed moderate and five severe intellectual impairment.

Four students (three with behaviour problems and one with Reye syndrome) did not use any form of alternative communication system. The others used different combinations of speech, letters, Blissymbols, pictures and objects. Four used manual signs as well. At present, there is only one student, a boy with athetoid cerebral palsy, who is using Blissymbols exclusively for communication. In 1995, 22 students were attending the Centre and there was a long waiting list.

Between 1983 and 1993, six persons collaborated on introducing augmentative and alternative communication on a volunteer basis, working in 'borrowed time', meaning time outside ordinary working hours and regular work settings. The process has been entirely dependent on the trainers' and trainees' dedication and enthusiasm, but the commitment and energy proved communicable and contagious. Today, the Centre has a paid staff of 14 members, twelve of them on a part time basis. During 1993–1995, the staff gave 30 lectures, seminars, presentations, etc, eight of them at international meetings. The Centre, however, has no permanent financing.

# Characteristics of the introduction of augmentative and alternative communication in Hungary

Despite the similarities with other countries introducing augmentative and alternative communication, the definitive cut-off between East and West resulted in marked differences from the earliest stages. Instead of official help and opportunities, personal ties and contacts, informal support, individual likes and dislikes, and information acquired through unofficial channels provided the basis for building a nation-wide network of teachers and different therapists. Today, one can hardly find a part of the country without somebody in the area who either has attended a full course, or has heard about augmentative communication through some other channel. Official recognition, however, at least in the form of moral support, did not arrive until the early nineties, and alternative communication intervention is still not considered as a part of habilitation and rehabilitation programmes. It is not financed by the national health insurance system, nor by any of the educational or health authorities.

The root of this still existing 'outlaw' situation of augmentative and alternative communication in Hungary may be found in general attitudes toward disability, sociological issues and the possibilities of communication aid technology in a former Soviet bloc country.

## General attitude toward disability

Socialism had several characteristic features in Hungary. One of them was to present only success, hiding problems and the darker sides of life. Living in this society meant that one had new factories and aeroplanes, and a tremendous breakthrough in agriculture and space science every other week, but people were not allowed to learn about problems like alcoholism, battered women, child abuse and drug addiction. In Hungary there were no beggars or homeless people in the streets, and unemployment was unknown. Deviant youngsters, psychiatric patients, old, demented and disabled people, and the other 'wastes' of life were not fit for the society to confront, and they were therefore kept in large institutions run by the state. These institutions were situated outside the big cities, for example in old castles, confiscated after the Second World War and absolutely unfit for this purpose. These residential settings were securely hidden behind beautiful parks, at the end of tiny little villages, or sometimes in the middle of nowhere.

The residents were more or less well cared for, well fed, regularly seen by doctors and nurses, properly medicated, and sometimes they even received some forms of intervention. The more serious their disability, the more hidden they were. Strolling in the streets of the big cities one would never see a severely disabled person. Children with well defined but single problems, such as deafness, blindness, motor impairment or intellectual impairment, had not only the right, but also the plight, of attending fairly good schools, designed especially for them. However, they would never meet peers without disabilities. Integration, even in the most remote sense of the word, was unknown and undesired. This tendency was reinforced by the fact that in Hungary segregated special schools had a 200-year-old history and that the training of special teachers was the monopoly of an independent, separate college, founded at the turn of the century, still not belonging to a university.

The tradition of keeping society in ignorance with regard to disability and its consequences and making decisions about disabled people without involving them in these decisions, meant a major obstacle for the spreading of alternative forms of communication in the country. One significant reason may have been that augmentative and alternative communication has important messages for the person and the society at large. For the person these messages imply self-worth and importance: 'You are important for us. You are a worthy person in your own right. We trust that you have the strength and ability to express your wishes about your own life'. For the society the message has a corresponding content: 'This is a person with thoughts, emotions and wishes like everybody else, who should be entitled to express himself in any way possible'. Promotion of learned dependency, ignorance, and authoritarian decisions stood on one side; independence, information, and freedom of choice on the other. As long as a disabled person was expected to accept what was provided for him, there was no need for augmentative and alternative communication.

In sum, augmentative and alternative communication was not simply another intervention approach or discipline to be introduced to enrich the field of habilitation and rehabilitation. With its emphasis on the individual's needs and rights, it proved at the same time to be a tool in the efforts for providing human rights for people with disabilities.

### Problems in service delivery

As already mentioned, in Hungary most severely and profoundly impaired people have been living in secluded residential institutions, even though recently their number has decreased somewhat, particularly for adults. In 1985, 5028 children and adolescents and 8198 adults were living in residential institutions. In 1994, the corresponding figures were reduced to 4632 and 2142 (Háztartásstatisztika 1985; Magyar Statisztikai Zsebkönyv 1994).

The fact that disabled people were not part of everyday life had some logical consequences. One of them was that, generally speaking, people were not accustomed to having people with disabilities in their surroundings. Teenagers in wheelchairs did not visit movies, swimming pools and ice cream parlours. Even if they had wanted to, it would not have been possible because of inaccessible buildings, poor quality wheelchairs, high kerbs, etc. Generations of children grew up without ever having met a blind, deaf, intellectually impaired or motor impaired peer. Without personal experiences, the necessary knowledge, empathy, acceptance and tolerance could not become part of their thinking. Most people never thought about a disabled individual as a person, demonstrated by the fact that they tended to call disabled people according to their impairment: 'this Down', 'that dummy', 'the limper', 'little bunny' (a child with cheilo-schisis), etc.

Another consequence of the fact that people with disabilities were not part of society was misconceptions about their lives in residential institutions. The institutions were not open to the public. There was often only one visit per month, restricted to close relatives and taking place in a designated area of the building. Sometimes the relatives were not allowed to see where the resident was sleeping, eating or playing. Accordingly, the general public had only vague ideas about life in institutions. They never heard about the impersonal and emotionally inadequate care provided by busy, overworked and sometimes untrained personnel for the hundreds of residents. They never learned about the emptiness of long, uniform and senseless days. Since they knew no better, most people were convinced that institutions were the only and best solution for the disabled people. 'What more could they want? They were fed, got heating, clean clothing, television and medical attention. What could be better for the poor souls?' Thus people fully accepted the choice of sending a relative to live in a residential setting for life.

A third consequence was the almost total lack of family support systems. Since most families chose to have disabled relatives in institutions, the necessary social network (home care services, relief or crisis intervention centres, etc.) had not yet been woven. If a family decided to keep its disabled member at home, it was regarded with suspicion and awe, and often the question was posed why they chose to destroy their own lives. Moreover, many families' economy was based on two salaries and if the mother stayed at home to care for the disabled person, the father had to work 12–15 hours per day to maintain the income. He lost touch with his children and the trivialities of everyday life. He would only rarely take part in the disabled member's care. Without any relief service or outside help, the mother might get burned out in a few years. The world was hostile: there were stairs everywhere, it was difficult to get on and off the buses, people stared if the child was drooling, etc. The family was outcast, people tended neither to invite nor visit them. The national health insurance system provided for only the most basic aids and parents could not afford expensive new services or Western products.

They thus became financially wasted, emotionally exhausted and socially impossible.

The situation may not have changed much. During 1993–1995, eighty-three parents filled out a questionnaire while attending the Centre for an assessment of their multiply impaired child with severe communication difficulties. These showed that 65 per cent of the fathers held a job outside their homes, compared to 27 per cent of the mothers. In Hungary, the employment rate is usually the same for men and women. Four per cent of the fathers stated that they spent all hours of the day with the disabled child, while 34 per cent of the mothers were in this situation. Most of the parents judged their own health to be average, but four per cent of the fathers and 19 per cent of the mothers thought that they had health problems as a result of their continuous care of the child. Future research will determine how the situation of parents with disabled children in Hungary differs from that of the population in general.

There are thus two typical situations. In the first, the disabled person lives in a residential setting run by the state, the municipality or some newly established private service provider and the rest of the family leads a separate life at home. In the second, the family keeps the disabled member at home and tries to survive under tremendous pressure.

Within this context, in spite of professional curiosity and recognition of the need for augmentative and alternative communication, it has been difficult to achieve acceptance by institutions and families. Professionals in the institutions argued that if there were no alternatives to the usual daily routine, the person did not need a communication tool. In the families, with their many financial, social and emotional problems, alternative communication systems came last on the list of priorities. They thought it was best to stick to the daily routines and do whatever was necessary as fast as possible. A communication board would only delay things. The families were simply reflecting the attitudes of society: it might be inconvenient if people with disabilities learned to express their needs and wants.

To sum up, until the nineties, the formerly prevalent attitude toward disabled persons and the general acceptance of residential care as the only practical solution for people needing continuous care had been working against a more widespread use of augmentative and alternative communication in Hungary.

## Technical opportunities

The East European countries still have lower standards of technology than most Western countries. Technology, especially technical goods of high quality, has not been part of everyday life in Hungary. A washing machine, a refrigerator, a radio, a black and white television and maybe a video player or a tape recorder comprise the average technical household equipment. The proportion of households who had a car increased from eight per cent in 1984 to 38 per cent in 1993. In 1980, there were 1272 computers in the whole country, while in 1994 the number had increased to 223140 computers, including six per cent of households (Háztartásstatisztika 1985; Magyar Statisztikai Zsebkönyv 1994). In 1983, when communication aids were first introduced, we even had problems finding photocopying machines and it was not until 1990 that the Bliss Foundation got a fax machine.

In Hungary people did not usually have a telephone. They had to wait eight to ten years, sometimes even longer, to get a phone. Communication was one way. Practically everybody had radio, television and newspapers, media controlled and censured carefully by those in power, but it was not felt important to ensure other channels of communication. This was also reflected in the fact that provision of better communication opportunities for disabled people was not among the favoured projects of the authorities. Technology for habilitation and rehabilitation had even lower standards, because through many decades the emphasis had been only on acute care. Institutions and technology for habilitation and rehabilitation were not properly supported and developed and hardly mentioned in the Hungarian medical textbooks. A few state-run companies produced various aids and tools, but there was such a huge need even for their poorest products that they were not motivated to improve their quality. High-technology aids have arrived only recently and have not yet become part of the education. Most teachers and interventionists have not been trained to use a computer and even young special education teachers may never have heard about high-technology communication aids and other types of electronic aids.

Until 1989, the group who had been introducing alternative communication systems in Hungary did not have a single high-technology aid. A scanning device with voice output, called *Augmentor*, has been developed, as well as two Hungarian-speaking programmes for IBM compatible computers; one based on Blissymbols, *Blissvox*, the other using the alphabet, *BlissABC* (Olaszy, Kalman and Olaszi, 1994). The Blissvox programme functions so that correct Hungarian sentences will be produced in synthetic speech, without regard to how 'telegraphic' or 'mosaic' the input of Blissymbols is. The group has also developed low-technology switches and toys. An educational programme, progressing from switch control to letter recognition, was developed during 1993–1995, and a test programme, simulating the Snijders-Oomen nonverbal intelligence test (Snijders, Tellegen and Laros, 1989) on an IBM compatible computer, is being prepared. In addition, as a result of generous help from a number of Western companies and agencies, the Centre is now in possession of several high-technology communication aids, as well as smaller electronic devices with digitised voice output, toys, switches and computer programmes.

In addition to the equipment of the Centre, three schools and institutions have received a few communication aids and some other technical equipment from Western donors. However, as a rule, acceptable and affordable communication aids are not part of Hungarian communication intervention programmes.

# How is it possible to overcome insurmountable obstacles?

When starting up in the eighties, it soon became clear that because of the financial and social disadvantages, special means and ways had to be found for the introduction of augmentative and alternative communication. New skills had to be acquired, as well as new knowledge and several new techniques. We had to learn to be creative (finding the simplest solutions), co-operate in the broadest sense of the word (with suspicious colleagues, hostile authorities, parents in despair and unmotivated students), and concentrate on areas not requiring too sophisticated devices and much funding. We also had to learn how to create a foundation, organise a nation-wide organisation, and raise funding.

While trying to balance the disadvantages detailed above, the lack of skills and the effects of counter forces (like protection of territory and lack of will to change), it seemed advisable to tackle this major challenge as a series of 'small' steps: firstly, finding the people in need of augmentative and alternative communication; secondly, training teachers to help these people; and thirdly, and importantly, trying to reach out to the families. These three steps will be discussed below.

## The need for augmentative and alternative communication intervention in Hungary

It was assumed that if the people who were in need of augmentative and alternative communication were found, the professionals working with them would be found as well. These professionals had to be the best candidates for training courses. However, as in most other countries, no statistics were available in Hungary about this kind of need. In the statistics, people without the ability to speak were included in categories like 'cerebral palsy', 'brain damage', 'Little disease', 'oligophrenia', etc.

In 1988–1989, a nation-wide survey of people with severe speech disorders was made (Kalman, 1989). Since at that time practically no people with severe and profound disabilities were living at home, the survey concentrated on residential settings only. The questionnaire used was compiled and distributed on the basis of representative information about institutions, gathered during 1985–1987. One hundred and eighty-one residential institutions were approached. In 107 of them, residents were adults who were either severely intellectually impaired or had other severe behaviour problems (schizophrenia, dementia of different etiologies, e.g. Korsakoff or Alzheimer disease, etc.). In 42 institutions the residents were severely multiply impaired children. The 32 remaining institutions were boarding schools and other residential settings for students with various disabilities.

Eighty-eight questionnaires (48.6%) were returned, of which 77 (42.5%) could be analysed. The information collected concerned 6728 residents, among them 1576 persons (23.4%) without functional speech. This would comprise 0.06 per cent of the population. According to this estimate, Hungary, with a population of ten million people, has 6000 people with unmet needs for alternative communication intervention. This number did not include hearing impaired people because they had their own schools and institutions, which were not part of this survey. Moreover, since at the time of the survey only psychiatrists used the diagnosis of autism, and children with autistic symptoms were generally considered psychiatric patients without specific descriptions of the nature of their problems, their number remained unknown as well. We did not get information about people with other acquired communication disorders like aphasia and laryngectomy, because people with these types of problems were not usually sent to institutions and the survey addressed residential settings only.

If the many problems of gathering information are taken into consideration – there was no information from families at all; 52 per cent of the questionnaires were not returned; there were substantiated suspicions about the credibility of some of the information, etc. – the estimate of 6000 people without functional speech may be rather low.

## Increasing awareness and disseminating knowledge

The first Hungarian training course in Blissymbolics was held in Budapest in October 1984. From then on, 2–4 three-day-long Blissymbolics courses have been held every year. They were attended by teachers, speech and language therapists, teachers trained in 'conductive' education (cf. Hári and Ákos, 1988), other professionals and parents, generally 20–30 people per course. In 1990, it became necessary to broaden the scope of the courses. The disadvantages of having Blissymbolics as the only alternative communication system with organised courses and available teaching material had become apparent. People had started to think about alternative communication as Blissymbolics only. When it turned out that it was not appropriate for everybody, many teachers became disappointed and gave up the efforts for their students. The almost exclusive insistence on Blissymbolics for such a long time was based on several practical reasons. The major reason was the scarcity of knowledge about other available methods. Another reason was the strong opposition, from parents and teachers alike, against using means other than speech or writing for communication. For forty years it was prohibited to teach or practise sign language for deaf children, and neither this nor any other manual sign system was part of the teachers' training. The teachers themselves convinced parents about the irredeemable consequences of using anything but speech or traditional orthography. Therefore, whenever we failed using Blissymbols, instead of adopting another, more feasible system, such as manual signs, pictographic systems or pictures, we had to start the explanations all over again.

A new and more comprehensive course was introduced in 1992, lasting six days (one day weekly for six weeks). In addition, there is now an information course for parents because the general course was considered too long and professional for them. In 1988, augmentative and alternative communication became a faculty subject, optional for students majoring in speech and language therapy at the Barczy Gusztav Teachers' Training College for Special Education in Budapest. As part of a curriculum reform in 1995, augmentative and alternative communication became part of the regular programme of some college departments. Practically all students have to attend at least one informative lecture during their college education.

Over the period 1984–1995, a total of 555 participants have attended training courses. Fifty per cent were special education teachers (85 per cent of them speech and language therapists), eleven per cent were college students, eleven per cent were primary care workers, eleven per cent were parents, nine per cent were 'conductors', seven per cent were nurses, and linguists, sociologists, and psychologists made up one per cent.

**Fostering attitudes**

Considering the local conditions and the prevalent educational attitudes, it seemed necessary not only to teach communication intervention but to convey some of the underlying messages as well. The aim was that the trainees should not only learn about augmentative and alternative communication, but also feel and experience the need for it. We wanted to deal with the psychological aspects of teaching students without functional speech. As soon as the individual's needs and personal characteristics take a leading role in the curriculum, the teacher's personality becomes of primary importance (Brocher, 1975). The unusual difficulties of communicating with a person without functional speech, such as the frequent misunderstandings and tiring find-out-what-I-think games, and the modified and sometimes distorted human relations and forms of communication, also made it imperative to deal with the teachers' special situations.

Since one's own experiences may leave a deeper impression than explanations addressed at the intellectual level only, the psychotherapeutic approach seemed appropriate to address these aims. An empathy-increasing experience group programme has been developed and made an inherent part of the training course in augmentative and alternative communication (Kalman and Pajor, 1987, 1989). The programme lasts four hours and uses carefully selected elements of different psychotherapeutic methods: free verbal interaction, sensitivity training, T-groups, encounter groups and psychodrama. It is goal oriented and thematic, and employs non-verbal elements for enhancing the intensity of the experience. The method belongs to the set of T-groups, Balint groups and encounter groups; in all of these, group methods are used as tools for general behaviour change.

The course was structured according to a series of different exercises, each introduced verbally by a therapist. Verbal and non-verbal exercises were offered in turn and the therapists emphasised the requirement that there should be no use of speech, except during the verbal practices and the discussions. Role playing was an important element. The participants worked in pairs, alternating between the role of a helper and that of a person with communication difficulties. Group sessions were followed by discussions of games presented, problems, topics, significant events, etc. Video recording was used occasionally, but considering the intimacies and emotional turmoil that sometimes occurred during sessions, no outside observer or video recording was allowed.

While the sessions followed a usual group pattern (cf. Hidas, 1984; Lewin, 1935, 1948; Liebermann, 1977), some modifications evolved. The warm-up period was rather short and during the busy work period, typical forms of resistance could be felt. Instead of discussing events and feelings related to the present situation, the trainees complained about their everyday struggles, or turned the group session into a case conference and asked for the therapists' advice about the communication problems of one of their students. The closing period also tended to be longer than expected, since the programme is a one-time event and the attachment-detachment circle must be closed within the given time frame.

The group sessions showed considerable similarities both in their dynamics and in the discoveries the participants made for themselves and formulated verbally at the end of the sessions. For many of the trainees, the most difficult experience encountered had been the glimpse of the 'other' side. Whilst it was simply in the form of a game, under artificial circumstances and for a little while only, the trainees still got a feeling of not being able to express themselves freely and the frustration related to this. They also had to face their own feelings while playing the role of the helper. The insight that followed from this was that living and working with a person who is incapable of verbal expression is emotionally overwhelming, and sometimes equally frustrating for both parties. Another recognition concerned the communication themes of the person without functional speech, which showed much greater variety than was expected by anybody. No matter how trivial this might sound, this recognition was a significant step in the process of gaining insight into the overall problems of a person without speech. The third discovery concerned the mirroring of the participants as they saw themselves as helpers. The picture in the mirror showed overprotective, arrogant and impatient professionals, posing rattling questions without providing the slightest chance for an answer. They recognised this one-way street, into which the person without sufficient communication was forced to retreat.

No evaluation has been made of the long-term effects of this group programme. However, in 1993, fifty teachers and speech therapists who had attended training courses in 1988–1992 were approached. Most of them remembered it as a useful experience, some stating that as a consequence of its deep influence, they definitely had changed their style of work. For almost half of them, it had been an unforgettable experience, and many would have wanted to share it with their colleagues as well. Some, however, felt it was a bad and unpleasant experience, and a few stated that the whole programme left them unaffected.

To sum up, it is our belief that the programme for increasing empathy and awareness has played an important part in the process of introducing augmentative and alternative communication in Hungary. This issue was emphasised, because we were convinced that no matter how technically or financially well off a country might be, the human side was still the most important factor. This, or a similar programme may be useful in other countries where a change of attitude seems to be desirable paralleling the introduction of new communication systems.

### Reaching out to families

From the earliest stage, parent involvement was also emphasised. This was an unusual approach in the eighties, and the teachers and speech and language therapists were sometimes quite surprised to meet parents at the training course. In acknowledgement of the new problems parents had to face after the positive but difficult changes of 1989, and the need for partners in implementing augmentative and alternative communication in the homes, a support-group programme was introduced in 1993 for parents with children at the Centre in Budapest. This free verbal interaction group was open and conducted in a semi-directed way by experienced psychotherapists.

One to six mothers participated in each group. With a few exceptions, fathers were not willing to participate. The themes discussed in the group sessions were generally the same as described in the literature; practical difficulties of everyday life, loss of self esteem, reconsideration of one's life goals, guilt, pain, permanent grief, etc. (cf. Noland, 1970; Paul, 1983). However, it was notable that these parents felt very lonely and deserted by society. They suffered because their child and their lives were so different from the 'norm'. Nearly all of them felt physically and emotionally drained. In the course of the group, two distinct types of maternal behaviour could be recognised: the young child's enthusiastic, ambitious, and overactive, almost 'agitated', mother; and the overtired, bitter and frustrated mother of the teenagers and young adults.

When the therapeutic group programme was started, the aim was to find intervention partners among the parents. As the group has developed, a new aim has appeared: to provide parents with support in both their own inner struggles and those of everyday life. It should be emphasised that the organisation of a support group for parents is not necessarily part of every communication training programme. In some circumstances it seemed necessary, because results could not be achieved without the effective cooperation of the family.

# Why is it not working?

Despite all the strenuous efforts directed at implementing augmentative and alternative communication over the years, desired results at the clinical level have not been reached. There may be at least two possible reasons for this. The first is related to the surprising discrepancy between the high number of trained teachers and the extremely low number of users. The question was why the teachers did not implement their expertise. The other possible cause for the failure was the poor co-operation between parents and professionals. In 1992, recognition of these issues led us to focus on the difficult problem of co-operation between parents and professionals.

### Why do teachers not teach?

There has always been a remarkable discrepancy between the high number of trained professionals and the fairly low number of students in actual programmes for alternative and augmentative communication. Therefore in 1989, 161 teachers who had attended Blissymbolics elementary training courses between 1984 and 1988 were asked about their teaching experience (Kalman, 1989). The answers showed that 59 per cent had never even attempted to apply their knowledge, and only 20 per cent worked regularly with one or more students without functional speech. There was hardly any difference between Budapest and other parts of the country. There were some minor differences with regard to workplace. Seventy-two per cent of those working in the health care system, 61 per cent of the primary child care workers, and 55 per cent of teachers in schools had never applied their knowledge.

The 95 former trainees who had never applied their knowledge professionally provided different reasons: for example 26 per cent had attended the training course out of personal interest with no desire to teach; 15 per cent had no direct contact with students or clients in their work; 13 per cent had either changed workplace or were assigned other duties; another 19 percent had personal reasons, eight per cent reported that their superiors did not give consent to augmentative communication programmes.

Sixty-six trainees had attempted to build up a communication programme, but in 1989 only 30 programmes had been continued. In one third of the cases, the programme was stopped because of the teacher's or speech and language therapist's personal reasons. In one quarter of the cases, there were other reasons, for example that the student was moved, the environment was against augmentative communication, use of Blissymbols was not adequate, or death or negatively progressing conditions made continuation impossible. In five cases, speech development made the programme redundant.

The ratio appears to be even worse today. We have knowledge of 30–35 teachers, 'conductors', therapists, etc. who are actually teaching or using augmentative and alternative communication methods. This is only 5–6 per cent of the professionals trained at the Centre.

The results are disturbing. There is no reason to doubt that most of the trainees had a positive and knowledgeable attitude towards communication and could easily have implemented and assisted local communication projects. Moreover, considering the human efforts, the costs of the training courses and the unmet needs for augmentative and alternative communication, a better result should have been achieved. The reasons reported for not teaching augmentative and alternative communication sometimes seemed quite trivial, except with regard to the limitations of the method used. They seem to call for more attention to selection of both trainees and students and the importance of the implementation strategies applied.

### Why are we not co-operating?

Within this field, success would mean well-worn communication charts used at every possible scene of the person's life – at school, in shops, in church, in swimming pools, etc. To achieve this, possibly because of lack of previous experience, was the goal of the group attempting to implement Blissymbolics in Hungary. But what happened was that parents brought their children to the Christmas party or anniversary celebration without the charts. They sent them to field trips and summer camps without communication boards. When asked about the use of the boards at home, except on rare occasions, a strong and convincing 'no' was usually the answer. 'We do not need it at home'. However, detailed interviews, home visits, discussions with the potential users and other family members proved that this was not really the case. The children appeared passive and dependent, surrounded by well-meaning, 'mind-reading' parents and grandparents, who consequently gave answers, thought and felt instead of the 'child' – who in some cases was 20–30 years old.

Thus the overwhelming lack of use of communication charts led to a change in approach. It was realised that, in many cases, the failure of the intervention was a result of the poor co-operation between parents and professionals. They talked *to* instead of *with* each other. The failures may have had several roots, but it seemed likely that the work had been made harder by the failure of the courses and the Centre to create a climate of real co-operation. Influenced by Gale and Grant (1990) it was recognised that knowing and understanding the context in which the desired change should have happened was essential, and our attention became focused on the sensitive relationship between parents and professionals. This attention might not seem fully relevant from the viewpoint of introducing augmentative and alternative communication in a country, but we wish to emphasise that it would not have been possible to implement augmentative and alternative communication through the ordinary educational channels within the context of traditional parent-professional interactions.

The complexity of the process also directed attention to the problems of parents of children who have chronic problems. These parents have a long-lasting relationship with the professional world (doctors, nurses, therapists, etc.) which may not be easy for either party. As has been frequently described, it may be very emotional, comprising anger, sympathy, hostility, frustration, love and hatred (Buscaglia, 1983). It may be like a sine wave, with ups and downs, and as a rule it is almost always asymmetric. It is our impression that there are three distinct phases in this relationship, related to the age of the child or the onset of the problem (see Table 21.1).

During the first phase, the child is usually young or the problem is new. The parents are full of hope, questions and doubts. Even though they are emotionally troubled, they want to try out everything and are willing to co-operate with enthusiastic helpers. In this period, a frequently overactive, emotionally hurt and imbalanced but trusting parent is the partner of a determined-to-help professional.

In the second phase the child is usually taking part in different interventions. The parents have already lost some hope and are confronted by the realities. Their life has been dramatically changed. They meet many controversial opinions and a future-oriented, sometimes superior,

Table 21.1 The disabled child, its parents and the professional: Changes in relationship over time

| Age of child and the characteristic problems of that age | Emotional state of the parents and their actual problems | The attitudes and ambitions of the professionals |
| --- | --- | --- |
| The young child is always `sweet' and helpless to the parents and other people. It is in need of constant protection. | Shock, pain, guilt, anger and high hopes. Discovery of disabled persons' world. Trust in professionals. Agitated shopping for opinions, and waiting for miracles to happen. | Almost aggressive diagnostic activity. Belief in the effectiveness of early intervention explains the therapeutic fervour. |
| The child is busy with education and diverse therapies. It slowly starts to realise that it is different from others, and learns to suffer as a consequence of this difference. | The parents are confronted with the realities. They are forced to give up their own life goals. Because of the many contradictory opinions, confidence in professionals is decreasing. | The initial fervour is already cooled by the realities. The professionals demand future-oriented hard work, but offer only small results in exchange. |
| Pressing questions concerning the future: love, marriage, work, independence? The security of the school years is gone. The future is bleak. | Total physical, emotional and financial exhaustion. Insecure future. The only goal is survival. There are no miracles, there is no use trying. | The professional's partners are the exhausted parents and the anxious young person. This therapeutic loneliness results in feelings of failure and frustration. |

professional attitude. At this point, not too trusting and disappointed parents and realistic professionals face each other.

The third phase is full of anxieties for the grown child, concerning independence, marriage, job, etc. The parents are bitter and exhausted, and have given up their last hopes. Their only concern is to provide a future for the child. They turn back to the original nurturing role and refuse to participate in any further intervention efforts. Frustrated professionals, on the other hand, finding no more challenge in the case, turn their attention towards younger children again.

If these impressions are correct, they might provide an explanation of frequently observed disharmonies between parents and professionals.

In order to explain and demonstrate the nature of the parent-professional relationship to teachers and parents, Berne's model of transactional analysis (Berne, 1961) was employed. Applying this model to the long term relationship between parents and professionals, we have found this relationship to be mostly unbalanced and asymmetric, based on 'games', according to Berne's use of this expression. Effective and mutually satisfactory co-operation can be expected only when, instead of games, real communication is taking place between parents and professionals, resulting in a well-balanced, symmetric relationship. However, in order to reach this symmetry, it is necessary that parents' involvement is based on sufficient information and understanding of the processes.

## Conclusions

It has been a challenge to introduce augmentative communication in a 'communication impaired' society, where communication blockages were the rule rather than the exception. Today, recognition of the new needs is present, even though the implementation of the necessary changes is hindered by old stereotypes and attitudes. All in all, in the last twelve years there has been a breakthrough in this area in Hungary. The 555 professionals who have participated in training courses and the hundreds of professionals who have attended informative lectures during the last three years, have created an opinion-forming power in the professional world. Articles published in popular magazines and references in radio and television programmes have added to the growing professional and public awareness of augmentative and alternative communication. Today, invitations to professional forums, symposia, meetings of disabled people's rights movement, etc. demonstrate that professionals working in the field of augmentative communication have become accepted partners in habilitation and rehabilitation work in Hungary. These are facts to treasure, but we are aware of the shortcomings as well. We still have a lot to learn, teaching strategies to refine, and implementation to improve, before those who need the services may get what they deserve.

## Acknowledgement

The chapter has been supported by the National Scientific Research Fund (OTKA), the National Committee for Technical Development (OMFB-MEC), the Mentalhygienic Board of the National Health Insurance, and the Public Education Funds of the Ministry for Education and Culture. The authors want to express their thanks to the many people who helped ease the introduction of augmentative and alternative communication in Hungary, in particular Shirley MacNaughton, Judy Wine and the late Karoly Galyas.

# References and Citation Index

Abbeduto, L., Furman, L. and Davies, B. (1989). Relation between receptive language and mental age of persons with mental retardation. American Journal on Mental Retardation 93: 535–543. **p.193.**

Abberley, P. (1987). The concept of oppression and the development of a social theory of disability. Disability, Handicap and Society 2: 5–19. **p.35.**

Abrahamsen, A.A., Lamb, M., Brown-Williams, J. and McCarthy, S. (1991). Boundary conditions on language emergence: Contributions from atypical learners and input. In P. Siple and S.D. Fischer (Eds.), Theoretical Issues in Sign Language Research. Volume 2: Psychology. Chicago: Chicago University Press, pp 231–254. **p.135, 215.**

Abrahamsen, A.A., Romski, M.A. and Sevcik, R. (1989). Concomitants of success in acquiring an augmentative communication system: Changes in attention, communication and sociability. American Journal on Mental Retardation 93: 475–496. **p.182.**

Adams, C. (1990). Syntactic comprehension in children with expressive language impairment. British Journal of Disorders of Communication 25: 149–171. **p.120.**

Albani, P. and Buonarotti, L. (1994). Aga Magera Difura. Dizionario delle lingue inesistenti (Aga Magera Difura. Vocabulary of Languages that Don't Exist). Bologna: Zanichelli. **p.185.**

Allen, W.H. (1975). Intellectual abilities and instructional media design. Audio Visual Communication Review 23: 139–170. **p.191.**

Alm, N., Arnott, J.L. and Newell, A.F. (1989). Discourse analysis and pragmatics in the design of a conversation prosthesis. Journal of Medical Engineering and Technology 13: 10–12. **pp.7, 179.**

Alm, N., Arnott, J.L. and Newell, A.F. (1992). Prediction and conversational momentum in an augmentative communication system. Communications of the ACM 35 (5): 46–57. **p.179.**

Alm, N., Brophy, B., Arnott, J.L. and Newell, A.F. (1988). Preliminary evaluation of a conversation aid based on speech acts. Presented at the Fifth International Conference of the International Society for Augmentative and Alternative Communication, Anaheim, California, October 1988. **p.179.**

Alm, N., Dye, R. and Harper, G. (1995). ALADIN – Advanced Language Device for Interaction. Proceedings of the Third European Conference on the Advancement of Rehabilitation Technology, Lisbon, October 1995. Lisbon: ECART. pp 150–151. **p.180.**

Alm, N., Nicol, M. and Arnott, J.L. (1993). The application of fuzzy set theory to the storage and retrieval of conversational texts in an augmentative communication system. In M. Binion (Ed.), Proceedings of RESNA 93, Washington, DC., June 1993. Washington, DC: The RESNA Press, pp 127–129. **p.180.**

Angelman, H. (1965). Puppet children. Developmental Medicine and Child Neurology 7: 681–687. **p.322.**

Anisfield, M. (1984). Language Development from Birth to Three. Hillsdale, New Jersey: Lawrence Erlbaum. **p.102.**

Anthony, A., Bogle, D., Ingram, T. and McIsaac, M. (1971). The Edinburgh Articulation Test. Edinburgh: Churchill Livingstone. **p.110.**

Archer, L.A. (1977). Blissymbolics – a non-verbal communication system. Journal of Speech and Hearing Disorders 42: 568–579. **p.189.**

Argyle, M. and Cook, M. (1976). Gaze and Mutual Gaze. Cambridge: Cambridge University Press. **p.50.**

Armstrong, D.F., Stokoe, W.C. and Wilcox, S.E. (1995). Gesture and the Nature of Language. Cambridge, UK: Cambridge University Press. **p.169.**

Arnott, J.L. (1990). The communication prosthesis: A problem of human-computer integration. Proceedings of ECART 1 – European Conference on the Advancement of Rehabilitation Technology, Maastricht, The Netherlands, November 1990. Hoensbroek, The Netherlands: ECART, pp 3.1.1–3.1.5. **p.181.**

Arthur, G. (1952). The Arthur Adaptation of the Leiter International Performance Scale. Washington: Psychological Service Center Press. **pp.235, 251.**

Arvio, M., Hautamäki, J. and Tiilikka, P. (1993). Reliability and validity of the Portage assessment scale for clinical studies of mentally handicapped populations. Child: Care, Health and Development 19: 89–98. **p.219.**

Atkinson, J. and Heritage, J. (Eds.) (1984). Structures of Social Action – Studies in Conversation Analysis. London: Cambridge University Press. **p.177.**

Atkinson, M. (1992). Children's Syntax: An Introduction to Principles and Parameter Theory. Oxford: Blackwell. **p.101.**

Aukrust, V.G. (1992). Fortellinger fra stellerommet. To-åringer i barnehage: En studie av språkbruk – innhold og struktur (Narratives from the nursing room. Two-year-olds in the preschool. A study of language use – content and structure). Dissertation, University of Oslo. **p.71.**

Austin, J.L. (1962). How to do Things with Words. Oxford: Clarendon Press. **p.179.**

Avent, J.R., Edwards, D.J., Franco, C.R. and Lucero, C.J. (1995). A verbal and non-verbal treatment comparison study in aphasia. Aphasiology 9: 295–303. **p.189.**

Azevedo, L. (1995). Assistive Technology Training. Brussels: The Commission of the European Communities. **p.344.**

Baker, B. (1982). Minspeak. Byte 7 (9): 186–202 **p.177.**

Baker, B. (1986). Using images to generate speech. Byte 11: 160–168. **p.6.**

Ballard, K.D. (1991). Assessment for early intervention: evaluating child development and learning in context. In D. Mitchell and R.I. Brown (Eds.), Early Intervention Studies for Young Children with Special Needs. London: Chapman and Hall, pp 127–159. **p.219.**

Baron-Cohen, S. (1989). Perceptual role taking and protodeclarative pointing in autism. British Journal of Developmental Psychology 7: 113–127. **p.52.**

Baron-Cohen, S. (1991). Precursors to a theory of mind: Understanding attention in others. In A. Whiten (Ed.), Natural Theories of Mind: Evolution, Development and Simulation of Everyday Mindreading. Oxford: Blackwell, pp 233–251. **p.53.**

Baron-Cohen, S. (1993). From attention-goal psychology to belief-desire psychology: The development of a theory of mind and its dysfunction. In S. Baron-Cohen, H. Tager-Flusberg and D. Cohen (Eds.), Understanding Other Minds: Perspectives from the Theory of Mind Hypothesis of Autism. Oxford: Oxford University Press, pp 59–82. **p.53.**

Baron-Cohen, S. (1995). Mindblindness: An Essay on Autism and Theory of Mind. Cambridge, Massachusetts: MIT Press. **p.55.**

Baron-Cohen, S. and Bolton, P. (1993). Autism: The Facts. Oxford: Oxford University Press .**p.56.**

Baron-Cohen, S., Leslie, A. M. and Frith, U. (1985). Does the autistic child have a 'theory of mind'? Cognition 21: 37–46. **p.53.**

Baron-Cohen, S., Tager-Flusberg, H. and Cohen, D.J. (Eds.) (1993). Understanding Other Minds. Oxford, UK: Oxford University Press. **p.265.**

Barthes, R. (1986). The Responsibility of Form: Critical Essays on Music, Art and Representation. Oxford, UK: Basil Blackwell. **p.191.**

Basil, C. (1992). Social interaction and learned helplessness in severely disabled children. Augmentative and Alternative Communication 8: 188–199, **pp.29, 68, 80, 87, 271, 310, 314, 346.**

Basil, C. (1994). Family involvement in the intervention process. In J. Brodin and E. Björck-Åkesson (Eds.), Methodological Issues in Research in Augmentative and Alternative Communication. Jönköping: Jönköping University Press, pp 89–95 **p.324.**

Basil, C. and Puig de la Bellacasa, R. (1988). Comunicación aumentativa (Augmentative Communication). Madrid: Inserso, **pp.312.313.**

Basso, A. (1981). Il paziente afasico. Guida pratica alla riabilitazione (The Aphasic Patient. A Practical Guide to Rehabilitation). Milano: Feltrinelli. **p.191.**

Basso, A. (1987). La riabilitazione del linguaggio (The Rehabilitation of Language). In A. Mazzucchi (Ed.), La riabilitazione neuropsicologica. Bologna: Il Mulino. pp 57–85. **p.191.**

Bates, E. (Ed.) (1979). The Emergence of Symbols: Cognition and Communication in Infancy. New York: Academic Press. **p.233.**

Bates, E. (1979). Intentions, conventions, and symbols. In E. Bates (Ed.), The Emergence of Symbols. Cognition and Communication in Infancy. New York: Academic Press, pp 33–42. **p.50.**

Bates, E., Bretherton, I. and Snyder, L. (1988). From First Words to Grammar: Individual Differences and Dissociable Mechanisms. Cambridge: Cambridge University Press. **pp.1, 102, 115, 119, 169.**

Bates, E., Camaioni, L. and Volterra, V. (1975). The acquisition of performatives prior to speech. Merrill-Palmer Quarterly 21: 205–224. **pp.214, 220.**

Bates, E., Camaioni, L. and Volterra, V. (1976). Sensorimotor performatives. In E. Bates (Ed.), Language and Context: The Acquisition of Pragmatics. New York: Academic Press. pp 49–71. **pp.50, 51.**

Bates, E. and MacWhinney, B. (1982). Functionalist approaches to grammar. In E. Wanner and L. Gleitman (Eds.), Language Acquisition: The State of the Art. Cambridge, Massachusetts: MIT Press. pp 173–218. **p.102.**

Bates, E., O'Connell, B. and Shore, C. (1987). Language and communication in infancy. In J.D. Osofsky (Ed.), Handbook of Infant Development. Second Edition. New York: Wiley. pp 149–203. **p.50.**

Bates, E., Shore, C., Bretherton, I. and McNew, S. (1983). Names, gestures and objects: Symbolization in infancy and aphasia. In K.E. Nelson (Ed.), Children's Language, Volume 4. Hillsdale, New Jersey: Lawrence Erlbaum, pp 59–123. **p.25.**

Baumgart, D., Johnson, J. and Helmstetter, E. (1990). Augmentative and Alternative Communication Systems for Persons with Moderate and Severe Disabilities. Baltimore: Paul H. Brookes. **p.56.**

Bedrosian, J.L. (1988). Adults who are mildly to moderately retarded: Communicative performance, assessment and intervention. In S.N. Calculator and J.L. Bedrosian

(Eds.), Communicative Assessment and Intervention for Adults with Mental Retardation. Austin, Texas: Pro-ed, pp 265–307. **p.198**.

Bedrosian, J.L. (1995). Limitations in the use of non-disabled subjects in AAC research. Augmentative and Alternative Communication 11: 6–10. **p.135**.

Bellugi, U. and Fischer, S.D. (1972). A comparison of sign language and spoken language. Cognition 1: 173–200. **pp.25, 237**.

Bellugi, U., Klima, E. and Siple, P. (1975). Remembering in signs. Cognition 3: 93–125. **p.191**.

Bellugi, U. and Studdert-Kennedy, M. (Eds.) (1980). Signed and Spoken Language: Biological Constraints on Linguistic Form. Basel: Verlag Chemie. **p.29**.

Benson, G., Abbeduto, L., Short, K., Nuccio, J.B. and Maas, F. (1993). Development of Theory of Mind in individuals with mental retardation. American Journal on Mental Retardation 98: 427–433. **p.265**.

Berg, Å. and Sørhuglen, M. (1980). Tegn med psykisk utviklingshemmede (Signs for the Intellectually Impaired). Bergen: Vestlandsheimen. **p.5**.

Berne, E. (1961). Transactional Analysis in Psychotherapy. New York: Ballantine Book. **p.371**.

Berry, D.C. and Dienes, Z. (1993a). Towards a working characterisation of implicit learning. In D.C. Berry and Z. Dienes (Eds.), Implicit Learning. Theoretical and Empirical Issues. Hove: Lawrence Erlbaum, pp 1–18. **p.46**.

Berry, D.C. and Dienes, Z. (1993b). Practical implications. In D.C. Berry and Z. Dienes (Eds.), Implicit Learning. Theoretical and Empirical Issues. Hove: Lawrence Erlbaum, pp 129–143. **p.46**.

Besio, S. and Chinato, M.G. (1991). F., l'integrazione linguistica a diciotto anni (F.: The linguistic Integration at Eighteen). Genova: University Press. **p.190**.

Besio, S. and Ferlino, L. (1992). Software and hardware for mobility disorders. Proceedings of the 3rd International Conference on Computers for Handicapped Persons, Vienna, July 1992. pp 22–30. **p.193**

Besio, S. and Ferlino, L. (1993). Blissymbolics software worldwide: From prototypes towards future optimized products. Proceedings of the 2nd European Conference on the Advancement of Rehabilitation Technology, Stockholm, May 1993. Vällingby, Sweden: The Swedish Handicap Institute, p 34.2. **p.193**.

Beukelman, D.R. and Ansel, B. (1995). Research priorities in augmentative and alternative communication. Augmentative and Alternative Communication 11: 131–134. **pp.291, 342**.

Beukelman, D.R. and Mirenda, P. (1992). Augmentative and Alternative Communication: Management of Severe Communication Disorders in Children and Adults. London: Paul H. Brookes. **pp.33, 177, 178, 271, 310, 319**.

Beukelman, D.R., Yorkston, K., Poblete, M. and Naranjo, C. (1984). Frequency of word occurrence in communication samples produced by adult communication aid users. Journal of Speech and Hearing Disorders 49: 360–367. **p.177**.

Biancardi, A. (1985). Gesti e segni per comunicare (Gestures and Signs for Communication). Torino: Omega. **pp.189, 192**.

Bickerton, D. (1990). Language and Species. Chicago: Chicago University Press. **p.31**.

Bishop, D. (1982). Comprehension of spoken, written and signed sentences in childhood language disorders. Journal of Child Psychology and Psychiatry 23: 1–20. **p.118**.

Bishop D. and Edmundson, A. (1987). Language-impaired 4-year-olds: Distinguishing transient from persistent impairment. Journal of Speech and Hearing Disorders 52: 156–173. **p.120**.

Bishop, D. and Mogford, K. (Eds.) (1993). Language Development in Exceptional Circumstances. Hove, UK: Lawrence Erlbaum. **p.29**.

Bjerregaard, M. and Nygaard, L. (1975). Tegnsprogets betydning for den verbalsproglige udvikling (The significance of sign language for language development). S.Å. Pædagogen 3 (9). **p.5.**

Björck-Åkesson, E. (Ed.) (1983). Kommunikationshjälpmedel för talhandikappade. Del I (Communication Aids for the Speech Impaired. Part I). Gothenburg: Rikscentralen för Pedagogiske Hjälpmedel för Rörelseshindrade. **p.5.**

Björck-Åkesson, E. (1986). Juegos con juguetes que funcionan con pilas (Play with Battery-operated Toys). Madrid: ATAM-FUNDESCO. (Swedish edition, 1984, Rikscentralen för Pedagogiske Hjälpmedel för Rörelseshindrade). **p.271.**

Björck-Åkesson, E. (1990). Communicative interaction of young physically disabled nonspeaking children and their parents. Presented at the Fourth Biennial Conference of the International Society of Alternative and Augmentative Communication, Stockholm, August 1990. **p.275.**

Björck-Åkesson, E. (1992). Kommunikation und interaktion zwischen Kleinkinder mit körperlicher Behinderung und ihren ersten Bezugspersonen (Communication and interaction between motor impaired children and their care-givers). Presented at Symposium of ARGE Frühförderung 'Behinderung - Interaktion; Interaktion - Behinderung; Beziehungsmuster in der frühen Kindheit', Wien, November 1992. **p.332.**

Björck-Åkesson. (1993). Communicative interaction between young non-speaking children with physical disabilities and their parents. Handicap Research Group, Report No. 13. Jönköping: Jönköping University. **p.332.**

Björck-Åkesson, E. and Granlund, M. (1995). Family involvement in assessment and intervention: Perceptions of professionals and parents in Sweden. Exceptional Children 61: 520–535. **p.326.**

Blackstone, S. (Ed.) (1986). Augmentative Communication: An Introduction. Rockville, Maryland: American Speech and Hearing Association. **p.177.**

Blackstone, S. (1991). Intervention with the partners of AAC consumers: Part I - Interaction. Augmentative Communication News 4 (2): 1–3. **p.171.**

Blackstone, S. and Williams, M. (1994). Family involvement in the AAC intervention process: Conceptual and methodological issues. In J. Brodin and E. Björck-Åkesson (Eds.), Methodological Issues in Research in Augmentative and Alternative Communication. Jönköping: Jönköping University Press, pp 82–88. **p.324.**

Blau, A.F. (1986). Communication in the back-channel: Social structural analyses of non-speech/speech conversations. Dissertation, City University of New York. **pp.7, 22, 32, 35, 68.**

Bliss, C. (1965). Semantography (Blissymbolics). Sydney: Semantography Publications. **pp.13, 15, 182–3.**

Blohm, W. and Mülbach, L. (1990). Videotelephony with high-resolution transmission of documents. Proceedings of the 13th International Symposium on Human Factors in Telecommunications, Torino, 1990 pp. 409–416. **p.206.**

Bloom, L. (1970). Language Development: Form and Function in Emerging Grammars. Cambridge, Massachusetts: MIT Press. **p.102.**

Bloom, L. (1973). One Word at a Time. The Hague: Mouton **pp.102, 132.**

Bloom, L. and Capatides, J.B. (1991). Language Development from 2 to 3. Cambridge, UK: Cambridge University Press. **pp.101, 115.**

Bloom, L. and Lahey, M. (1978). Language Development and Language Disorders. New York: John Wiley. **pp.159, 197.**

Bloom, L., Lightbown, P. and Hood, L. (1975). Structure and variation in early child language. Monographs of the Society for Research in Child Development 40: Serial No. 160. **pp.102, 113.**

Bloom, P. (Ed.) (1993). Language Acquisition: Core Readings. Cambridge, Massachusetts: MIT Press. p.138.

Bomers, A.J.A.M. and Mugge, A.M. (1982). Reynell Taalontwikkelingstest, Nederlandse instructie (Reynell's Developmental Language Scales, Dutch instructions). Nijmegen, The Netherlands: Berkhout. p.236.

Bondurant, J.L., Romeo, D.J. and Kretschmer, R. (1983). Language behaviors of mothers of children with normal and delayed language. Language, Speech, and Hearing Services in Schools 14: 233–242. p.44.

Bondy, C., Cohen, R., Eggert, D. and Lüer, G. (1975). Testbatterie für geistig behinderte Kinder, TBGB (Test Battery for Intellectually Impaired Children). Weinheim: Beltz. p.294.

Bonfantini, M. (1987). La semiosi e l'abduzione (Semiotics and Abduction). Milano: Bompiani. p.185.

Bonvillian, J.D. and Blackburn, D.W. (1991). Manual communication and autism: Factors relating to sign language acquisition. In P. Siple and S.D. Fischer (Eds.), Theoretical Issues in Sign Language Research. Volume 2: Psychology. Chicago: Chicago University Press, pp 255–277. p.266.

Bonvillian, J.D. and Nelson, K.E. (1982). Exceptional cases of language acquisition. In K.E. Nelson (Ed.), Children's Language, Volume 3. London: Lawrence Erlbaum, pp 322–391. pp.3, 6.

Bonvillian, J.D., Nelson, K.E. and Rhyne, J.M. (1981). Sign language and autism. Journal of Autism and Developmental Disorders 11: 125–137. p.56.

Bourdieu, P. (1977). Outline of a Theory of Practice. Cambridge, UK: Cambridge University Press. pp.249, 266.

Bowerman, M. (1994). From universal to language-specific in early grammatical development. Philosophical Transactions of the Royal Society of London, B 346: 37–45. p.119.

Bowman, S.N. (1984). A review of referential communication skills. Australian Journal of Human Communication Disorders 12: 93–112. p.125.

Braun, U. (1994). Kleine Einführung in unterstützte Kommunikation. (A short introduction to augmentative communication). In U. Braun (Ed.), Unterstützte Kommunikation. Düsseldorf: Verlag Selbstbestimmtes Leben, pp 3–9 .pp.5, 292.

Bray, M. and Woolnough, L. (1988). The language skills of children with Down's syndrome aged 12 to 16 years. Child Language Teaching and Therapy 4: 311–324. pp.214, 215.

Bridges, A. (1984). Preschool children's comprehension of agency. Journal of Child Language 11: 593–610. p.102.

Brien, D. (1992). A Dictionary of British Sign Language. London: Faber and Faber. p.115.

Brocher, T. (1975). Csoportdinamika és felnőttoktatás (Group Dynamics and Adult Education). Budapest: Tankönyvkiadó. p.364.

Brodin, J.M. (1993). Telefax för personer med förståndshandikapp (Telefax for People with Intellectual Impairment). Stockholm: Swedish Telecom. p.200.

Brodin, J.M. (1994). Videotelephony for two persons with moderate mental retardation. International Journal of Rehabilitation Research 17: 357–363. p.196.

Brodin, J.M. and Alemder, I. (1995). Videotelephones: A tool for facilitating communication and social integration for persons with moderate mental retardation. Research report 13. Stockholm: Stockholm Institute of Education. pp.206, 208.

Brodin, J.M. and Björck-Åkesson, E. (1991). Evaluation of Still Picture Telephone for Mentally Retarded Persons. Stockholm: Swedish Telecom.pp.201, 202.

Brodin, J.M. and Björck-Åkesson, E. (1992). Still Picture Telephones for People with

Profound Mental Retardation Stockholm: Swedish Telecom. **p.205.**

Brodin, J.M. and Björck-Åkesson, E. (1995). Still picture telephone use by persons with profound retardation: A pilot study. European Journal of Special Needs Education, 10: 31–39. **pp.201, 202.**

Brodin, J.M., Fahlén, M. and Nilsson, S-H. (1993). Minitrial. A limited-study of the use of videotelephony. Report No. 7, Stockholm University, Department of Education. **p.208.**

Broumley, L. (1994). Talksback: The use of social knowledge in an augmentative communication system. Dissertation, University of Dundee, UK. **p.180.**

Broumley, L., Cairns, A.Y. and Arnott, J.L. (1990). TalksBack: An application of AI techniques to a communication prosthesis for the non-speaking. Proceedings of the 9th European Conference on Artificial Intelligence, Stockholm, August 1990. pp 117–119. **p.179.**

Brown, C. (1954). My Left Foot. London: Secker and Warburg. **p.3.**

Brown, R. (Ed.) (1970). Psycholinguistics. New York: The Free Press. **p.1.**

Brown, R. (1973). A First Language: The Early Stages. Cambridge, Massachusetts: Harvard University Press. **pp.101, 102, 111.**

Brown, R. (1978). Why are signed languages easier to learn than spoken languages?. The Bulletin of the American Academy of Arts and Sciences 32: 25–44 **p.191.**

Bruner, J.S (1975). The ontogenesis of speech acts. Journal of Child Language 2: 1–19. **pp.59, 86.**

Bruner, J.S. (1983). Child's Talk. Oxford: Oxford University Press. **pp.1, 50.**

Bruno, J. (1989). Customising a Minspeak system for a preliterate child: A case example. Augmentative and Alternative Communication 5: 89–100. **p.119.**

Bruno, J. and Bryen, D.N. (1986). The impact of modelling on physically disabled non-speaking children's communication. Presented at the Second Biennial Conference on Augmentative and Alternative Communication, Cardiff, September 1986. **p.77.**

Bryen, D.N., Goldman, A. and Quinlisk-Gill, S. (1988). Sign language with students with SPMR: How effective is it? Education and Training of the Mentally Retarded 23: 123–137. **p.105.**

Bryen, D.N. and Joyce, D.G. (1985). Language intervention with the severely handicapped: A decade of research. The Journal of Special Education 19: 7–39. **p.266.**

Bryen, D.N. and McGinley, V. (1991). Sign language input to community residents with SPMR: How effective is it? Education and Training of the Mentally Retarded 23: 129–137. **p.33.**

Burack, J.A. (1994). Selective attention in persons with autism: Preliminary evidence of an inefficient attentional lens. Journal of Abnormal Psychology 103: 535–543. **p.54**

Burgermeister, B., Blum, L. and Lorge, I. (1972). Colombia Mental Maturity Scales. Cleveland: The Psychological Corporation. **p.293.**

Buscaglia, L. (1983). The Disabled and Parents. Thorofare, New Jersey: Holt, Rinehart and Winston. **p.369.**

Butterworth, B., Hine, R.R. and Brady, K.D. (1977). Speech and interaction in sound-only communication channels. Semiotica 20: 81–99. **p.197.**

Byrne, B. and Davidson, E. (1985). On putting the horse before the cart: Exploring conceptual bases of word order via acquisition of a miniature artificial language. Journal of Memory and Language 24: 377–389. **p.102.**

Cadman, D., Goldsmith, C. and Bashim, P. (1984). Values, preferences and decisions in the care of children with developmental disabilities. Developmental and Behavioral Pediatrics 5: 60-64. **p.329.**

Calculator, S.N. (1988). Evaluating the effectiveness of AAC programmes for persons with severe handicaps. Augmentative and Alternative Communication 4: 177–179. **p.177.**

Calculator, S. and Luchko, C. (1983). Evaluating the effectiveness of a communication board training program. Journal of Speech and Hearing Disorders 47: 281–287. **p.139.**

Camarata, S., Nelson, K. and Camarata, M. (1994). Comparison of conversational recasting and imitative procedures for training grammatical structures in children with specific language impairment. Journal of Speech and Hearing Research 37: 1414–1423. **p.120.**

Campbell, D.T. (1975). 'Degrees of freedom' and the case study. Comparative Political Studies 8: 178–193. **p.9.**

Canal, A. and Riviére, A. (1993). La conducta comunicativa de los niños autistas en situaciónes naturales de interacción (The communicative behaviour of autistic children in natural interaction situations). Estudios de Psicología 50: 49–74. **p.54.**

Cannao, M. (1991). Comunicazione alternativa e ritardo mentale (Alternative communication and mental retardation). In M.L. Gava and D. Montalto (Eds.), La comunicazione alternativa. Sistemi comunicativi nelle disabilità verbali. Milano: Franco Angeli, pp 111–130. **pp.189, 190.**

Cannao, M. and Moretti, G. (1982). Il grave handicappato mentale (The Severely Intellectually Impaired). Roma: Armando. **p.191.**

Cardoso-Martins, C. and Mervis, C.B. (1985). Maternal speech to prelinguistic children with Down syndrome. American Journal of Mental Deficiency 89: 451–458. **p.214.**

Cardoso-Martins, C., Mervis, C.B. and Mervis, C.A. (1985). Early vocabulary acquisition by children with Down syndrome. American Journal of Mental Deficiency 90: 177–184. **p.214.**

Caselli, M.C. and Volterra, V. (1990). From communication to language in hearing and deaf children. In V. Volterra and C.J. Erting (Eds.), From Gesture to Language in Hearing and Deaf Children. New York: Springer-Verlag, pp 263-277. **pp.101, 118, 127.**

Casto, G. (1987). Plasticity and the handicapped child. A review of efficacy research. In J.J. Gallagher and C.T. Ramey (Eds.), The Malleability of Children. Baltimore: Paul H. Brookes, pp 103–113. **p.213.**

Chevigny, H. (1962). My Eyes have a Cold Nose. New Haven, Connecticut: Yale University Press. **p.175.**

Chomsky, N. (1959). A review of B.F. Skinner's 'Verbal behavior'. Language 35: 26–58. **p.5.**

Chomsky, N. (1968). Language and Mind. New York: Harcourt Brace Jovanovich. **pp.5, 128.**

Chueca y Mora, F.A. (1988). La normalización del deficiente: Actitudes del profesorado (Teachers' Attitudes toward Mainstreaming Handicapped Children in Spain). (Bilingual volume). Ann Arbor: University of Michigan Press. **p.310.**

Ciesielski, K.T., Courchesne, E. and Elmasian, R. (1990). Effects of focused selective attention tasks on event-related potentials in autistic and normal individuals. Electroencephalography and Clinical Neurophysiology 75: 207–220. **p.54.**

Clark, C.R. (1984). A close look at the standard Rebus system and Blissymbolics. Journal of the Association for Persons with Severe Handicaps 9: 37–48. **p.15.**

Clark, E.V. (Ed.) (1993). The proceedings of the Twenty-fourth Annual Child Language Research Forum. Stanford: Center for the study of Language and Information. **p.138.**

Clark, H.H. (1992). Arenas of Language Use. Chicago: University of Chicago Press. **p.93.**

Clark, H.H. and Brennan, S.E. (1991). Grounding in communication. In L.B. Resnick, J. Levine and S.D. Terasley (Eds.), Perspectives on Socially Shared Cognition. Washington, DC: American Psychological Association, pp 127–149. **pp.98, 99.**

Clark, H.H. and Carlson, T.B. (1982). Hearers and speech acts. Language 58: 332–373. **p.137.**

Clark, H.H. and Marshall, C.R. (1981). Definite reference and mutual knowledge. In A.K. Joshi, B. Webber and I. Sag (Eds.), Linguistic Structure and Discourse Setting. Cambridge, UK: Cambridge University Press. pp 10–63. **p.137.**

Clark, H.H. and Schaefer, E.F. (1989). Contributing to discourse. Cognitive Science 13: 259–294. **pp.93, 143.**

Clark, H.H. and Wilkes-Gibbs, D. (1986). Referring as a collaborative process. Cognition 22: 1–39. **p.93.**

Clark, R. (1982). Theory and method in child-language research: Are we assuming too much? In S. Kuczaj, II (Ed.), Language Development, Volume 1: Syntax and Semantics. Hillsdale, New Jersey: Lawrence Erlbaum. pp.1–36. **p.85.**

Coerts, J. and Mills, A. (1994). Early sign combinations of deaf children in sign language of the Netherlands. In I. Ahlgren, B. Bergman and M. Brennan (Eds.), Perspectives on Sign Language Structure. Durham, UK: ISLA, pp 319–332. **p.102.**

Collins, S. (1994). Venturing into problematic talk. Communication Matters 8 (3): 27–30. **p.172.**

Collins, S. and Marková, I. (1995). Complementarity in the construction of a problematic utterance in conversation. In I. Marková, C.F. Graumann. and K. Foppa (Eds.), Mutualities in Dialogue. Cambridge: Cambridge University Press, pp 238–263. **p.89.**

Colombo, J. (1993). Infant Cognition. London: Sage. **p.230.**

Cook, A.M. and Coleman, C.L. (1987). Selecting augmentative communication systems by matching client skills and needs to system characteristics. Seminars in Speech and Language 8: 153–167. **p.65.**

Cook, A.M. and Hussey, S.M. (1995). Assistive technologies: Principles and Practice. St. Louis: Mosby Yearbook Publishers. **p.311.**

Copeland, K. (1974). Aids for the Severely Handicapped. London: Spector. **p.6.**

Couturat, L. and Leau, L. (1903). Histoire de la langue universelle (History of the Universal Language). Paris: Hachette. **p.183.**

Crain, S. (1993). Language acquisition in the absence of experience. In P. Bloom (Ed.), Language Acquisition: Core readings. London: Harvester Wheatsheaf, pp 364–419. **p.119.**

Cromer, R.F. (1991). Language and Thought in Normal and Handicapped Children. Oxford: Basil Blackwell. **p.161.**

Cruickshank, W.M., Morse, W.C. and Grant, J.O. (1990). The Individual Education Planning Committee: A Step in the History of Special Education. Ann Arbor: University of Michigan Press. **p.310.**

Crystal, D. (1986). ISAAC in chains: The future of communication systems. Augmentative and Alternative Communication 2: 140–145. **p.9.**

Crystal, D. (1987). Concepts of language development: A realistic perspective. In W. Yule and M. Rutter (Eds.), Language Development and Disorders. London: MacKeith, pp 42–52 **p.1.**

Crystal, D. (1991). A Dictionary of Linguistics and Phonetics (3rd edition). Oxford: Basil Blackwell **pp.25, 114.**

Cubelli, R. (1986). Le variabili che influenzano il recupero dell'afasia (The variables that influence the recovery of aphasia). Europa Medicophysica 22: 81–91 **p.193.**

Cubelli, R., Foresti, A., Consolini, T. (1988). Re-education strategies in conduction aphasia. Journal of Communication Disorders 21: 239–249. **p.193.**

Cullen, K., Ollivier, H., Kubitschke, L., Clarkin, N., Darnige, A., Robinson, S. and Dolphin, C. (1995). Connecting to the information superhighway: Access issues for elderly and people with disabilities. In P.R.W Roe (Ed.), Telecommunications for All. Luxembourg: Office for Official Publications of the European Communities, pp 233–244. pp.199,200.

Cunningham, C.C. (1988). Early intervention: Some results from the Manchester Down's syndrome cohort study. Paper based on a talk given to The Fundacion Catalana per a la Sindrome de Down. Santander, Spain, March 1988. pp.213, 229.

Curcio, F. (1978). Sensorimotor functioning and communication in mute autistic children. Journal of Autism and Childhood Schizophrenia 8: 281–292. pp.52, 57.

Dalgarno, G. (1661). Ars signorum, vulgo character universalis et lingua philosophica (The Art of Signs, which is also named Universal Character and Philosophical Language). London: Hayes. p.183.

Daniloff, J.K. and Shafer, A. (1981). A gestural communication program for severely and profoundly handicapped children. Language, Speech and Hearing Services in Schools 12: 258–268. p.106.

Darwin, C. (1871). The Descent of Man, and Selection in Relation to Sex. London: Murray. p.22.

Dawson, G. and Adams, A. (1984). Imitation and social responsiveness in autistic children. Journal of Abnormal Child Psychology 12: 209–226. p.53.

Deich, R.F. and Hodges, P.M. (1977). Language Without Speech. London: Souvenir Press. p.5.

de L'Epée, C.M. (1776). Institution des sourd-muets par la voie des signes méthodique (Education of the deaf-mute via methodological signs). Paris: Nyon. (Extracts published in American Annals of the Deaf, 1861 13: 8–29). pp.3, 12.

de Loache, J. and Burns, N.M. (1994). Early understanding of the representational function of pictures. Cognition 52: 83–110. p.126.

Deloche, G., Dordain, M. and Kremin, H. (1993). Rehabilitation of confrontation naming in aphasia. Relations between oral and written modalities. Aphasiology 7: 201–216. p.195.

del Rio, M.J. (1986). La adquisicion del lenguaje: Un analisis interaccional (The acquisition of language: an interactional analysis). Dissertation, University of Barcelona. p.346.

del Rio, M.J. (Ed.) (1995). Interacción y desarrollo del lenguaje en personas con necesidades especiales (Interaction and Language Development in Persons with Special Needs). Barcelona: Martinez-Roca. p.345.

Delvert, J. (1989). Video Communication for Deaf People in their Working Lives. Borlänge: Kaljedo. p.206.

Demorest, A., Silberstein, L., Gardner, H. and Winner, E. (1983). Telling it as it isn't: Children's understanding of figurative language. British Journal of Developmental Psychology 1: 121–134. p.138.

Dennis, R., Reichle, J., Wiliams, W. and Vogelsberg, R.T. (1982). Motoric factors influencing the selection of vocabulary for sign production programs. Journal of the Association for Persons with Severe Handicaps 7: 20–32 p.28.

de Saussure, F. (1977). Course in General Linguistics. Glasgow: Fontana/Collins (first published in French in 1916). pp.25, 36, 85, 186.

de Villiers, J.G. and de Villiers, P. (1973). Development of the use of word order in comprehension. Journal of Psycholinguistic Research 2: 331–341. p.102.

Dexter, L.A. (1958). A social theory of mental deficiency. American Journal of Mental Deficiency 62: 918–931. p.175.

Dienes, Z. (1993). Implicit concept formation. In D.C. Berry and Z. Dienes (Eds.),

Implicit Learning. Theoretical and Empirical Issues. Hove: Lawrence Erlbaum, pp 37–61. **p.46.**

Dockrell, J. and McShane, J. (1993). Children's Learning Difficulties: A Cognitive Approach. Oxford: Basil Blackwell. **p.29.**

Donaldson, M. (1993). Sense and sensibility – some thoughts on the teaching of literacy. In R. Beard (Ed.), Teaching Literacy: Balancing Perspectives. London: Hodder and Stoughton. pp 35–60 **pp.20, 23.**

Dopping, O. (1991). Videotelephony on 2 Mbit/s for deaf people in their working lives. In S. von Tetzchner (Ed.), Issues in Telecommunication and Disability. Luxembourg: Office for Official Publications of the European Communities, pp 386–394. **p.206.**

Downing, J. (Ed.) (1973). Comparative Reading. New York: Macmillan. **p.13.**

Dunn, J. (1988). The Beginnings of Social Understanding. Oxford: Basil Blackwell. **p.63**

Dunst, C., Trivette, C. and Deal, A. (1988). Enabling and Empowering Families. Cambridge: Brookline Books. **p.67.**

Dykens, E.M., Hodapp, R.M. and Evans, D.W. (1994). Profiles and development of adaptive behavior in children with Down syndrome. American Journal on Mental Retardation 98: 580–587. **p.214.**

Eco, U. (1971). Le forme del contenuto (Forms of Meaning). Bologna: Zanichelli. **p.187.**

Eco, U. (1975). Trattato di semiotica generale (Theory of Semiotics). Milano: Bompiani. (English version, 1977, Macmillan). **pp.182, 186–8.**

Eco, U. (1993). La ricerca della lingua perfetta (In Search of the Perfect Language). Roma-Bari: Laterza. **pp.183, 185.**

Edgerton, R.B. and Gaston, M.A. (1991). "I've seen it all". Lives of older Persons with Mental Retardation in the Community. Baltimore, Maryland: Paul H. Brookes. **p.198.**

Ekman, P. (1975). Movements with precise meanings. Journal of Communication 26: 14–26. **p.33.**

Emiliani, P.L. and Stephanidis, C. (1995). Multimedia services and applications in a broadband environment. In P.R.W. Roe (Ed.),Telecommunications for All. Luxembourg: Office for Official Publications of the European Communities, pp 245–261. **p.200.**

Engberg-Pedersen, E., Hansen. B. and Sørensen, R.K. (1981). Døves tegnsprog (Sign Language of the Deaf). Århus, Denmark: Arkona. **pp.5, 12.**

Fehr, B.J. and Exline, R.V. (1987). Social visual interaction: A conceptual and literature review. In A.W. Siegman and S. Feldstein (Eds.), Non-verbal Behavior and Communication. Second Edition. Hillsdale, New Jersey: Lawrence Erlbaum, pp 225–326. **p.50.**

Fenn, G. and Rowe, J. (1975). An experiment in manual communication. British Journal of Disorders of Communication 10: 3–16. **pp.102, 106, 108, 112.**

Ferguson, C. (1959). Diglossia. Word 15: 469–480. **p.34.**

Ferreira, J.M., Teixeira, A.C., Ramalho, J.L. and Lourenço, M.L. (1994). A portable device to improve the communication ability of people with cerebral palsy. ISAAC'94 Conference Book and Proceedings. Hoensbroek, The Netherlands: Institute for Research, Development and Knowledge Transfer in the Field of Rehabilitation and Handicap. pp 446–448. **p.344.**

Ferreira, M.C., da Ponte, M.M., Azevedo, L.M. and Carvalho, M.R. (1995). Inovaçào curricular na implementaçào de meios alternativos de comunicaçào em crianças com deficiência neuromotora grave (Curricular Innovation in the Implementation of Alternative Communication Systems for Children with Motor Impairments). Lisbon: Centro de Reabilitaçào de Paralisia Cerebral Calouste Gulbenkian. **p.344.**

Fey, M., Cleave, P., Long, S. and Hughes, D. (1993). Two approaches to the facilitation of grammar in children with language impairment: An experimental evaluation. Journal of Speech and Hearing Research 36: 141–157. **p.120.**

Fischer, M.A. (1987). Mother-child interaction in pre-verbal children with Down syndrome. Journal of Speech and Hearing Disorders 52: 179–190. **p.214.**

Fischer, S., Metz, D.E., Brown, P.M. and Caccamise, F. (1991). The effects of bimodal communication on the intelligibility of sign and speech. In P. Siple and S. Fischer (Eds.), Theoretical Issues in Sign Language Research. Volume 2: Psychology. Chicago: University of Chicago Press, pp 135–147. **p.129.**

Fodor, J.A. (1983). The Modularity of Mind. Cambridge, Massachusetts: MIT Press. **p.27.**

Fodor, J.A., Bever, T.G. and Garrett, M.F. (1974). The Psychology of Language: An Introduction to Psycholinguistics and Generative Grammar. Toronto: McGraw-Hill. **p.154.**

Fowler, A., Gelman, R. and Gleitman, L. (1994). The course of language learning in children with Down syndrome. In H. Tager-Flusberg (Ed.), Constraints on Language Acquisition: Studies of Atypical Children. London: Lawrence Erlbaum. pp 91–140, **pp.103, 117.**

Franzkowiak, T. (1994). Verständigung mit grafischen Symbolen (Understanding with graphic symbols). In U. Braun (Ed.), Unterstützte Kommunikation. Düsseldorf: Verlag Selbstbestimmtes Leben, pp 22–32. **p.16.**

Frawley, W. (1992). Linguistic Semantics. Hove, UK: Lawrence Erlbaum **pp.168, 169.**

Frazier, L. (1995). Issues of representation in psycholinguistics. In J.L. Miller and P.D. Eimas (Eds.), Language, Speech and Communication. New York: Academic Press, pp 1–27. **p.29.**

Frederiksen, J., Martin, M., Puig de la Bellacasa, R. and von Tetzchner, S. (Eds.) (1989). Use of Telecommunication: The Needs of People with Disabilities. Madrid: Fundesco. **p.196.**

Friedman, L. (Ed.) (1977). On the Other Hand. London: Academic Press. **pp.5, 86.**

Fried-Oken, M. and More, L. (1992). Initial vocabulary for non-speaking preschool children based on developmental and environmental language samples. Augmentative and Alternative Communication 8: 1–16. **p.79.**

Fristoe, M. and Lloyd, L.L. (1980). Planning an initial expressive sign lexicon for persons with severe communication impairment. Journal of Speech and Hearing Disorders 45: 170–180. **p.79.**

Frith, U. (1989). Autism: Explaining the Enigma. Oxford: Blackwell. **p.53.**

Fuller, D., Lloyd, L.L. and Schlosser, R. (1992). Further development of an AAC symbol taxonomy. Augmentative and Alternative Communication 8: 67–74. **p.26.**

Fuller, P. and Wright, A. (1994). The beauty of the unspoken: The development of language without either recognition or production of speech. ISAAC'94 Conference Book and Proceedings. Hoensbroek The Netherlands: Institute for Research, Development and Knowledge Transfer in the Field of Rehabilitation and Handicap. pp 89–91. **pp.22, 31, 32.**

Fulwiler, R.L. and Fouts, R.S. (1976). Acquisition of American sign language by a non-communicating autistic child. Journal of Autism and Childhood Schizophrenia 6: 43–51. **p.5.**

Fundudis, T., Kolvin, I. and Garside, R. (Eds.) (1979). Speech Retarded and Deaf Children: Their Psychological Development. London: Academic Press. **p.44.**

Gale, R. and Grant, J. (1990). Managing Change in a Medical Context: Guidelines for Action. London: The Joint Centre for Educational Research and Development in Medicine. **pp.355, 369.**

Gangkofer, M.H. (1989). Zum Stand der Forschung über die Bliss-Symbol-Kommunikationsmethode (The state of the art of research on the Blissymbol communication method). Zeitschrift für Heilpedägogik 40: 300–305. **p.297.**

Gangkofer, M.H. (1993). Bliss und Schriftsprache (Blissymbolics and Literacy). Bottighofen, Switzerland: Libelle. **p.297.**

Garfinkel, H. (1967). Studies in Ethnomethodology. New Jersey: Prentice Hall. **p.177.**

Garton, A.F. (1992). Social Interaction and the Development of Language and Cognition. Hove, UK: Lawrence Erlbaum. **p.65.**

Gava, M.L. (1991). Comunicazione alternativa. Dieci anni di esperienze: Risultati e prospettive (Alternative communication. Ten years of experience: Results and prospects). In M.L. Gava, and D. Montalto (Eds.), La comunicazione alternativa. Sistemi comunicativi nelle disabilità verbali. Milano: Franco Angeli, pp 131–150. **p.193.**

Gava, M.L. and Montalto, D. (Eds.) (1991). La comunicazione alternativa. Sistemi comunicativi nelle disabilità verbali (Alternative Communication. Communication Systems in Language Disabilities). Milano: Franco Angeli. **pp.182, 190.**

Gerber, S. and Kraat, A.W. (1992). Use of a developmental model of language acquisition: Application to children using AAC systems. Augmentative and Alternative Communication 8: 19–32. **pp.119, 234.**

Gibbon, F. and Grunwell, P. (1990). Specific developmental language learning disabilities. In P. Grunwell (Ed.), Developmental Speech Disorders. Edinburgh: Churchill Livingstone. pp 135–161. **p.40.**

Gibson, D. and Harris, A. (1988). Aggregated early intervention effects for Down's syndrome persons: Patterning and longevity of benefits. Journal of Mental Deficiency Research 32: 1–17. **p.229.**

Givón, T. (1984). Syntax: A Functional-typological Introduction, Volume I. Amsterdam: Benjamins. **p.169.**

Gjessing, H.-J. and Nygaard, H.D. (1975). Illinois Test of Psycholinguistic Abilities håndbok (Manual). Oslo: Universitetsforlaget. **p.251.**

Glennen, S.L. and Calculator, S. N. (1985). Training functional communication board use: a pragmatic approach. Augmentative and Alternative Communication 1: 134–142. **p.271.**

Glucksberg, S. and Krauss, R.M. (1967). What do people say after they have learned to talk? Studies of the development of referential communication. Merrill-Palmer Quarterly 13: 309–316. **p.140.**

Glucksberg, S., Krauss, R.M. and Weisberg, R. (1966). Referential communication in nursery school children: Method and some preliminary findings. Journal of Experimental Child Psychology 3: 333–342. **p.124.**

Goffman, E. (1959). The Presentation of Self in Everyday Life. London: Penguin. **pp.174, 175, 268.**

Goffman, E. (1963). Stigma: Notes on the Management of Spoiled Identity. London: Penguin. **pp.174–6.**

Goffman, E. (1969). Strategic Interaction. Philadelphia: University of Pennsylvania Press. **p.194.**

Goffman, E. (1974). Frame Analysis. New York: Harper and Row **pp.29, 71.**

Goffman, E. (1981). Forms of Talk. Philadelphia: University of Pennsylvania Press. **p.194.**

Goldberg, H. and Fenton, J. (1960). Aphonic Communication for those with Cerebral Palsy: Guide for the Development and Use of a Conversation Board. New York:

United Cerebral Palsy of New York State. **p.4.**

Goldin-Meadow, S. and Morford, M. (1990). Gesture in early child language. In V. Volterra and C.J. Erting (Eds.), From Gesture to Language in Hearing and Deaf Children. New York: Springer-Verlag, pp 249–262. **p.214.**

Goldin-Meadow, S. and Mylander, C. (1990). Beyond the input given: The child's role in the acquisition of language. Language 66: 323–355. **p.105.**

Gómez, J.C. (1991). Visual behaviour as a window for reading the minds of others in primates. In A. Whiten (Ed.), Natural Theories of Mind: Evolution, Development and Simulation of Everyday Mindreading. Oxford: Basil Blackwell, pp 195–207. **pp.51, 55.**

Gómez, J.C. (1995). Eye gaze, attention and the evolution of mindreading in primates. Presented at the 25th Meeting of the Jean Piaget Society, Berkeley, California, June 1995. **p.57.**

Gómez, J.C., Sarriá, E. and Tamarit, J. (1993). The comparative study of early communication and theories of mind: Ontogeny, phylogeny and pathology. In S. Baron-Cohen, H. Tager-Flusberg, and D. Cohen (Eds.), Understanding Other Minds: Perspectives from Autism. Oxford: Oxford University Press, pp 397–426. **pp.51, 54, 55.**

Gómez, J.C., Sarriá, E., Tamarit, J., Brioso, A. and León, E. (1995). Los inicios de la comunicación: Estudio comparado de niños y primates no humanos e implicaciones para el autismo (The Beginnings of Communication: A Comparative Study of children and Non-human Primates and its Implications for Autism). Madrid: M.E.C. **p.54,55.**

Goossens', C.A. (1989). Aided communication intervention before assessment: A case study of a child with cerebral palsy. Augmentative and Alternative Communication 5: 14–26. **p.271.**

Goossens', C.A. and Crain, S. (1986). Augmentative Communication: Intervention Resource. Wauconda, Illinois: Don Johnston Developmental Equipment. **p.128.**

Gràcia, M. and Urquía, B. (1994). Interacción comunicativa y lingüística madre-nino y maestro-nino en poblaciones con retraso mental (Communicative and linguistic interaction between mother and child, and teacher and child, in populations with intellectual impairment). Revista de Logopedia y Fonoaudiologia 14: 137–147. **p.346.**

Granlund, M. (1988). Behandlingsarbete (Intervention Work). Stockholm: Stiftelsen ALA. **p.327.**

Granlund, M. (1993). Communicative competence in persons with profound mental retardation. Acta Universitatis Upsaliensis: Studia Psychlogica Clinica Upsaliensia 3. **p.197, 324.**

Granlund M. and Björck-Åkesson, E. (in press). Inservice training of pre-school consultants in family-oriented intervention–training process and outcome. British Journal of Developmental Disabilities. **p.336.**

Granlund, M., Björck-Åkesson, E., Brodin, J. and Olsson, C. (1995). Communication intervention for persons with profound disabilities: A Swedish perspective. Augmentative and Alternative Communication 11: 49–59. **p.324.**

Granlund, M. and Karlan, G.R. (1985). The Social and Physical Environment Survey (SPES). Stockholm: Stiftelsen ALA. **p.337.**

Granlund, M., Olsson, C., Andersson, M. and von Dardel, T. (1990). Parents, group home staff, and school staff working together around children with profound multiple disabilities. British Journal of Mental Subnormality 36: 94–113. **p.329.**

Granlund, M., Steensson, A.-L., Sundin, M. and Olsson, C. (1992). Inservice training in collaborative problem solving and goal setting for special education teacher consultants working with profoundly impaired persons. British Journal of Mental Subnormality 38: 94–113. **pp.326, 331.**

Granlund, M., Terneby, J. and Olsson, C. (1992a). Subject characteristics and the communicative environment of profoundly retarded adults. Scandinavian Journal of Educational Research 36: 323–338 **p.335.**

Granlund, M., Terneby, J. and Olsson, C. (1992b). Creating communicative opportunities through a combined inservice training/supervision package. European Journal of Special Needs Education 7: 229–252. **pp.335, 336.**

Gresham, F.M. (1989). Assessment of treatment integrity in school consultation and prereferral intervention. School Psychology Review 18: 37–50. **p.331.**

Grice, P. (1975). Logic and conversation. In P. Cole and J.L. Morgan (Eds.), Syntax and Semantics. Volume 3: Speech Acts. London: Academic Press, pp 41–58. **p.26.**

Grove, N. (1990). Developing intelligible signs with learning-disabled students: A review of the literature and an assessment procedure. British Journal of Disorders of Communication 25: 265–294. **p.28.**

Grove, N. (1993). Good with their hands? Analysing the skills of signers with learning disabilities. In J. Clibbens and B. Pendleton (Eds.), CLS '93: Proceedings of the Child Language Seminar. Plymouth: University of Plymouth. pp 209–218. **p.109.**

Grove, N. and McDougall, S. (1991). Exploring sign use in two settings. British Journal of Special Education 18: 149–156. **pp.33, 106.**

Grove, N. and Walker, M. (1990). The Makaton Vocabulary: Using manual signs and graphic symbols to develop interpersonal communication. Augmentative and Alternative Communication 6: 15–28. **pp.5, 6, 108.**

Gudi, S.P. and Gore, G.B. (1993). Language therapy for aphasics. Recent trends. Indian Journal of Disability and Rehabilitation 7: 27–36. **p.191.**

Guillaume, P. (1971). Imitation in Children. Chicago: Chicago University Press. **p.40.**

Gumperz, J. (1982). Discourse Strategies. London: Cambridge University Press. **p.178.**

Gutfreund, M., Harrison, M. and Wells, G. (1989). Bristol Language Development Scales. Windsor, UK: NFER-Nelson. **p.131.**

Habermas, J. (1984). The Theory of Communicative Action, Volume 1. Boston: Beacon Press. **p.10.**

Habermas, J. (1987). The Theory of Communicative Action, Volume 2. Boston: Beacon Press. **p.10.**

Hamers, J.F. and Blanc, M.H.A. (1989). Bilinguality and Bilingualism. Cambridge, UK: Cambridge University Press. **p.24.**

Hamers, J.H.M., Sijtsma, K. and Ruijssenaars, A.J.J.M. (1993). Learning Potential Assessment. Amsterdam: Swets and Zeitlinger. **p.38.**

Happé, F.G.E. (1993). Communication competence and theory of mind in autism: A test of relevance theory. Cognition 48: 101–119. **p.27.**

Happé, F.G.E. (1994). Autism: An Introduction to Psychological Theory. London: University College of London Press. **p.198**

Hári, M. and Ákos, K. (1988). Conductive Education. London: Routledge. (Hungarian version, 1971, Tankönyvkiado). **p.363.**

Harris, D. (1982). Communicative interaction processes involving non-vocal physically handicapped children. Topics in Language Disorders 2: 21–37. **pp.68, 131, 232, 314.**

Harris, J. (1983). What does mean length utterance mean? Evidence from a comparative study of normal and Down's syndrome children. British Journal of Disorders of Communication 1, 8: 153–169. **p.114.**

Harris, M. (1992). Language Experience and Early Language Development: Fran

Imput to Uptake. Cambridge, Mass: MIT Press. **pp.26, 30.**

Harris, M. and Beech, J. (1995). Reading development in pre-lingually deaf children. In K. Nelson and Z. Reger (Eds.), Children's Language, Volume 8. Hillsdale, New Jersey: Lawrence Erlbaum, pp 181–202. **p.110.**

Hartje, W. and Sturm, W. (1987). La riabilitazione non-verbale delle afasie (The non-verbal rehabilitation of aphasia). In A. Mazzucchi (Ed.), La riabilitazione neuropsicologica. Bologna: Il Mulino. pp 87–114. **p.191.**

Háztartásstatisztika 1985 (Home Statistics 1985) (1986). Budapest: Központi Statisztikai Hivatal. **pp.358, 361.**

Hedelin, L. and Hjelmquist, E. (1991). Children's referential communication in a game situation. In J. Verschueren (Ed.), Pragmatics at Issue. Amsterdam: John Benjamins, pp 191–209. **p.143.**

Heim, M.J.M. (1989). Kommunikatieve vaardigheden van niet of nauwelijks sprekende kinderen met infantiele encephalopathie (Communicative skills of non-speaking children with cerebral palsy). Manuscript, Institute for General Linguistics, University of Amsterdam. **p.237.**

Heim, M.J.M. (1990). Communicative skills of non-speaking CP-children: A study on interaction. Presented at the Fourth Biennial Conference of the International Society for Augmentative and Alternative Communication, Stockholm, August 1990. **p.232.**

Heim, M.J.M. and Mills, A.E. (1992). Effects of partner instruction on the communicative development of non-speaking CP toddlers. Presented at the Fifth Biennial Conference of the International Society for Augmentative and Alternative Communication, Philadelphia, August 1992. **p.235.**

Heritage, J. (1984). Garfinkel and Ethnomethodology. Cambridge, UK: Polity Press. **p.89.**

Hidas, G. (Ed.) (1984). A csoportpszichoterápia elméleti és gyakorlati kérdései (Practical and Theoretical Aspects of Group Psychotherapy – essays). Budapest: Akadémia Kiadó. **p.365.**

Higginbotham, D.J. (1989). The interplay of communication device output mode and interaction style between non-speaking persons and their speaking partners. Journal of Speech and Hearing Research 54: 320–333. **p.138.**

Higginbotham, D.J. (1995). Use of non-disabled subjects in AAC research: Confessions of a research infidel. Augmentative and Alternative Communication 11: 2–5. **p.135.**

Higginbotham, D.J., Mathy-Laikko, P. and Yoder, D.E. (1988). Studying conversations of augmentative communication system users. In L.E. Bernstein (Ed.), The Vocally Impaired: Clinical Practice and Research. Philadelphia: Grune and Stratton. pp 265–294. **p.89.**

Hind, M. (1989). SYNREL: Programs to teach sequencing of Blissymbols. Communication Outlook 10 (4): 6–9. **p.190.**

Hiraga, M.K. (1994). Diagrams and metaphors: Iconic aspects in language. Journal of Pragmatics 22: 5–21. **p.25.**

Hjelmquist, E., Sandberg, A.D. and Hedelin, L. (1994). Linguistics, AAC, and metalinguistics in communicatively handicapped children. Augmentative and Alternative Communication 10: 169–183. **p.137.**

Hobson, P. (1993). Autism and the Development of Mind. Hillsdale, New Jersey: Lawrence Erlbaum. **p.55.**

Hockett, C.F. (1960). The origin of speech. Scientific American 203: 88–96. **pp.20, 186.**

Hodapp, R.M. and Burack, J.A. (1990). What mental retardation teaches us about typical development: The examples of sequences, rates and cross-domain relations. Development and Psychopathology 2: 213–216. **p.114.**

Hodges, P. and Schwethelm, B. (1984). A comparison of the effectiveness of graphic symbol and manual sign training with profoundly retarded children. Applied Psycholinguistics 5: 223–253. **p.106.**

Hoffmeister, R. and Farmer, A. (1972). The development of manual sign language in mentally retarded deaf individuals. Journal of Rehabilitation of the Deaf 6: 19–26. **p.106.**

Holand, U., von Tetzchner, S. and Steindal, K. (1991). Two field trials with videotelephones in psychiatric and habilitative work. In S. von Tetzchner (Ed.), Issues in Telecommunication and Disability. Luxembourg: Office for Official Publications of the European Communities, pp 372–378. **p.211.**

Holgersen, A. (1996). "Skulle alle muligheter taes fra meg, med en unntagelse, da ville jeg beholde muligheten til å kommunisere, for med den ville jeg snart overvinne resten" (Should all possibilities be taken away from me, with exception of one, then I would keep the possibility to communicate, because with this, I would soon win over the others"). CP-Bladet 42:31–33. **p.5.**

Holm, J.A. (1993). Installering og opplæring i bruk av telefonen for å gi en psykisk utviklingshemmet mann økt sosial tilpasning (Installation and teaching use of the telephone for increasing the social integration of an intellectually impaired man). In K.B. Nilsson and S. von Tetzchner (Eds.), Telekommunikasjon for mennesker med psykisk utviklingshemning. Oslo: Rådet for tekniske Tiltak for Funksjonshemmede, pp 23–28. **p.195.**

Holmgren, B. (1984). Illinois Test of Psycholinguistic Abilities (Swedish translation and standardisation). Stockholm: Psykologiförlaget. **p.140.**

Holtz, K.-L., Eberle, G., Hillig, A. and Marker, K.R. (1984). Handbuch für Heidelberger-Kompetenz-Inventar für geistig Behinderte. Heidelberg: Edition Schindele. **p.393.**

Hornby, G. (1991). Parent involvement. In D. Mitchell and R.I. Brown (Eds.), Early Intervention Studies for Young Children with Special Needs. London: Chapman and Hall. pp 206–225. **p.229.**

Howlin, P. and Yates, P. (1989). Treating autistic children at home: A London based programme. In C. Gillberg (Ed.), Diagnosis and Treatment of Autism. New York: Plenum Press. pp 307–322. **p.56.**

Hunt, P. and Goetz, L. (1988). Teaching spontaneous communication in natural settings through interrupted behaviour chains. Topics in Language Disorders 9: 58–71 **p.90.**

Iacono, T. (1992). Individual language learning styles and augmentative and alternative communication. Augmentative and Alternative Communication 8: 33–40. **pp.119, 234.**

Iacono, T. (1994). Language development research: Theoretical concerns and future challenges. In J. Brodin and E. Björck-Åkesson (Eds.), Methodological Issues in Research in Augmentative and Alternative Communication. Jönköping: Jönköping University Press. pp 11–17. **p.9.**

Iacono, T. and Parsons, C.L. (1986). A comparison of techniques for teaching signs to intellectually disabled individuals using an alternating treatment design. Australian Journal of Human Communication Disorders 14: 23–34. **p.41.**

Ingram, D. (1989). First language acquisition: Method, Description and Explanation. Cambridge, UK: Cambridge University Press. **pp.101, 112, 119, 132.**

Iverson, J.M., Capirci, O. and Caselli, M.C. (1994). From communication to language in two modalities. Cognitive Development 9: 23–43. **pp.239, 246.**

Jackendoff, R. (1989). Consciousness and the Computational Mind. Cambridge, Massachusetts: MIT Press. **p.169, 170.**

Jaroma, M. (1992). Blissymbolics in Dysphatic School Children. Kuopio: Kuopio University Printing Office. **p.5.**

Jensen, K. (1992). Hjemlig omsorg i offentlig regi (Home-oriented Public Care). Oslo: Universitetsforlaget. p.249.

Johansen-Horbach, H., Cegla, B., Mager, U. Schempp, B. and Wallesch, C. (1985). Treatment of global aphasia with a non-verbal communication system. Brain and Language 24: 74–82. p.182.

Johansson, I. (1987). Tecken - en genväg till tal (Signs - a shortcut to speech). Down syndrom: Språk och tal nr. 7. Umeå University, Department of Phonetics. Publication 28 p.215.

Johansson, I. (1988). Språkutveckling hos handikappade barn (Language Development in Disabled Children). Lund, Sweden: Studentlitteratur. p.324.

Johansson, I. (1990). Contributions of language to cognitive development. Paper at The Fourth Biennial Conference of the International Association for Augmentative and Alternative Communication, Stockholm, August 1990. p.226.

Johnson, R. (1981). The Picture Communication Symbols. Solana Beach, California: Mayer-Johnson. p.15.

Johnson, R. (1985). The Picture Communication Symbols - Book II. Solana Beach, California: Mayer-Johnson. p.15.

Johnson-Laird, P. (1993). The Computer and the Mind: an Introduction to Cognotive Science. Cambridge, Massachusetts: MIT Press. p.169

Jolleff, N., McConachie, H., Winyard, S., Jones, S., Wisbeach, A. and Clyton, C. (1992). Communication aids for children: Procedures and problems. Developmental Medicine and Child Neurology 34: 719–730. p.66

Jones, A.A., Blunden, R., Coles, E., Evans, G. and Porterfield, J. (1987). Evaluating the impact of training, supervisory feedback, self-monitoring and collaborative goal-setting on staff and client behaviour. In J. Hoggs and P. Mittler (Eds.), Staff Training in Mental Handicap. Beckenham: Croom Helm, pp 213–300. p.326

Jones, P.R and Cregan, A. (1986). Sign and Symbol Communication for Mentally Handicapped People. London: Croom Helm. p.16, 184

Jonker, V.M. and Heim, M.J.M. (1994). Implementation of an intervention programme for non-speaking children and their partners: In-service training. ISAAC'94 Conference Book and Proceeding. Hoensbroek, The Netherlands: Institute for Research, Development and Knowledge Transfer in the Field of Rehabilitation and Handicap. pp 410–412. p.324

Jordan, R. and Powell, S. (1995). Understanding and Teaching Children with Autism. Chichester: John Wiley. P.56.

Kahn, J.V. (1975). Relationship of Piaget's sensorimotor period to language acquisition of profoundly retarded children. American Journal of Mental Deficiency 79: 296–303 p.38

Kahn, J.V. (1981). A comparison of sign and verbal language training with non-verbal retarded children. Journal of Speech and Hearing Research 46: 113–119. p.106

Kallen, J.L. and Smith, M.M. (1992). Irish language acquisition and speech/language therapy: Principles and needs. In D.P.Ó. Baoill (Ed.), Acquisition of Irish as a First Language. Dublin: IRAAL, pp 26–42. p.6.

Kalman, S. (1989). A Bliss-nyelv bevezetése, oktatásának és alkalmazásának eddigi eredményei Magyarországon. (Introduction of Blissymbolics in Hungary, present results of its teaching and implementation.) Dissertation, University of Budapest. pp.362, 367.

Kalman, S. and Pajor, A. (1987). Enhancement of communication sensitivity by drama play. Proceedings of the Congress of the World Association of Social Psychiatry, Budapest 1987. Budapest: Magyar Pszichológiai Társaság p 85. p.365

Kalman, S. and Pajor, A. (1989). Psychological impact of teaching augmentative communication. Augmentative and Alternative Communication - Journal of the

Society for the Development of Blissymbols in Israel 5 (5): 31–32. **p.365.**

Kamhi, A. and Masterson, J. (1989). Language and cognition in mentally handicapped people: Last rites for the difference-delay controversy. In M. Beveridge, G. Conti-Ramsden and I. Leudar (Eds.), Language and Communication in Mentally Handicapped People. London: Chapman and Hall, pp 83–111.**p.114.**

Kangas, K.A. and Lloyd, L.L. (1988). Early cognitive skills as prerequisites to augmentative and alternative communication use: What are we waiting for? Augmentative and Alternative Communication 4: 211–221. **p.270.**

Karlan, G.R., Brenn-White, B., Lentz, A., Hodur, P., Egger, D. and Frankoff, D. (1982). Establishing generalised productive verb-noun phrase usage in a manual language system with mentally handicapped children. Journal of Speech and Hearing Disorders 47: 431–442. **p.107.**

Karlan, G.R. and Lloyd, L.L. (1983). Considerations in the planning of communication intervention: Selecting a lexicon. Journal of the Association for the Severely Handicapped 8: 13–25. **p.79.**

Karmiloff-Smith, A. (1979). A Functional Approach to Child Language: A Study of Determiners and Reference. Cambridge, UK: Cambridge University Press. **p.104.**

Kates, B. and McNaughton, S. (1975). The First Application of Blissymbolics as a Communication Medium for Non-speaking Children: Historical Development, 1971-1974. Don Mills, Ontario: ESCI. **p.182.**

Kavanagh, J.F. and Venezky, A.L. (1980). Orthography, Reading and Dyslexia. Baltimore: University Park Press. **p.39.**

Kaye, K. (1982). The Mental and Social Life of Babies. Chicago: University of Chicago Press. **p.288.**

Kaye, K. and Charney, R. (1981). Conversational asymmetry between mothers and children. Journal of Child Language 8: 35–49. **p.288.**

Kendon, A. (1973). Some functions of gaze-direction in social interaction. In M. Argyle (Ed.), Social Encounters: Readings in Social Interaction. Harmondsworth, UK: Penguin. pp 76–92. **p.131.**

Kent, L. (1983). El niño que no se comunica. Bases teóricas y practicas para la intervención (The child who does not communicate. Theoretical and practical bases of intervention). Revista de Logopedia y Foniatria 3: 78–95. **p.313.**

Kiernan, C. (1983). The use of non-vocal communication techniques with autistic individuals. Journal of Child Psychology and Psychiatry 24: 339–375. **p.56**

Kiernan, C., Reid, B. and Jones, L. (1982). Signs and Symbols: Use of Non-vocal Communication systems. London: Heinemann. **pp. 3, 5, 6, 33, 101, 103, 105, 226, 343.**

Kikuchi, T., Yamashita, Y., Sagawa, K. and Wake, T. (1979). An analysis of tactile letter confusions. Perception and Psychophysics 26: 295–301. **p.29.**

Kipila, E.L. and Williams-Scott, B. (1988). Cues, speech and speech reading. Volta Review 90: 179–189. **p.28.**

Kiresuk, T., Smith, A. and Cardillo, J. (1994). Goal Attainment Scaling: Applications, Theory, and Measurement. London: Lawrence Erlbaum. **p.332.**

Kirk, S.A., McCarthy, J.J. and Kirk, W.D. (1968). Examiner's Manual. Illinois Test of Psycholinguistic Abilities. Urbana, Illinois: University of Illinois Press. **p.140.**

Kirman, B.H. (1985). Mental Retardation: Medical aspects. In M. Rutter and L. Hersov (Eds.), Child and Adolescent Psychiatry. Oxford: Blackwell. pp 650–660. **p.197.**

Kirsner, K. (1986). Lexical functioning: Is a bilingual account necessary? In J. Vaid (Ed.), Language Processing in Bilinguals: Psycholinguistic and Neuropsychological Perspectives. Hillsdale, New Jersey: Lawrence Erlbaum. pp 21–45. **p.31.**

Kleinke, C.L. (1986). Gaze and eye contact: A research review. Psychological Bulletin 100: 78–100. **p.50.**

Klima, E. and Bellugi, U. (1979). The Signs of Language. London: Harvard University Press. **pp.5, 86, 121.**

Knoors, H. (1991). Use of spatial syntax by non-native signing deaf children: Occurrence, frequency, structure. Presented at the conference 'Growing Up in Sign and Word', University of Bristol, November 1991. **p.104.**

Koegel, R.L. and Johnson, J. (1989). Motivating language use in autistic children. In G. Dawson (Ed.) Autism: Nature, Diagnosis, and Treatment. New York: The Guildford Press. pp 310–325. **p.56.**

Koegel, R.L., O'Dell, M.C. and Koegel M.K. (1987). A natural language teaching paradigm for non-verbal autistic children. Journal of Autism and Developmental Disorders 17: 187–200. **p.56.**

Koerselman, E. (1994). It all started with Bliss. The ISAAC Bulletin, 37: 6–7. **pp.5, 23.**

Konstantareas, M.M., Oxman, J. and Webster, C.D. (1978). Iconicity: Effects on the acquisition of sign language with autistic and other severely dysfunctional children. In P. Siple (Ed.), Understanding Language through Sign Language Research. New York: Academic Press, pp 213–237. **p.262.**

Kopchick, G., Rombach, D. and Smilovitz, R. (1975). A total communication environment in an institution. Mental Retardation 13: 13–33. **p.106.**

Koppenhaver, D. and Yoder, D. (1992). Literacy issues in persons with severe physical and speech impairments. In R. Gaylord-Ross (Ed.), Issues in Research and Special Education, Volume 2. New York: Teacher's College Press, pp 156–201. **p.297.**

Kraat, A.W. (1985). Communication Interaction between Aided and Natural Speakers: A State of the Art Report. Toronto: Canadian Rehabilitation Council for the Disabled. **pp.7, 32, 89, 172, 177, 271.**

Kraat, A.W. (1991). Methodological issues in the study of language development among children using aided language. Reactant Paper 1. In J. Brodin and E. Björck-Åkesson (Eds.), Methodological Issues in Research in Augmentative and Alternative Communication. Stockholm: Swedish Handicap Institute, pp 118–123. **pp.119, 120.**

Kyle, J.G. and Woll, B. (Eds.) (1983). Language in Sign: An International Perspective on Sign Language. London: Croom Helm. **pp.86, 121.**

Kyle, J.G., Woll, B. and Ackerman, J. (1989). Gesture to sign and speech. Final report to the Economic and Social Research Council. **p.103.**

LaCour, G., Freund, A.M. and Nielsen, F. (1979). Bliss Symbol Systemet (Blissymbolics). Dansk Audiologopædi 15 (1): 11–24. **p.3.**

Lahey, M. (1988). Language Disorders and Language Development. New York: Macmillan. **pp.102, 112, 113, 117.**

Lane, H. (1977). The Wild Boy of Aveyron. London: George Allen and Unwin. **p.3.**

Lane, H. (1984). When the Mind Hears. Harmondsworth, UK: Penguin. **p.24.**

Langacker, R. (1987a). Foundations of Cognitive Grammar. I: Theoretical Prerequisites. Stanford, California: Stanford University Press. **p.169.**

Langacker, R. (1987b). Nouns and verbs. Language 63: 53–94. **p.169.**

Layton, T.L. and Savino, M.A. (1990). Acquiring a communication system by sign and speech in a child with Down syndrome: A longitudinal investigation. Child Language Teaching and Therapy 6: 59–76. **p.215.**

Le Guern, M. (1975). Sémantique de la metaphore et de la metonymie (Semantics of Metaphor and Metonymy). Paris: Larousse. **p.187.**

Leitão, A.R. (1994). Interacção mae-criança e acticidade simbólica (Mother-child Interaction and Symbolic Activity). Lisbon: Secretariado Nacional de Reabilitação. **p.313.**

Lenneberg, E.H. (1962). Understanding language without ability to speak. Journal of Abnormal and Social Psychology 65: 419–425. **p.4.**

Lenneberg, E.H. (1967). Biological Foundations of Language. New York: Wiley. **pp.5, 22.**

Leonard, L.B., Schwartz, R.G., Folger, K.M. and Wolcox, M.J. (1978). Some aspects of child phonology in imitative and spontaneous speech. Journal of Child Language 5: 403–415. **p.26.**

Leopardi, G. (1956-1966). Opere (Works). Milano: Ricciardi. (English version, 1983, Colombia University Press). **p.188.**

Le Prevost, P. (1983). Using the Makaton vocabulary in early language learning with a Down's baby. Mental Handicap 11: 28–29. **p.215.**

Leslie, A.M. and Happé, F. (1989). Autism and ostensive communication: The relevance of metarepresentation. Development and Psychopathology 1: 205–212. **p.52.**

Levelt, W.J.W. (1989). Speaking. From Intention to Articulation. Cambridge, Massachusetts: MIT Press. **p.160.**

Levelt, W.J.M. (1994). What can a theory of normal speaking people contribute to AAC? ISAAC'94 Conference Book and Proceedings. Hoensbroek, The Netherlands: Institute for Research, Development and Knowledge Transfer in the Field of Rehabilitation and Handicap. pp 18–20. **pp.30, 153, 160.**

Levinson, S.C. (1979). Activity types and language. Linguistics 17: 356–399. **p.96.**

Levinson, S.C. (1983). Pragmatics. Cambridge: Cambridge University Press. **p.177.**

Levy-Shiff, R. (1986). Mother-father-child interactions in families with a mentally retarded young child. American Journal of Mental Deficiency 91: 141–149. **p.214.**

Lewin, K. (1935). A Dynamic Theory of Personality. New York: McGraw-Hill. **p.365.**

Lewin, K. (1948). Resolving Social Conflicts. London: Harper and Row. **p.365.**

Lewy, A.L. and Dawson, G. (1992). Social stimulation and joint attention in young autistic children. Journal of Abnormal Child Psychology 20: 555–566. **p.56.**

Liebermann, A. (1977). Small Groups - Theory and Practice. Chicago: University of Chicago Press. **p.365.**

Light, J. (1985). The Communicative Interaction Patterns of Young Non-speaking Physically Disabled Children and their Primary Caregivers. Toronto: Blissymbolics Communication Institute. **pp.7, 87, 271, 286.**

Light, J. (1988). Interaction involving individuals using augmentative and alternative communication systems: State of the art and future directions. Augmentative and Alternative Communication 4: 66–82. **pp.7, 151, 154, 172, 177.**

Light, J. (1989). Toward a definition of communicative competence for individuals using augmentative and alternative communication systems. Augmentative and Alternative Communication 5: 137–144. **p.154.**

Light, J. and Collier, B. (1986). Facilitating the development of effective initiation strategies by non-speaking, physically disabled children. In S. W. Blackstone (Ed.), Augmentative Communication: An Introduction. Rockville, Maryland: American Speech and Hearing Association, pp 197–266. **p.271.**

Light, J., Collier, B. and Parnes, P. (1985a). Communicative interaction between young non-speaking physically disabled children and their primary caregivers: Part 1 - Discourse patterns. Augmentative and Alternative Communication 1: 74–83. **pp.67, 68, 75, 119, 138, 142, 151, 271.**

Light, J., Collier, B. and Parnes, P. (1985b). Communicative interaction between young non-speaking physically disabled children and their primary caregivers: Part 2 - Communicative function. Augmentative and Alternative Communication

1: 98–107. **pp.119, 138, 142, 151.**

Light, J., Collier, B. and Parnes, P. (1985c). Communicative interaction between young non-speaking physically disabled children and their primary caregivers Part 3 - Modes of communication. Augmentative and Alternative Communication 1: 125–134. **pp.138, 142, 151, 232, 246–8.**

Light, J., Dattilo, J., English, J. and Gutierrez, L. (1992). Instructing facilitators to support the communication of people who use augmentative communication systems. Journal of Speech and Hearing Research 35: 865–875. **p.139.**

Light, J., McNaughton, D. and Parnes, P. (1986). A protocol for the assessment of communication interaction skills of non-speaking severely handicapped adults and their facilitators. Toronto: Hugh McMillan Centre. **pp.324, 333.**

Light, P., Remington, B., Clarke, S. and Watson, J. (1989). Signs of language. In M. Beveridge and G. Conti-Ramsden (Eds.), Language and Communication in Mentally Handicapped People. London: Chapman and Hall, pp 57–79. **pp.105, 107.**

Lindblom, B. (1990). On the communication process: Speaker-listener interaction and the development of speech. Augmentative and Alternative Communication 6: 20–230. **pp.139, 151.**

Lindström, J.-I. and Pereira, L.M. (1995). Videotelephony. In P.R.W. Roe (Ed.), Telecommunications for All. Luxembourg: Office for Official Publications of the European Communities. pp 110–118. **p.206.**

Linell, P. (1991). Dialogism and the orderliness of conversation disorders. In J. Brodin and E. Björck-Åkesson (Eds.), Methodological Issues in Research in Augmentative and Alternative Communication. Stockholm: The Swedish Handicap Institute, pp 9–21. **p.89.**

Linell, P. and Korolija, N. (1995). On the division of communicative labour within episodes in aphasic discourse. International Journal of Psycholinguistics 11: 143–165. **p.91.**

Lloyd, L.L. and Fuller, D.R. (1986). Toward an augmentative and alternative symbol taxonomy: A proposed superordinate classification. Augmentative and Alternative Communication 2: 165–171. **p.10.**

Lloyd, L. and Karlan, G. (1984). Non-speech communication symbols and systems: Where have we been and where are we going? Journal of Mental Deficiency Research 38: 3–20. **p.38.**

Lloyd, L.L., Quist, R.W. and Windsor, J. (1990). A proposed augmentative and alternative communication model. Augmentative and Alternative Communication 6: 172–183. **pp.21, 22, 27, 28, 105.**

Lock, A. (1980). The Guided Reinvention of Language. London: Academic Press. **pp.1, 38, 59, 65, 271, 290, 291, 345.**

Loew, R. (1980). Learning American sign language as a first language: Roles and reference. Presented at the Third International Symposium on Sign Language Research and Teaching, Boston, 1980. **p.81.**

Lombardino, L. and Langley, M.B. (1989). Strategies for assessing severely multihandicapped children for augmentative and alternative communication. European Journal of Special Needs Education 4: 157–170. **pp.38, 39.**

Loncke, F., Quertinmont, S., Ferreyra, P. and Counet, A.-F. (1986). Sign order in children and adolescents. In B. Tervoort (Ed.), Signs of Life: Proceedings of the 2nd European Congress on Sign Language Research. Amsterdam: Institute for General Linguistics, pp 182–193. **p.104.**

Lord, C. and Magill, J. (1989). Methodological and theoretical issues in studying peer-directed behaviour and autism. In G. Dawson (Ed.), Autism: Nature, Diagnosis and Treatment. New York: Guildford Press, pp 326–345. **p.53.**

Loveland, K. and Landry, S. (1986). Joint attention in autistic and language delayed children. Journal of Autism and Developmental Disorders 16: 335–350. **pp.52, 53.**

Luchsinger, R. and Arnold, G.E. (1965). Voice – Speech – Language. New York: Wadsworth. **pp.40, 45.**

Luckman, T. (1990). Social communication, dialogue and conversation. In I. Marková and K. Foppa (Eds.), The Dynamics of Dialogue. London: Harvester-Wheatsheaf. pp 45–61. **p.65.**

Luria, A.R. and Yudovich, F.I. (1959). Speech and the Development of Mental Processes in the Child. London: Staples. **p.19.**

Lyons, J. (1977). Semantics, Volume 1. Cambridge, UK: Cambridge University Press.

Magyar Statisztikai Zsebkönyv 1994 (Hungarian Statistics 1994) (1995). Budapest: Központi Statisztikai Hivatal. **pp.358, 361.**

Maharaj, S.C. (1980). Pictogram Ideogram Communication. Regina, Canada.: The George Reed Foundation for the Handicapped. **p.15.**

Mann, V.A. and Brady, S. (1988). Reading disability: The role of language deficiencies. Journal of Consulting and Clinical Psychology 56: 811–816. **p.294.**

Manschot, W. and Bonnema, J. (1974). Peabody Picture Vocabulary Test. Lisse, The Netherlands: Swets and Zeitlinger. **p.236.**

Marcell, M.M. and Weeks, S.L. (1988). Short-term memory difficulties and Down's syndrome. Journal of Mental Deficiency Research 32: 153–162. **p.214.**

Marková, I. (1995). Asymmetry and intersubjectivity in dialogue involving non-speaking people. In J. Rönnberg and E. Hjelmquist (Eds.), Proceedings from the International Symposium on Communicative Disability: Compensation and Development. Linköping: Linköping University. pp 67–78. **pp.32, 68.**

Marková, I., Graumann, C. and Foppa, K. (Eds.) (1995). Mutualities in Dialogue. Cambridge, UK: Cambridge University Press. **p.1.**

Marriner, N., Yorkston, K. and Farrier, L. (1984). Transcribing and coding communication interaction between speaking and non-speaking individuals. In A.W. Kraat, Communication Interaction between Aided and Natural Speakers. Toronto: Canadian Rehabilitation Council for the Disabled, pp 330-355. **p.237.**

Martinsen, H. (1980). Biologiske forutsetninger for kulturalisering (The biological bases for culturalisation). Tidsskrift for Norsk Psykologforening, Monografiserien 6: 122–129. **p.271.**

Martinsen, H., Nordeng, H. and von Tetzchner, S. (1985). Tegnspråk (Sign Language). Oslo: Universitetsforlaget. **pp.5, 12.**

Martinsen, H. and von Tetzchner, S. (1988). The development of intended communication. Presented at the Third European Conference on Developmental Psychology, Budapest, August 1988. **p.57.**

Martinsen, H. and von Tetzchner, S. (1989). Imitation at the onset of speech. In S. von Tetzchner, L.S. Siegel and L. Smith (Eds.), The Social and Cognitive Aspects of Normal and Atypical Language Development. New York: Springer-Verlag. pp 51–68. **pp.76, 78, 102, 132.**

Mathisen, K.O. (1991). Teleteknikk og telenett (Teletechnique and telecommunication networks). In K.O. Mathisen, T. Rasmussen and S. von Tetzchner (Eds.) Nye nettverk. Telekommunikasjon og samfunn. Oslo: Ad Notam Gyldendal, pp 43–68. **p.200.**

Maurer, H. and Sherrod, K. (1987). Context directives given to young children with Down syndrome and non-retarded children: development over two years. American Journal of Mental Deficiency 91: 579–590. **p.214.**

Maxwell, M., Bernstein, M.E. and Mear, K.M. (1991). Bimodal language production.

In P. Siple and S. Fischer (Eds.), Theoretical Issues in Sign Language Research. Volume 2: Psychology. Chicago: University of Chicago Press, pp 171–190. **p.127.**

McConachie, H.R. (1991). Home-based teaching: What are we asking parents? Child: Care, Health and Development 17: 123-136. **p.272.**

McCoy, K.F., McKnitt, W.M., Peischl, D.M., Pennington, C.A., Vanderheyden, P.B. and Demasco, P.W. (1994). AAC-user therapist interactions: Preliminary linguistic observations and implications for compansion. RESNA'94 Proceedings. Arlington, Virginia: RESNA. pp 129–131. **pp.162, 167.**

McEwan, J. (1995). TeleCommunities. An interim report of the results of the RACE project R2033, TeleCommunity for the year 1994. Framlingham: Northwold System and Services. **p.207.**

McEwen, I. and Lloyd, L.L. (1990). Some considerations about the motor requirements of manual signs. Augmentative and Alternative Communication 6: 207–216. **p.28.**

McGregor, A. (1991). I'm in prison. Communication Outlook 12 (3): 21. **p.174.**

McIntire, M. (1977). The acquisition of American sign language hand configurations. Sign Language Studies 16: 247-266. **p.28.**

McKinlay, A. (1991). Using a social approach in the development of a communication aid to achieve perceived communicative competence. In J. Presperin (Ed.), Proceedings of RESNA '91 Conference, Kansas City. Washington, DC: The RESNA Press, pp 204–206. **p.177.**

McNaughton, S. (1985). Communicating with Blissymbolics. Toronto: Blissymbolics Communication Institute. **p.186.**

McNaughton, S. (1990). Gaining the most from AAC's growing years. Augmentative and Alternative Communication 6: 2–14. **pp.3, 4.**

McNaughton, S. and Kates, B. (1974). Visual symbols: Communication system for the pre-reading physically handicapped child. Presented at the American Association on Mental Deficiency Annual Meeting, Toronto, 1974. **pp.5, 13.**

McNaughton, S. and Kates, B. (Eds.) (1978). Handbook of Blissymbolics. Toronto: Ontario Crippled Children's Centre. **p.177.**

McNeill, D. (1987). Psycholinguistics: A New Approach. New York: Harper and Row. **p.29.**

McNeill, D. (1992). Hand and Mind. Chicago: University of Chicago Press. **pp.33, 81, 104, 118.**

McTear, M. (1985). Children's Conversations. Oxford: Basil Blackwell. **p.71.**

Meier, R.P. (1990). Person deixis in American sign language. In S.D. Fischer and P. Siple (Eds.), Theoretical Issues in Sign Language Research. Volume 1: Linguistics. Chicago: University of Chicago Press. pp 175–190. **p.81.**

Meier, R. and Newport, E. (1990). Out of the hands of babes: On a possible sign advantage in language acquisition. Language 66: 1–23. **p.102.**

Meisels, S.J. and Shonkoff, J.P. (Eds.) (1990). Handbook of Early Intervention. Cambridge, UK: Cambridge University Press. **p.311.**

Merchen, M. (1990). Some reasons for being passive from a personal perspective. Communication Outlook 12 (1): 10–11. **pp.171, 172.**

Meshcheryakov, A. (1979). Awakening to Life. Moscow: Progress. **p.3.**

Miller, J.L. and Eimas, P.D. (Eds.) (1995). Language, Speech and Communication. New York: Academic Press. **p.19, 29.**

Mills, A. (1994). AAC and linguistic theory: The robustness of the language faculty. In J. Brodin and E. Björck-Åkesson (Eds.), Methodological Issues in Research in Alternative and Augmentative Communication. Jönköping: Jönköping University Press, p 2. **p.31.**

Mirenda, P.L., Donnellan, A.M. and Yoder, D.E. (1983). Gaze behaviour: A new look at an old problem. Journal of Autism and Developmental Disorders 13: 397–410. **p.53.**

Mitchell, D. and Brown, R.I. (Eds.) (1991). Early Intervention Studies for Young Children with Special Needs. London: Chapman and Hall. **p.213.**

Mittler, P. (1987). Staff development; changing needs and service context in Britain. In J. Hoggs and P. Mittler (Eds.), Staff Training in Mental Handicap. Beckenham: Croom Helm, pp.31–61. **p.335.**

Moerk, E.L. (1988). Procedimentos y processos de aprendizaje y enseñanza del primer lenguaje (Developments and processes of teaching and learning the first language). Revista de Logopedia y Fonoaudiologia 8: 72–83 **p.352.**

Moerk, E. (1992). A First Language Taught and Learned. Baltimore: Paul H. Brooks. **p.291.**

Morford, J., Singleton, J. and Goldin-Meadow, S. (1994). From homesign to ASL: Identifying the influence of a self-generated system upon language proficiency in adulthood. Presented at the 19th Annual Conference on Child Language Development, Boston University, November 1994. **p.105.**

Morris, C., Newell, A.F., Booth, L. and Arnott, J.J. (1991). Syntax PAL: A system to improve the syntax of those with language dysfunction. In J. Presperin (Ed.), Proceedings of RESNA '91 Conference, Kansas City. Washington, D.C.: The RESNA Press, pp 105–106. **p.177.**

Moscovici, S. (1967). Communication processes and the properties of language. Advances in Experimental Psychology 3: 225–270. **p.196.**

Mundy, P., Kasari, C., Sigman, M. and Ruskin, E. (1995). Non-verbal communication and early language acquisition in children with Down syndrome and in normally developing children. Journal of Speech and Hearing Research 38: 157–167. **p.214.**

Mundy, P., Sigman, M. and Kasari, C. (1993). Theory of mind and joint attention deficits in autism. In S. Baron-Cohen, H. Tager-Flusberg and D. Cohen (Eds.), Understanding Other Minds: Perspectives from Autism. Oxford, UK: Oxford University Press, pp 181–203. **pp.52, 53, 54.**

Mundy, P., Sigman, M., Ungerer, J. and Sherman, T. (1986). Defining the social deficits of autism: the contribution of non-verbal communication measures. Journal of Child Psychology and Psychiatry 27: 657–669. **pp.52, 53.**

Murphy, J., Collins, S. and Moodie, E. (1994). The limited use of AAC systems: why the current situation is problematic and how it can be improved. Communication Matters 8 (3): 9–12. **pp.171, 172.**

Musselwhite, C.R. (1986). Adaptative Play for Special Needs Children. San Diego: College-Hill Press. (Spanish translation, 1990, INSERSO). **p.271.**

Musselwhite, C.R. and St. Louis, K.W. (1988). Communication Programming for Persons with Severe Handicaps. Boston: College-Hill. **pp.79, 193.**

Myklebust, H.R. (1960). The Psychology of Deafness. New York: Grune and Stratton. **p.25.**

Møllerbråten, B. (1991). The development of videotelephony. In S. von Tetzchner (Ed.), Issues in Telecommunication and Disability. Luxembourg: Office for Official Publications of the European Communities. pp 306–318. **p.200.**

Nakken, H. (1993). Perspectives and goals: central issues in intervention. Issues in Special Education and Rehabilitation 8: 37–44. **p.330.**

Nelson, N.W. (1992). Performance is the prize: Language competence and perfor- mance among AAC users. Augmentative and Alternative Communication 8: 3–19. **pp.119, 234.**

Newell, A. F. (1984). Do we know how to design communication aids? Proceedings of the Second Annual Conference on Rehabilitation Engineering, Ottawa, June 1984. Bethesda, Maryland: Rehabilitation Engineers Society of North America, pp 345–346. **p.177.**

Newell, A.F. and Alm, N. (1994). Developing AAC technologies: a personal story and philosophy. European Journal of Disorders of Communication 29: 399–411. **p.178.**

Newell, A.F., Alm. N.A. and Arnott J.L. (1993). An integrated strategy for improving communication systems for severely physically impaired non-speaking people. In I. Plancencia Porrero and R. Puig de la Bellacasa (Eds.), Rehabilitation Technology - Strategies for the European Union. Amsterdam: IOS Press, pp 249–253. **p.178.**

Newell, A.F., Arnott, J.L., Booth, L., Beattie, W., Brophy, B. and Ricketts, I.W. (1992). Effect of the 'Pal' word prediction system on the quality and quantity of text generation. Augmentative and Alternative Communication 8: 304–311. **p.28.**

Newman, H. (1982). The sounds of silence in communicative encounters. Communication Quarterly 30 (2): 142–149. **p.173.**

Nippold, M.A. (Ed.) (1988). Later Language Development: Ages Nine Through Nineteen. AustinTexas: Pro-Ed. **p.119.**

Noland, R.L. (1970). Counselling Parents of the Mentally Retarded. Springfield, Illinois: Charles C. Thomas. **p.367.**

Norsk tegnordbok (Norwegian Sign Dictionary) (1988). Bergen: Døves Forlag. **p.12.**

Olaszy, G., Kalman, S. and Olaszi, P. (1994). Blissvox - Beszélô kommunikációs rendszer (Blissvox - A Speaking Communication system). In M. Gósy (Ed.), Beszédkutatás. Budapest: Magyar Tudományos Akadémia Nyelvtudományi Intézete, pp 228–236. **p.361.**

Oliver, M. (1986). Social policy and disability: Some theoretical issues. Disability, Handicap and Society 1: 5–17. **p.35.**

Olson, D.R. (1993). How writing represents speech. Language and Communication 13: 1–17. **pp.34, 298.**

O'Neill, Y.V. (1980). Speech and Speech Disorders in Western Thought Before 1600. London: Greenwood Press. **pp.3, 37.**

Osgood, C.E. (1957). A behavioristic analysis of perception and language as cognitive phenomena. In J.S. Bruner, E. Brunswick, L. Festinger, F. Heider, K.F. Muenzinger and C.E. Osgood (Eds.), Contemporary Approaches to Cognition. Cambridge, Massachusetts: Harvard University Press, pp 75 –118. **p.28.**

Ottenbacher, K.J. and Cusick, A. (1993). Discriminative versus evaluative assessment: Some observations on goal attainment scaling. American Journal of Occupational Therapy 47: 349–354. **p.332.**

Paget, R. (1936). Sign language as a form of speech. Nature 137: 384–388. **p.12.**

Paget, R., Gorman, P. and Paget, P. (1976). The Paget Gorman Sign System (6th Edition). London: Association for Experiment in Deaf Education. **pp.12, 121.**

Paivio, A. (1986). Mental Representations. A Dual Coding Approach. Oxford: Oxford University Press. **p.29.**

Paul, J.L. (1983). The Exceptional Child. Syracuse, New York: Syracuse University Press. **p.367.**

Peirce, C.S. (1931-1958). Collected Papers, Volume 1-8. Cambridge, Massachusetts: Harvard University Press. **pp.10, 186.**

Pellerey, R. (Ed.) (1992a). Le lingue perfette (The perfect languages). Versus. Quaderni di Studi Semiotici 29: 61–63. **p.185.**

Pellerey, R. (1992b). Le lingue perfette nel secolo dell'utopia (Perfect Languages in the Century of Utopia). Roma-Bari: Laterza. **pp.185, 186.**

Pembrey, M. (1992). Genetics and language disorder. In P. Fletcher and D. Hall (Eds.), Specific Speech and Language Disorders in Children. London: Whurr, pp 51–62. **p.323.**

Perälä, J. and Lounela, L. (1991). Videotelephone-based support services for elderly and mobility disabled people. In S. von Tetzchner (Ed.), Issues in Telecommunication and Disability. Luxembourg: Office for Official Publications of the European Communities, pp 379–385. **p.207.**

Pereira, L.M., Matos, M.G., Purificação, J. and Lebre, P. (1992). Videotelephony and People with Mental Impairment. Lisbon: Technical University of Lisbon. **p.206.**

Pereira, L.M., Rocha, N., Cidade, C., Lebre, P. and Purifição, M.J. (1993). Visual, Mental Impaired, Elderly People and Picture Communication. Lisbon: Technical University of Lisbon. **p.207.**

Pereira, L.M., Vieira, F., Rocha, N. and Cidade, C. (1994). Videotelephony and remote learning for mentally impaired people. In L.M. Pereira and J.-I. Lindström (Eds.), Videotelephony for Disabled and Elderly People. Brussels: Commission of the European Communities, DG XIII, pp 42–46. **p.207.**

Pettygrove, W.B. (1985). A psychosocial perspective on the glossectomy experience. Journal of Speech and Hearing Disorders 50: 107–109. **p.176.**

Phillips, W., Gómez, J.C., Baron-Cohen, S., Laá, M.V. and Riviére, A. (1995). Treating people as objects, agents or 'subjects': How young children with and without autism make requests. Journal of Child Psychology and Psychiatry 36: 1383–1389. **p.53.**

Piaget, J. (1951). Play, Dreams and Imitation. New York: Norton. (First published in French in 1945). **p.191.**

Piaget, J. (1952). The Origins of Intelligence in Children. New York: International Universities Press. (First published in French in 1936). **pp.38, 293.**

Pine, J.M. (1992). Maternal style at the early one-word stage: re-evaluating the stereotype of the directive mother. First Language 12: 169–186. **p.214.**

Pinker, S. (1994). The Language Instinct. London: Penguin. **p.29.**

Plotkin, H. (1994). Darwin Machines and the Nature of Knowledge. London: Penguin. **p.4.**

Poizner, H. (1983). Perception and movements in American sign language: Effects of linguistic structure and the linguistic experience. Perception and Psychophysics 33: 215–231. **p.28.**

Pradatdiehl, P. and Bergego, C. (1994). Neuropsychological rehabilitation after stroke. Circulation et Métabolisme du Cerveau 11: 129–134. **p.191.**

Premack, D. (1974). Teaching visual language to apes and language deficient persons. In R.L. Schiefelbusch and L.L. Lloyd (Eds.), Language Perspectives - Acquisition, Retardation and Intervention. London: University Park Press, pp 347–375. **p.5.**

Premack, D. and Premack, A.J. (1972). Teaching language to an ape. Scientific American 227 (4): 92–99. **p.13.**

Prutting, C.A. and Elliott, J.B. (1979). Synergy: Toward a model of language. In N.J. Lass (Ed.), Speech and Language, Volume 1. New York: Academic Press, pp 337–365. **p.27.**

Pueschel, S.M., Gallagher, P.L., Zartler, A.S. and Pezzullo, J.C. (1987). Cognitive and learning processes in children with Down syndrome. Research of Developmental Disabilities 8: 21–37. **p.214.**

Raanaas, R.K. (1993). Bruk av bilder som kommunikasjonsmedium (The use of pictures as a medium for communication). Dissertation, University of Trondheim. **pp.30, 80.**

Radford, A. (1992). Syntactic Theory and the Acquisition of Syntax. Oxford, UK: Basil Blackwell. **pp.25, 102, 115, 119.**

Radutzky, E. (1981). Iconicità e arbitrarietà (Iconicity and arbitrariness). In V. Volterra (Ed.), I segni come parole: la comunicazione dei sordi. Torino: Boringhieri. pp 39–48. **p.186.**

Raghavendra, P. and Fristoe, M. (1995). 'No shoes; They walked away?': Effects of enhancement on learning and using Blissymbols by normal 3-year-old children. Journal of Speech and Hearing Research 38: 174–188. **p.126.**

Ramer, A. (1976). Syntactic styles in emerging language. Journal of Child Language 3: 49–62. **pp.102, 112.**

Rappaport, J. (1981). In praise of paradox: A social policy of empowerment over prevention. American Journal of Community Psychology 9: 1–25. **p.325.**

Rappaport, J. (1987). Terms of empowerment/exemplars of prevention: Toward a theory for community psychology. American Journal of Community Psychology 15: 121–148. **pp.325, 326.**

Raven, J.C. (1965). Guide to using the Coloured Progressive Matrices. London: H.K. Lewis. **pp.140, 293.**

Reddy, V. (1991). Playing with others' expectations: Teasing and mucking about in the first year. In A. Whiten (Ed.), Natural Theories of Mind: Evolution, Development and Simulation of Everyday Mindreading. Oxford: Basil Blackwell,pp 143–158. **p.63.**

Reichle, J. (1991). Developing communicative exchanges. In J. Reichle, J. York, and J. Sigafos (Eds.), Implementing Augmentative and Alternative Communication. Baltimore: Paul H. Brookes. pp 133–156. **p.41.**

Reichle, J. and Karlan, G. (1985). The selection of an augmentative communication system in communication intervention: A critique of decision rules. Journal of the Association for Persons with Severe Handicaps 10: 146–156. **p.38.**

Reichle, J., Piché-Cragoe, L., Sigafoos, J. and Doss, S. (1988). Optimizing functional communication for persons with severe handicaps. In S.N. Calculator and J.L. Bedrosian (Eds.), Communication Assessment and Intervention for Adults with Mental Retardation. Austin, Texas: Pro-ed, pp 239–264. **p.40.**

Reichle, J., York, J. and Sigafoos, J. (1991). Implementing Augmentative and Alternative Communication: Strategies for Learners with Severe Disabilities. Baltimore: Paul H. Brookes. **p.271.**

Remington, B. and Clarke, S. (1993). Simultaneous communication and speech comprehension, 1: A comparison of two methods of teaching expressive signing and speech comprehension skills. Augmentative and Alternative Communication 9: 36–48. **p.114.**

Renfrew, C.E. (1989). Action Picture Test. Oxford, UK: C.E. Renfrew. **p.122.**

Riviére, A. (1990). Procesos pragmáticos y atribución de estados mentales: Un análisis de las deficiencias sociales severas en humanos y de las peculiaridades comunicativas en otros primates (Pragmatic processes and attribution of mental states: An analysis of severe social deficits in humans and the communicative peculiarities of other primates). In Actas del II Congreso del Colegio Oficial de Psicólogos, Valencia, April 1990. Valencia: Colegio Oficial de Psicólogos, pp 94–99. **p.52.**

Riviére, A., Belinchón, M., Pfeiffer, A. and Sarriá, E. (1988). Evaluación y alteraciones de las funcionees psicológicas en autismo infantil (Assessment and Change of the Psychological Functions of Infantile Autism). Madrid: CIDE. **pp.52,53.**

Rockey, D. (1980). Speech Disorders in the Nineteenth Century in Britain. London: Croom Helm. **pp.3, 38.**

Roe, P.R.W. (Ed.) (1995). Telecommunications for All. Luxembourg: Office for Official Publications of the European Communities. **p.196.**

Roe, P.R.W., Sandhu, L., Delaney, L., Gill, J.M. and Mercinelli, M. (1995). Consumer overview. In P.R.W Roe (Ed.), Telecommunications for All. Luxembourg: Office for Official Publications of the European Communities, pp 9–27. **p.196.**

Rommetveit, R. (1974). On Message Structure. New York: Wiley. **p.151.**

Romski, M.A. and Ruder, K. F. (1984). The effects of speech and speech and sign instruction on oral language learning and generalisation of Action + Object combinations by Down's syndrome children. Journal of Speech and Hearing Disorders 49: 293–302. **pp.105, 107.**

Rondal, J.A. (1983). Lenguaje y deficiencia mental: Datos recientes y perspectivas (Language and intellectual impairment: Recent findings and perspectives). Revista de Logopedia y Foniatria 3: 67–77. **p.313.**

Rondal, J. (1988a). Down's syndrome. In D. Bishop and K. Mogford (Eds.), Language development in exceptional circumstances. Edinburgh: Churchill Livingstone, pp 165–176. **pp.345, 352.**

Rondal, J.N. (1988b). Estratégias de enseñanza adoptadas por los padres y aprendizaje del lenguaje (Teaching strategies adopted by parents and language learning). Revista de Logopedia y Fonoaudiologia 8: 11–22. **pp.345, 352.**

Rosenberg, S. and Abbeduto, L. (1993). Language and Communication in Mental Retardation. Hillsdale, New Jersey: Lawrence Erlbaum. **pp.103, 114, 197, 198.**

Ross, A.J. (1974). A study of the application of Blissymbolics as a means of communication for a young brain damaged adult. British Journal of Disorders of Communication 14: 103–119. **pp.182, 190, 191.**

Rutter, D.R. (1987). Communicating by Telephone. Oxford: Pergamon Press. **p.197.**

Rutter, S. and Buckley, S. (1994). The acquisition of grammatical morphemes in children with Down's Syndrome. Research and Practice, 2: 76–82. **p.103.**

Ryan, J. (1977). The silence of stupidity. In J. Morton and J.C. Marshall (Eds.), Psycholinguistic Series, Vol 1. Developmental and Pathological. London: Elek Science. pp 99–124. **pp.271, 290, 345.**

Sameroff, A.J. (1987). The social context of development. In N. Eisenberg (Ed.). Contemporary Topics in Developmental Psychology. New York: Wiley. pp 273–291. **p.326.**

Sameroff, A.J. and Chandler, M.J. (1975). Reproductive risk and the continuum of caretaking casualty. In F.D. Horowitz (Ed.), Review of Child Development Research, Volume 4. Chicago: Chicago University Press, pp 187–244. **pp.1, 65.**

Sameroff, A.J. and Fiese, B.H. (1990). Transactional regulation and early intervention. In S.J. Meisels and J.P. Shonkoff (Eds.). Handbook of Early Intervention. Cambridge: Cambridge University Press, pp 119–149. **pp.1, 329.**

Sanders, D.A. (1976). A model for communication. In L.L. Lloyd (Ed.), Communication Assessment and Intervention Strategies. Baltimore: University Park Press, pp 1–32. **p.27.**

Sansone, G. and Tagliapietra, L. (1983). L'apprendimento della comunicazione nei soggetti con handicap grave (Communication learning in subjects with severe disabilities). Udine: Dispensa Scuola Biennale di Specializzazione, C.A.M.P.P. **pp.182, 191.**

Sarriá, E. and Riviére, A. (1986). Análisis comparativo de la conducta de niños autistas, deficientes y normales en una situación de interacción (A comparative analysis of autistic, intellectually impaired and normal children in an interaction situation). Infancia y Aprendizaje 33: 77–98. **p.53.**

Sarriá, E. and Riviére, A. (1991). Desarrollo cognitivo y comunicación intencional preverbal: Un estudio longitudinal multivariado (Cognitive development and preverbal intentional communication: A multivariate longitudinal study). Estudios de Psicología 46: 35–52. **p.51.**

Schaeffer, B. (1978): Teaching spontaneous sign language to non-verbal children: Theory and method. Sign Language Studies 21: 317–352. **p.59.**

Schaeffer, B., Musil, A. and Kollinzas, G. (1980). Total Communication. Champaign, Illinois: Research Press. **pp.41, 46.**

Schaeffer, B., Raphael, A. and Kollinzas, G. (1994). Signed Speech for Non-verbal Students. Seattle, Washington: Educational Achievement Systems. **pp.59, 60.**

Schaerlaekens, A.M. and Gillis, S. (1987). De taalverwerving van het kind. Een hernieuwde orientatie in het Nederlandstalig onderzoek (The Language Development of the Child. A Renewed Orientation of Dutch Research). Groningen, The Netherlands: Wolters-Noordhoff. **p.159.**

Schaffer, H.R. (1989). Language development in context. In S. von Tetzchner, L.S. Siegel and L. Smith (Eds.), The Social and Cognitive Aspects of Normal and Atypical Language Development. New York: Springer-Verlag, pp 1–22. **p.65.**

Schaffer, H.R. (1992). Joint involvement episodes as context for development. In H. McGurk (Ed.), Childhood Social Development. Hove, UK: Lawrence Erlbaum, pp 99–129. **pp.284, 291.**

Schaffer, H.R., Collis, G.M. and Parson, G. (1977). Vocal interchange and visual regard in verbal and pre-verbal children. In H.R. Schaffer (Ed.), Studies in Mother-infant Interaction. London: Academic Press, pp 291–324. **p.275.**

Schank, R.C. and Abelson, R.P. (1977). Scripts, Plans, Goals, and Understanding. Hillsdale, New Jersey: Lawrence Erlbaum. **p.29.**

Scherz, J.W. and Beer, M.M. (1995). Factors affecting the intelligibility of synthesized speech. Augmentative and Alternative Communication 11: 74–78. **p.28.**

Schiefelbusch, R.L. and Hollis, J.H. (1980). A general system for non-speech language. In R.L. Schiefelbusch (Ed.), Non-speech Language and Communication. Baltimore: University Park Press, pp 5–23. **p.28.**

Schjølberg, S. (1984). Forståelighet av talen til barn med språkvansker (The intelligibility of the speech of language disordered children). Dissertation, University of Oslo. **p.44.**

Schlenck, C., Schlenck, K.J. and Springer, L. (1995). Die Behandlung des schweren Agrammatismus. Reduzierte-Syntax-Therapie (REST) (Treatment of Severe Agrammatism. Reduced Syntax Therapy). Stuttgart: Thieme. **p.128.**

Schlesinger, I.M. (1970). The grammar of sign language and the problems of language universals. In J. Morton (Ed.), Biological and Social Factors in Psycholinguistics. Urbana-Champaign: University of Illinois Press, pp 98–121. **p.20.**

Schlesinger, I.M. and Namir, L. (Eds.) (1978). Sign Language of the Deaf. London: Academic Press. **p.5.**

Schulte-Sasse, H. (1994). Anforderung an den Computer in der Kommunikation mit Bliss (Computer options for communicating with Blissymbols). In H. Becker and M.H. Gangkofer (Eds.), Das Bliss-System in Praxis und Forschung. Heidelberg: Julius Groos Verlag, pp 79–103. **p.300.**

Scollon, R. (1976). Conversations with a One-year-old. Honolulu: University of Hawaii Press. **pp.83, 132.**

Scollon, R. and Scollon, S.W. (1994). Intercultural Communication: A Discourse Approach. Oxford: Blackwell. **p.71.**

Searle, J. (1969). Speech Acts. London: Cambridge University Press. **p.179.**

Seibert, J.M. and Hogan, A.E. (1982). Procedures Manual for the Early Social Communication Scales (ESCS). Miami: University of Miami Mailman Center for Child Development. **p.333.**

Seidenberg, M.S. (1995). Visual word recognition: An overview. In J.L. Miller and P.D. Eimas (Eds.), Language, Speech and Communication. New York: Academic Press, pp 137–179. **p.29.**

Service, V., Lock, A. and Chandler, P. (1989). Individual differences in early communicative development: a social constructivist perspective. In S. von Tetzchner, L.S. Siegel and L. Smith (Eds.), The Social and Cognitive Factors of Normal and Atypical Language Development. New York: Springer-Verlag, pp 23–49. **pp.1, 38.**

Sevcik, R.A., Romski, M.A. and Wilkinson, K.M. (1991). Roles of graphic symbols in augmented language acquisition process with severe cognitive disabilities. Augmentative and Alternative Communication 7: 161–170. **p.154.**

Shane, H.C. (1980). Approaches to assessing the communication of non-oral persons. In R.L. Schiefelbusch (Ed.), Non-speech Language and Communication. Baltimore: University Park Press. pp 197–224. **p.27.**

Shane, H.C. and Bashir, A.S. (1980). Election criteria for the adoption of an augmentative communication system: Preliminary considerations. Journal of Speech and Hearing Disorders 45: 408–414. **pp.38, 65.**

Shannon, C.E. and Weaver, W.W. (1949). The Mathematical Theory of Communication. Urbana, Illinois: University of Illinois. **p.28.**

Shonkoff, J.P. and Hauser-Cram, P. (1987). Early intervention for disabled infants and their families: A quantitative analysis. Pediatrics 80: 650–658. **p.326.**

Short, J., Williams, E. and Christie, B. (1976). The Social Psychology of Telecommunications. London: John Wiley. **p.196.**

Siegel-Causey, E. and Ernst, B. (1989). Theoretical orientations and research in nonsymbolic development. In E. Siegel-Causey and D. Guess (Eds.), Enhancing Nonsymbolic Communication Interactions among Learners with Severe Disabilities. Baltimore: Paul H. Brookes, pp 15–54. **p.271.**

Sigafoss, J., Kignre, J., Holt, K., Doss, S. and Mustone, L. (1991). Improving the quality of written developmental indices for adults with intellectual disabilities. British Journal of Mental Subnormality 37: 35–46. **p.330.**

Sigman, M. and Mundy, P. (1989). Social attachments in autistic children. Journal of the American Academy of Child Psychiatry 28: 74–81. **p.53.**

Simeonsson, R. (1995). Intervention in communicative disability: Evaluation issues and evidence. In J. Rönnberg and E. Hjelmquist (Eds.), Proceedings from the international symposium on communicative disability: Compensation and development. Linköping: Linköping University Press, pp 79–96. **p.331.**

Simeonsson, R. and Bailey, D.B. (1988). Abilities Index. Chapel Hill, North Carolina: Frank Porter Graham Child Development Centre. **p.333.**

Singleton, J., Goldin-Meadow, S. and McNeill, D. (1995). The cataclysmic break between gesticulation and sign: Evidence against a unified continuum of gestural communication. In K. Emmorey and J. Reilly (Eds.), Language, Gesture and Space. Hove, UK: Lawrence Erlbaum, pp 287–312. **p.104.**

Singleton, J. and Newport, E.L. (1992). When learners surpass their models: The acquisition of American Sign Language from impoverished input. Manuscript, University of Illinois. **p.31.**

Siple, P. and Fischer, S.D. (Eds.) (1991). Theoretical Issues in Sign Language Research. Volume 2: Psychology. Chicago: University of Chicago Press. **pp.29, 86.**

Skinner, B.F. (1957). Verbal Behavior. New York: Appleton-Century-Crofts. **p.5.**

Skovlund, D. (1983). Reynells Sprogudviklingsskalaer (Reynell's developmental language scales). København: Dansk Psykologisk Forlag. p.251.

Slobin, D.I. (1979). Psycholinguistics. London: Scott, Forsman. pp.1, 29.

Smith, L. and Hagen, V. (1984). Relationship between the home environment and sensorimotor development of Down syndrome and non-retarded infants. American Journal of Mental Deficiency 89: 124–132. pp.214, 229.

Smith, L. and von Tetzchner, S. (1986). Communicative, sensorimotor, and language skills of young children with Down syndrome. American Journal of Mental Deficiency 91: 57–66. p.214.

Smith, L., von Tetzchner, S. and Michaelsen, B. (1988). The emergence of language skills in young children with Down syndrome. In L. Nadel (Ed.), The Psychobiology of Down Syndrome. Cambridge, Massachusetts: MIT Press, pp 145–165. p.228.

Smith, M. (1991). Assessment of interaction patterns and AAC use: A case study. Journal of Clinical Speech and Language Studies 1: 76–102. pp.8, 67, 70.

Smith, N. and Tsimpli, I.-M. (1995). The Mind of a Savant. Oxford, UK: Basil Blackwell. p.29.

Snijders, J.T.H. and Snijders-Oomen, S.O. (1976). Non-verbal Intelligence Scale. Windsor: NFER Nelson. p.109.

Snijders, J.T., Tellegen, P.J. and Laros, J.A. (1989). Snijders-Oomen Non-verbal Intelligence Test. S.O.N.-R $5^{1}/_{2}$-17. Groningen, The Netherlands: Wolters-Noordhoff. p.361.

Snow, C.E. (1986). Conversations with children. In P. Fletcher and M. Garman (Eds.), Language Acquisition, Second edition. Cambridge: Cambridge University Press. pp 69–89. p.75.

Snow, C.E. and Ferguson, C.A. (Eds.) (1977). Talking to Children. Cambridge: Cambridge University Press. p.85.

Snyder-McLean, L.K., Solomonson, B., McLean, J.E. and Sack, S. (1984). Structuring joint attention action routines: A strategy for facilitating communication and language development in the classroom. Seminars in Speech and Language 5: 213–228. p.275.

Soro, E. and Basil, C. (1993). Estratégias para facilitar las iniciativas de interacción en hablantes asistidos (Strategies for facilitating communicative initiatives among aided speakers). Infancia y Aprendizaje 94: 29–48. pp.271, 346.

Soro-Camats, E. and Basil, C. (in press). Desarrollo de la comunicación y el lenguaje en niños con discapacidad motora y plurideficiencia (Communication and language development in children with motor and multiple impairments). In M.J. del Rio (Ed.), Interacción y adquisición del lenguaje en niños con necesidades especiales. Barcelona: Martinez-Roca. p.271.

Soro-Camats, E., Duarte, C. and Mendes, E. (1995). Linguagens alternativas e novas tecnologias ao serviço da integração (Alternative Language and New Technology in the Promotion of Integration). Lisbon: FENACERCI. pp.344, 345.

Soto, G. and Olmstead, W. (1993). A semiotic perspective for AAC. Augmentative and Alternative Communication 9: 134–141. pp.29, 130.

Soto, G. and Toro-Zambrana, W. (1995). Investigation of Blissymbol use from a language research paradigm. Augmentative and Alternative Communication 11: 118–130. pp.119, 127.

Sperber, D. and Wilson, D. (1986). Relevance: Communication and Cognition. Oxford, UK: Basil Blackwell. p.26.

Spiegel, B., Benjamin, B.J. and Spiegel, S. (1993). One method to increase spontaneous use of an assistive communication device: A case study. Augmentative and

Alternative Communication 9: 111–117. **pp.120, 126.**

Spradlin, J.E. (1963). Language and communication of mental defectives. In N.R. Ellis (Ed.), Handbook of Mental Deficiency: Psychological Theory and Research. New York: McGraw-Hill. pp 512–555. **p.191.**

Steenbuch, R. (1957). Jeg lever også (I live too). Oslo: Land og Kirke. **p.3.**

Steindal, K. (1993). Bruk av bildetelefon i veiledning av nærpersoner til barn med autisme (Use of videotelephones in supervision of significant persons in the environment of children with autism). In K.B. Nilsson and S. von Tetzchner (Eds.), Telekommunikasjon for mennesker med psykisk utviklingshemning. Oslo: Rådet for Tekniske Tiltak for Funksjonshemmede, pp 67–71. **p.211.**

Stella, G. and Biancardi, A. (1987). Elementi per una riflessione clinica sui problemi di apprendimento. (Elements for a clinical reflection about learning problems). Giornale di Neuropsichiatria dell'Età Evolutiva 7: 287–294. **p.191.**

Stokoe, W., Casterline, D.C. and Croneberg, C.G. (1965). A Dictionary of American Sign Language on Linguistic Principles. Washington, DC: Gallaudet College Press. **p.108**

Stubbs, M. (1983). Discourse Analysis - The Sociolinguistic Analysis of Natural Language. Oxford: Basil Blackwell. **p.177.**

Supalla, S.J. (1991). Manually Coded English: The modality question in signed language development. In P. Siple and S. Fischer (Eds.), Theoretical Issues in Sign Language Research. Volume 2: Psychology. Chicago: University of Chicago Press, pp 85-109. **pp.121, 135.**

Sutton, A.C. (1982). Augmentative communication systems: The interaction process. Paper presented at the Annual Convention of the American Speech-Language-Hearing Association, Toronto, 1982. **p.68.**

Sutton, A.E. and Gallagher, T.M. (1993). Verb class distinctions and AAC language-encoding limitations. Journal of Speech and Hearing Research 36: 1216–1226. **p.119.**

Swift, J. (1970). Gulliver's Travels. London: Norton. (First published in 1726). **p.2.**

Syse, A. (1992). Psykisk utviklingshemmetes rettsstilling (The judicial status of people with intellectual impairment). In S. Eskeland and A. Syse (Eds.), Psykisk utviklings-hemmedes rettsstilling. Oslo: Ad Notam Gyldendal. pp 15–46. **p.198.**

Tager-Flusberg, H. (1993). What language reveals about the undestanding of minds in children with autism. In S. Baron-Cohen, H. Tager-Flusberg and D.J. Cohen (Eds), Understanding other minds. Oxford: Oxford University Press, pp 138–157. **p.27.**

Tager-Flusberg, H. (Ed.) (1994). Constraints on Language Acquisition: Studies of Atypical Children. Hove, UK: Jersey: Lawrence Erlbaum. **pp.1, 29.**

Tamarit, J. (1993). La aportación del programa de comunicación total de Schaeffer y sus colaboradores a la educación especial en nuestro país (The contribution of the total communication approach of Schaeffer and his associates to special education in our country). In R. Canal (Ed.), El autismo 50 años después de Kanner (1943). Salamanca, Spain: Amarú, pp 199–204. **p.56.**

Tannen, D. and Saville-Troike, M. (Eds.) (1985). Perspectives on Silence. New Jersey: Ablex. **p.173.**

Tiilikka, P. and Hautamäki, J. (1986). Portaat - varhaiskasvatusohjelma. Helsinki: The National Welfare Association for the Mentally Retarded. (The Finnish edition of Portage Guide to Early Education). **p.219.**

Trevarthen, C. (1986). The structure of motives for human communication in infancy: A ground-plan for human ethology. In J. Lecamus and J. Cosnier (Eds.), Ethology and Psychology. Toulouse: Privat, pp 91–100. **p.55.**

Tyler, A.A. and Sandoval, K.T. (1994). Preschoolers with phonological and language disorders: Treating different linguistic domains. Language Speech and Hearing

Services in Schools 25: 215–234. **p.126.**

Udwin, O. and Yule, W. (1990). Augmentative communication systems taught to cerebral palsy children - A longitudinal study. 1: The acquisition of signs and symbols and syntactic aspects of their use over time. British Journal of Disorders of Communication 25: 295–309. **pp.67, 106, 120, 126, 234.**

Udwin, O. and Yule, W. (1991a). Augmentative communication systems taught to cerebral-palsied children - A longitudinal Study. 2. Pragmatic features of sign and symbol use. British Journal of Disorders of Communication 26: 137–148. **p.182.**

Udwin, O. and Yule, W. (1991b). Augmentative communication systems taught to cerebral-palsied children - A longitudinal study. 3. Teaching practices and exposure to sign and symbol use in schools and homes. British Journal of Disorders of Communication 26: 149–162. **p.182.**

Ur, P. (1981). Discussions that Work: Task-centred Fluency Practice. Cambridge: Cambridge University Press. **p.91.**

Vaid, J. (Ed.) (1986). Language Processing in Bilinguals: Psycholinguistic and Neuropsychological Perspectives. Hove, UK: Lawrence Erlbaum. **p.30.**

Vallini, S. (1981). Il metodo Bliss e la riabilitazione (The Blissymbolics method and rehabilitation). Quaderni AITR 6 (2). **p.189.**

van Balkom, H. (1991). The Communication of Language Impaired Children. A Study of Discourse Coherence of Specific Language Impaired and Normal Language Acquiring Children with their Primary Caregivers. Amsterdam: Swets and Zeitlinger. **p.138.**

van Balkom, H. and Welle Donker-Gimbrère, M. (1994). Kiezen voor Communicatie. Een handboek over de communicatie van mensen met een motorische of meervoudige handicap (Choosing for Communication. A Handbook of Communication for People with Physical and Multiple Impairments). Nijkerk, The Netherlands: INTRO. **pp.154, 155, 161.**

van den Meulen, B.F. and Smrkovsky, M. (1983). Bayley Ontwikkelingsschaal, BOS 2-30. Lisse, The Netherlands: Swets and Zeitlinger. **p.235.**

vander Beken, K., Geysels, G., Tollens and Loncke, F. (1994). Manual communication as facilitator for developing less accessible modalities. ISAAC'94 Conference book and proceedings. Hoensbroek, The Netherlands: Institute for Research, Development and Knowledge Transfer in the Field of Rehabilitation and Handicap. pp 287–288. **p.23.**

Vanderheiden, D.B., Brown, W.P., MacKenzie, P., Reinen, S. and Scheibel, C. (1975). Symbol communication for the mentally handicapped. Mental Retardation 13: 34–37. **p.65.**

Vanderheiden, G.C. and Grilley, K. (Eds.) (1977). Non-vocal Communication Techniques and Aids for the Severely Physically Handicapped. Baltimore: University Park Press. **p.193.**

Vanderheiden, G.C. and Lloyd, L.L.(1986). Communication systems and their components. In S.W. Blackstone (Ed.), Augmentative Communication: An Introduction. Rockville, Maryland: American Speech and Hearing Association. pp 49–161. **p.13.**

Vanderheyden, P.B., Pennington, C.A., Peischl, D.M., McKnitt, W.M., McCoy, K.F., Demasco, P.W., van Balkom, H. and Kamphuis, H. (1994). Developing AAC Systems that model intelligent partner interactions: Methodological considerations. RESNA'94 proceedings. Arlington, Virginia: RESNA, pp 126–128. **p.162.**

van Dijk, J. (1966). First steps of the deaf-blind child toward language. International Journal for the Education of the Blind 15: 112–114. **p.3.**

van Dijk, T.A. and Kintsch, W. (1983). Strategies of Discourse Comprehension. New York: Academic Press. **p.71.**

van Oosterom, J. and Devereux, K. (1985). Learning with Rebus glossary. Back Hill, UK: Earo, The Resource Centre. **p.15.**

Varnhagen, C.K., Das, J.P. and Varnhagen, S. (1987). Auditory and visual memory span: cognitive processing by TMR individuals with Down syndrome and other etiologies. American Journal of Mental Deficiency 91: 398–405. **p.214.**

Veneziano, E., Sinclair, H. and Berthoud, I. (1990). From one word to two words: repetition patterns on the way to structured speech. Journal of Child Language 17: 633–650. **p.102.**

Venkatagiri, H.S. (1994). The effect of sentence length and exposure on the intelligibility of synthesized speech. Augmentative and Alternative Communication 10: 96–104. **p.28.**

Volterra, V., Beronesi, S. and Massoni, P. (1990). How does gestural communication become language? In V. Volterra and C. Erting (Eds.), From Gesture to Language in Hearing and Deaf Children. Berlin: Springer-Verlag, pp 205–213. **p.104.**

Volterra, V. and Iverson, J.M. (1995). When do modality factors affect the course of language acquisition? In K. Emmorey and J.S. Reilly (Eds.), Language, Gesture and Space. Hove, UK: Lawrence Erlbaum, pp 371–390. **pp.234, 247.**

von Tetzchner, S. (1984). Facilitation of early speech development in a dysphatic child by use of signed Norwegian. Scandinavian Journal of Psychology 25: 265–275. **p.43.**

von Tetzchner, S. (1985). Words and chips - pragmatics and pidginization of computer-aided communication. Child Language Teaching and Therapy 1: 295–305. **pp.30, 31.**

von Tetzchner, S. (1987). Testprogrammer for barn med bevegelsesheming (Test Programmes for Motor Impaired Children). Oslo: Sentralinstituttet for Cerebral Parese. **p.67.**

von Tetzchner, S. (1988). Aided communication for handicapped children. In A. Mital and W. Karwowski (Eds.), Ergonomics in Rehabilitation. New York: Taylor and Francis. pp 233–252. **p.24.**

von Tetzchner, S. (1990). Tilbakeblikk (Looking back). CP-Bladet 36 (4): 5–9. **pp.3, 4, 5.**

von Tetzchner, S. (1991a). Methodological issues in the study of language development among children using aided language. In J. Brodin and E. Björck-Åkesson (Eds.), Methodological Issues in Research in Augmentative and Alternative Communication. Stockholm: Swedish Handicap Institute, pp 113-117. **p.119.**

von Tetzchner, S. (Ed.) (1991b). Issues in Telecommunication and Disability. Luxembourg: Office for Official Publications of the European Communities. **p.200.**

von Tetzchner, S. (1991c). The use of 64 kbit/s videotelephones for sign language. In S. von Tetzchner (Ed.), Issues in Telecommunication and Disability. Luxembourg: Office for Official Publications of the European Communities. **pp.327-339. p.200.**

von Tetzchner, S. (1992). Å vokse opp med funksjonshemning (Growing up with disability). In S. von Tetzchner and H. Schiørbeck, Habilitering. Oslo: Ad Notam Gyldendal, pp 9–19. **p.10.**

von Tetzchner, S. (1993a). The use of manual signs for non-deaf people in Norway. The ISAAC Bulletin 35: 5–6. **p.6.**

von Tetzchner, S. (1993b). Desarrollo del lenguaje asistido. (Development of aided language). Infancia y Aprendizaje 94: 9–28. **pp.31, 271, 283, 312, 314, 346.**

von Tetzchner, S. (1993c). Et kommunikasjonshjelpemiddel for en jente med Spielmeyer-Vogt-sykdommen (A communication aid for a girl with the Spielmeyer-Vogt disease). In K.B. Nilsson (Ed.), Tale- og språkvansker. Oslo:

Rådet for Tekniske Tiltak for Funksjonshemmede. pp 74–78. **p.72.**

von Tetzchner, S. (1995). Habilitation of young children using communication aids. In J. Rönnberg and E. Hjelmquist (Eds.), Proceedings from the International Symposium on Communicative Disability: Compensation and Development. Linköping: Linköping University. pp 118–129. **pp.66, 87, 80, 266, 329.**

von Tetzchner, S. (in press). The use of graphic language intervention among young children in Norway. European Journal of Disorders of Communication. **pp.8. 67.**

von Tetzchner, S. (in preparation). Communication skills of females with Rett syndrome. Paper to be presented at the 26th International Congress of Psychology, Montreal, August 1996. **p.58.**

von Tetzchner, S., Hesselberg, F. and Langeland, H. (1991). Supervision of habilitation via videotelephone. In S. von Tetzchner (Ed.), Issues in telecommunication and disability. Luxembourg: Office for Official Publications of the European Communities, pp 360–371. **p.209.**

von Tetzchner, S. and Martinsen, H. (1992). Introduction to Sign Teaching and the Use of Communication Aids. London: Whurr (Norwegian edition, 1991, Gyldendal; North American edition, 1992, Singular; Spanish edition, 1993, Aprendizaje-Visor). **pp.13, 32, 34, 43, 56, 87, 124, 270, 271, 286, 290, 310, 311, 312, 315, 342, 346.**

von Tetzchner, S. and Nordby, K. (1991). Telecommunication behaviour. In S. von Tetzchner (Ed.), Issues in Telecommunication and Disability. Luxembourg: Office for Official Publications of the European Communities. pp 26–38. **p.209.**

von Tetzchner, S. and Smith, L. (1986). Mødres tale til tre år gamle barn med Down syndrom (Mothers' speech to three-year-old children with Down syndrome). In P.E. Mjaavatn and L. Smith (Eds.), Barnespråk. Trondheim: NAVF's Senter for Barneforskning, pp 43–58. **pp.44, 214.**

Vriesema, P., Miedema, S. and VanBlokland, R. (1992). Prevention of non-motor developmental delay in infants and toddlers with neuromotor disabilities by means of a home-based early intervention programme. In H. Nakken, G.H. VanGemert and T. Zandberg (Eds.), Research on Intervention in Special Education. Lampeter: The Edwin Mellen Press, pp 255–276. **p.332.**

Vygotsky, L. (1962). Thought and Language. Cambridge, Massachusetts: MIT Press. **pp.1, 19, 38, 177, 293, 345.**

Walker, M. (1976). The Makaton Vocabulary (Revised). London: Royal Association in Aid of the Deaf and Dumb. **pp.234, 344.**

Walker, M. (1977). Teaching sign language to deaf mentally handicapped adults. In IMS Conference proceedings, 3, Language and the mentally handicapped. London: British Institute for Learning Disabilities, pp 3–25. **p.108.**

Walker, M., Parson, P., Cousins, S., Carpenter, B. and Park, K. (1985). Symbols for Makaton. Back Hill, UK: Earo, The Resource Centre. **p.15.**

Wasow, T. (1973). The innateness and grammatical relations. Synthese 26: 38–56. **p.25.**

Wathen-Dunn, W. (Ed.) (1967). Models for the Perception of Speech and Visual Form. Cambridge: Massachusetts, MIT Press. **p.29.**

Watson, J. (1986). Matrix training and sign language for the mentally handicapped. Dissertation, University of Southampton. **p.107.**

Weiner, P.S. (1986). The study of child language disorders: Nineteenth century perspectives. Journal of Communication Disorders 19: 1–47. **pp.3, 37.**

Weinert, F.E. (1990). How European is developmental psychology in Europe? In P.J.D. Drenth, J.A. Sergeant and R.J. Takens (Eds.), European Perspectives in Psychology, Volume 1. Chichester, UK: John Wiley, pp 153–170. **p.3.**

Weingart, P. (1989). Ist der Sprachenstreit ein Streit um die Sprache? (Is the language battle about language?) Psychologische Rundschau 40: 96–98. **p.3**.

Weir, R.H. (1962). Language in the Crib. The Hague: Mouton. **p.26**.

Welle Donker-Gimbrère, M. (1994). Neurology, psycholinguistics, semiotics system theory, and the study of graphic symbol communication in AAC. In J. Brodin and E. Björck-Åkesson (Eds.), Methodological Issues in Research in Alternative and Augmentative Communication. Jönköping: Jönköping University Press. pp 20–26. **p.20**.

Welle Donker-Gimbrère, M. and van Balkom, H. (1995). Grafische symbolen in ondersteunde communicatie (Graphic Symbols in Augmentative Communication). Baarn, The Netherlands: INTRO. **pp.13, 15, 155, 158**.

Welle Donker-Gimbrère, M., van Blom, K., van 't Hoofd, W. and van Balkom, H. (1991). GRASYCOM. Project report. IRV/6 Doc(91). Hoensbroek, The Netherlands: Institute for Research, Development and Knowledge Transfer in the Field of Rehabilitation and Handicap. **pp.155, 158**.

Wellman, H.M. (1990). The Child's Theory of Mind. Cambridge, Massachusetts: MIT Press. **p.265**.

Wetstone, H. and Friedlander, B. (1973). The effect of word order on young children's response to simple questions and commands. Child Development 44: 734–740. **p.102**.

Whybray, M. (1991.) Visual telecommunication for deaf people at 14.4 Kbit/s on the Public Switched Telephone Network. In S. von Tetzchner (Ed.), Issues in Telecommunication and Disability. Luxembourg: Office for Official Publications of the European Communities, pp 340–349. **p.206**.

Wilbur, R.B. (1976). The linguistics of manual languages and manual systems. In L. Lloyd (Ed.), Communication Assessment and Intervention Strategies. Baltimore: University Park Press, pp 423–500. **p.121**.

Wilkes-Gibbs, D. and Clark, H.H. (1992). Coordinating beliefs in conversation. Journal of Memory and Language 31: 183–194. **p.93**.

Wilkinson, K.M., Romski, M.A. and Sevcik, R.A. (1994). Emergence of visual-graphic symbol combinations by youth with moderate or severe mental retardation. Journal of Speech and Hearing Research 37: 883–895. **p.234**.

Wilson, B. (1987). La riabilitazione dei disturbi di memoria (The rehabilitation of memory deficits). In A. Mazzucchi (Ed.), La riabilitazione neuropsicologica. Bologna: Il Mulino, pp 219–248. **p.191**.

Windsor, J. and Fristoe, M. (1989). Key word signing: Listeners' classification of signed and spoken narratives. Journal of Speech and Hearing Disorders 54: 374–382. **p.227**.

Witt, J. and Martens, B. (1988). Problems with problem solving consultation: re-analysis of assumptions, methods, and goals. School Psychology Review 17: 211–226. **p.331**.

Wittgenstein, L. (1953). Philosophical Investigations. Oxford: Basil Blackwell. **p.177**.

Wodlinger-Cohen, R. (1991). The manual representation of speech by deaf children, their mothers and their teachers. In P. Siple and S. Fischer (Eds.), Theoretical Issues in Sign Language Research. Volume 2: Psychology. Chicago: University of Chicago Press, pp 149–169. **p.127**.

Woll, B. and Grove, N. (1995). On language deficits and modality in children with Down syndrome: A case study. Presented at the 20th Annual Boston University Conference on Language Development, November 1995. **p.117**.

Woll, B. and Kyle, J.G. (1989). Communication and language development in children of deaf parents. In S. von Tetzchner, L.S. Siegel and L. Smith (Eds.), The

Social and Cognitive Aspects of Normal and Atypical Language Development. New York: Springer-Verlag, pp 129–144. **p.103.**

Woll, B., Kyle, J. and Deuchar, M. (Eds.) (1981). Perspectives on British Sign Language and Deafness. London: Croom Helm. **p.5.**

Woodcock, R.W., Clark, C.R. and Davies, C.O. (1969). Peabody Rebus Reading Program. Circle Pines: American Guidance Service. **p.15.**

Worth, S. (1975). Pictures can't say ain't. Versus. Quaderni de studi Semiotico 12: 85–105. **p.188.**

Wrightsman, L.S. (1972). Social Psychology. Monterey, California: Wadsworth. **p.346.**

Yamada, J. (1990). Laura: A Case for the Modularity of Language. Cambridge, Massachusetts: MIT Press. **pp.1, 29.**

Yin, R.K. (1989). Case Study Research: Design and Methods. Newbury Park, California: Sage. **p.9.**

Yin, R.K. (1993). Applications of Case Study Research. Newbury Park, California: Sage. **p.10.**

Yoder, P.J. and Warren, S.F. (1993). Can developmentally delayed children's language development be enhanced through prelinguistic intervention? In A.P. Kaiser and D.B. Gray (Eds.), Enhancing Children's Communication. Research Foundations for Intervention. Baltimore: Paul H. Brookes, pp 35–61. **p.40.**

Yorkston, K., Honsinger, M.J., Dowden, P. and Marriner, N. (1989). Vocabulary selection: A case report. Augmentative and Alternative Communication 5: 101–108. **p.128.**

Yovetich, W.S. and Young, T.A. (1988). The effects of representativeness and concreteness on the 'guessability' of Blissymbols. Augmentative and Alternative Communication 4: 35–39. **p.28.**

Zangari, C., Lloyd, L. and Vicker, B. (1994). Augmentative and Alternative Communication: An historic perspective. Augmentative and Alternative Communication 10: 27–59. **pp.2, 3, 6, 119.**

Zimmerman, I.L., Steiner, V.G. and Pond, R.E. (1992). Preschool Language Scales - 3. New York: Harcourt Brace Jovanivich. **p.126.**

Zinna, A. (1993). Glossematica dell'Esperanto (Glossematics of Esperanto). Lecture at Collège de France, Paris, May 18th, 1993. **p.183.**

# Subject index